JN118324

Contents

＜本書は問題の解答や日本語訳は付属しておりません。あらかじめご了承ください＞

Introduction

Disease is part of life. I doubt if there is a person who, by the age of 50, has not had a serious illness, or whose life has never been touched by the illness of a family member, relative, or close friend. In this book there are five chapters, each one on a medical condition that I have encountered during my five decades of life. In writing these chapters, I have referred to numerous books and online sources and have asked questions of several medical specialists. The topics of the chapters are as follows:

Chapter 1: Diabetes mellitus

Chapter 2: Chronic kidney disease

Chapter 3: Inflammatory bowel disease

Chapter 4: Stroke

Chapter 5: Pneumonia

はじめに

　病気は人生の一部です。50 歳を過ぎて大病を患ったことのない人、あるいは家族や親戚、親しい友人の病気に触れたことのない人はいないのではないでしょうか。本書には 5 つの章があり、それぞれ、私が 50 年の人生で遭遇した病気・病状について説明しています。これらの章を書くにあたり、私は数多くの専門的な関連書を読み、オンラインの情報源を参照したり、何人かの医療専門家に質問してまとめました。各章のテーマは次の通りです。

　第 1 章　糖尿病

　第 2 章　慢性腎臓病

　第 3 章　炎症性腸疾患

　第 4 章　脳卒中

　第 5 章　肺炎

本書の使用方法

　この本は大学生向けの医療英語のテキストですが、医学に興味のある方なら、医学のトピックを扱ったエッセイ集として楽しんでいただけると思います。教科書として使うのであるなら、薬学部や医学部で学ぶ学生に最適です。わたしの勤める名城大学薬学部では本書を次のように使う予定なので、ぜひ参考にしてください。

・この本は、薬学部 1 年生から 5 年生までの薬学英語の授業で使用します。使い方次第で、どの年次にも対応できるようになっています。

・わたしが教えている学生にとって、1 章全部を読んでもらうのは負担が大きすぎます。そこで「エッセイ」のところと、「11 の語源を詳しく」「12 の話題を詳しく」をいくつか読むように指示します。

- エッセイの段落にはすべて番号がふられ、「11 の語源を詳しく」「12 の話題を詳しく」にも番号がふられています。このため、学生にどのセクションを読めばいいのか、正確に指示することができます。
- 1 章のまとめとして、学生がきちんと理解しているのかを確認するために、また学生に理解するための動機付けを与えるために、テキストの内容についての確認問題を作成いたしました。これを学生に解答してもらいます。学期末試験では、これらの確認問題のなかから問題が出題されます。
- ミニテストは、「ナビボキャ60」に載っている単語や、名城大学 根岸隆之先生が描いてくれたイラストから出題されます。

Abbreviations and symbols used in this book （この本で用いる略語と記号）

	Meaning （意味）	Example （例）
i.e.,	Stands for the Latin *id est*, meaning "that is." It introduces a word or sentence that restates or clarifies what has just been said. 「i.e.」はラテン語の "id est" で、"that is"（すなわち）" という意味です。前の文章で言っていることを明確にしたり、言い換えたりするときに使われています。	I am a pescatarian (i.e., a person who eats fish but not meat).
e.g.,	Stands for *exempli gratia*, a Latin phrase meaning "for example." これはラテン語の "exempli gratia" の略で "for example"（例えば）"を意味します。	Eating high-fiber foods (e.g., fruit, vegetables, legumes, oats) helps prevent constipation.
&	Introduces an example sentence. 例文を示しています。	The word root *spek* in "**retrospective study**" means "to observe." Words with this root include **spectrum**, **speculate**, and **circumspect**. *& Doctors should be more **circumspect** in prescribing antidepressants because of the risk of dependence and questions over their efficacy.*
/	or　または	*epi~* (= "on/upon")
=	means/which means 〜を意味する。	"Asymptomatic" means showing no symptoms of a particular disease (*a~* = "not/without").
→	changes to 〜に代わる。	*Syn~* (= "together") → *sym~* before "p"; e.g., **syn**chronize, **sym**pathy
lit.	literally 文字通りの意味	Drugs and other substances that cause birth defects are described as *teratogenic* (lit. "monster-producing").

Before turning to Chapter 1, it would be wise to read the following section. Doing so will make it easier for you to understand the many medical terms in this book.

What is in this book?　（この本の内容）

Each chapter consists of the following parts:

illustrations

- A page of **illustrations** related to the topic of the chapter. They are drawn by Takayuki Negishi, D.V.M., Ph.D., a teacher of anatomy and physiology in the Faculty of Pharmacy, Meijo University.

NAVvocab 60　（案内役の単語 60）

- **NAVvocab 60**, short for "navigational vocabulary," is a list of 60 key vocabulary items, with a Japanese translation. This vocabulary will help you on your reading-journey through the Essay. Many words and phrases in this book are in bold print. Some of these words are listed in NAVvocab 60, but because of **space constraints** in this book, many are not. However, with a smartphone, you can easily check the meaning of any word that you do not know. For example, some readers may not know what "constraint" means. If you are one of those, check the meaning now. And while you are on your smartphone, you could also check its etymology.

Essay

- An **Essay** on a particular disease. Within the essay, you will see that some words and phrases are in bold and underlined with a superscript "E" or "D"; for example:

COVID-19[D1] vaccine-related **myocarditis**[E1] has been reported worldwide.

Eleven Etymologies　（11 の単語を詳しく）

- The superscript [E] indicates that this is discussed in the **Eleven Etymologies** section. This section includes information on the word's structure and etymology.

Dozen in Detail　（12 の話題を詳しく）

- The superscript [D] indicates that this topic is discussed in the **Dozen in Detail** section.

SD　（追記）

- Interspersed within the *Eleven Etymologies* and the *Dozen in Detail* sections are **Slight Detours**, or **SD** for short. The information in each SD is related, albeit sometimes **tangentially**, to the chapter's topic.

Well, what do you know?　（どのくらいわかるようになったか試してみよう）
- These are questions to test and **consolidate** your knowledge of the chapter's content.

May Jo's Health-Podcast　（メイ・ジョーの健康ポッドキャスト）
- Since 2005, I've been an **avid** listener of podcasts provided by the BBC and other radio stations. **May Jo's Health-Podcast** is a dialogue inspired by the hundreds of medical-related podcasts I have listened to. The fictional presenter is a women called May Jo, a doctor turned journalist. If you are using this book in a classroom, you can practice these dialogues with a classmate.

Introducing medical English　（医療英語とは何か?）

Medical terminology can be **daunting**. The specialist terms used by healthcare professionals are often long and unfamiliar (I bet you didn't learn "**esophagogastroduodenoscopy**" in high school English lessons). Learning medical vocabulary is a challenge not only for Japanese students, but also for native English speakers. However, swimming through the sea of medical vocabulary becomes much easier if you have some knowledge of the SEA, that is, the **Structure** and **Etymology** of medical words, and how **Abbreviations** are used. Let's look at SEA in more detail.

・STRUCTURE　（医療用語の構造）
Medical words are built from parts. In this book, these parts are called **word-forming elements**, or **WFEs**（単語を構成する要素）for short. For example, the word **hypothermia** is built from three parts: *hypo~* + *therm* + *~ia*. The WFE *hypo~* is a **prefix** meaning "below normal"; *therm* is a word root that means "heat"; and *~ia* is a suffix indicating a "disease or condition." Medical words can be composed of four parts:

1) Prefix:　（接頭辞）
A prefix usually appears before a word root to modify its meaning. This book indicates prefixes by a ~ (tilde) after the prefix (e.g., *re~*).

2) Root:　（語根）
The root (or **word root**) is the main idea or concept of a word. Most medical terms contain at least one root. Unlike prefixes and suffixes, a root can appear in any position in a word; for example, the root *gen* (= "born/produced") can start a word (**gen***der*, **gen***etic*), come in the middle (e.g., *endo***gen***ous*, *de***gen***erate*), or be at the end of a word (e.g.,

pathogen, *carcinogen*). In everyday English, roots are often complete words. For example, *myth* is a Greek root for "story," and *form* is the Latin root meaning "shape." But in medical English, most roots are not complete words and must be used in combination with one or more WFEs. For example, the roots *nephr* (= "kidney"), *melan* (= "black"), and *onych* (= "nail") only become words when other WFEs are attached (e.g., **nephritis**, **melanoma**, **onychophagia**; *~itis* = "inflammation"; *~oma* = "tumor"; *phag* = "eat" + *~ia*). Onychophagia is the medical term for "nail biting," which is often a stress-related habit. I hope this book does not cause this condition in any of my students!

3) Suffix: （接尾辞）

The suffix is always at the end of a word. It often indicates a procedure, a condition, or a disease. The suffix may simply make the word a noun or adjective. In this book, suffixes are indicated by a ~ (tilde) before the suffix (e.g., *~ia*).

4) Combining vowel: （連結母音）

The word **arthroscope** is composed of the root *arthr* (= "joint") and *~scope* (= "to view"). The "o" between the root and another WFE is called a **combining vowel**. Two examples of words with the root for blood are **hematopoiesis** (*hemat* = "blood" + o + *poiesis* = "to make") and **hemophilia** (*hem* = "blood" + o + *phil* = "affinity for" + *~ia* = "condition"). The most common combining vowel is "o," but other vowels are sometimes used. A combining vowel is not used if the suffix begins with a vowel; for example, the term for "joint inflammation" is **arthritis** (*not* "arthroitis").

5) Combining form: （連結形）

The combination of a root and a combining vowel is called a **combining form**; for example: *gastr* (= "stomach") is sometimes written with its combining form as *gastro*, or with a forward slash as **gastr/o**; *oste* (= "bone") can be written as **oste/o**; and *hepat* (= "liver") can be written as **hepat/o**.

The above explanation of medical-word structure has probably left you with a few questions. Let me try to predict some of the questions you may have.

Q. Are all medical words made up of a prefix, suffix, and a root?

（すべての医学用語は、接頭辞、接尾辞、語根でできている?）

No. Many words do not have a prefix. For example, **cardiopulmonary** is composed of two roots (*cardi* = "heart" + o + *pulmon* = "lung") and the suffix *~ary* meaning "related to." The term for nerve pain, **neuralgia**, also has two roots (*neur* = "nerve" +

alg = "pain") and the suffix *~ia*, used here to indicate a pathological condition.

Some words consist only of a root and suffix; for example, **immunology** (*immune* + *o* + *logy*), **gastric** (*~ic* is a suffix that forms adjectives from nouns), and **rhinorrhea** (*rhin/o* = "nose" + *~rrhea* = a suffix meaning "flow/discharge"). Rhinorrhea is the medical term for "runny nose." (You will notice that in *rhinorrhea* there are two "r's"; when you add a suffix beginning with "rh" to a root, the "r" is doubled; other examples include **hemorrhage**, and **menorrhea**.)

In general English (i.e., the English used in everyday, not specialist, communication) there are many words with more than one prefix (e.g., **inconsiderate**: *in~* = "not" + *con~* = "together") or more than one suffix (e.g., **beautifully**: *~ful* = "full of" + *~ly* = a suffix forming an adverb). Such words also exist in medical English; for example, in **epidemiological**, *~logy* and *~cal* are both suffixes (*epi~* + *demi* + *o* + *logy* → *logi* + *~cal*). Medications used to treat depression are called **antidepressants**, and this word has two prefixes: *anti~* (= "against") and *de~* (= "down").

The word **anemia** could be considered to be composed of a prefix and suffix without a root. The prefix *an~* (= "not/without") and *~emia* a suffix meaning "condition of the blood". I write "could be considered" because some websites list *emia* as a root.

There are even a few cases of a prefix being used alone:

*& She suffered a **hypo** that made her lose consciousness.*

Hypo, a prefix meaning "below normal," is used as a short way to say "**hypoglycemic attack**" (*hypo~* + *glyc* = "sweet/sugar" + *em* = "blood" + *~ic* = a suffix to form adjectives). During a hypo, blood glucose levels fall below normal to levels that are dangerous.

Q. What is the function of combining vowels?　（連結母音は何のためにある？）

A combining vowel links a root with other word parts, like a **coupling** connects railway cars in a train, which makes long medical terms easier to pronounce. Of the following words, which is easier to say?

(A) gastrenterlogy　　　**(B) gastroenterology**

The combining vowels in (B) help with pronunciation and also make the word more **euphonic** (*eu~* = "good" + *phon* = "voice" + *~ic*). **Gastroenterology** is a branch of medicine concerned with diseases of the digestive system.

Q. Is there more than one WFE for "blood"?

（「血液」を言い表す"単語の構成要素"は複数ある？）

（WFE は"word-forming element"の省略。例えば、接頭語、接尾辞、語幹）

Yes, in the following words, mentioned above, the underlined parts all have the meaning of "blood": <u>**hemo**philia</u>, <u>**hemato**poiesis</u>, <u>an**emia**</u>. All three are derived from *haima*, the Greek word for blood. Roots often have several **variants** with different forms, but which are derived from the same root. Here are three examples:

- Drugs, hormones, neurotransmitters, and other molecules that bind to a receptor are called **ligands**. The Latin root *ligare* contained in ligand, means "to bind/to tie." You can see *liga* in words such as **ligament** and **ligature**, but *li* (e.g., **oblige**) and *ly* (e.g., **ally**) are variants.

- In the word **receptor**, the root *cept* means "catch/hold/grasp." It is derived from the root *cipere*. Variants of this root are *cip* (e.g., recipient), and *ceive* (e.g., receive).

- An **insidious disease** is a disease that develops slowly and does not have obvious symptoms at first (e.g., hypertension is an insidious condition). The root *sid* is a variant of *sed*, meaning "to sit." (An insidious disease "sits in" your body, waiting silently.) Words with *sed* include **sedentary**, **sedative** (a drug to treat anxiety), and **obsession** (*ob~* = "next to"; so, an obsession literally "sits next [to you])."

Many prefixes also have variants; for example:

- *Syn~*, meaning "with/together," is in words such as **syndrome** (*drome* means "to run," so a syndrome is composed of various symptoms that "run together"), and **synchronized**. But before a WFE beginning with "b," "p," "m," and some other letters, it changes to *sym~* (e.g., **symbiosis**, **symptom**, **symmetry**).

- The prefix *en~*, meaning "in," changes to *em~* before "p," "b," "m," and some other letters; for example, **ensure**, and **anencephaly**, but **empirical**, **embryo**, and **embolism**. (Anencephaly is a serious birth defect in which a baby is born without parts of the brain and skull. This word has two prefixes, *an~* meaning "without," and *en~* meaning "in," and the root *ceph*, meaning "head").

- The prefix *sub~*, meaning "under/below/from beneath" is in words such as **subcutaneous** (lit. "under the skin"; *cutis* = "skin") and **sublingual** (lit. "under the tongue"; some medications are administered **sublingually**). But the "b" of *sub~* changes depending on the first letter of the root. For example, we do not write "subfix," "subgest," "subport," or "substain," but **suffix, suggest, support, and sustain**. The word sustain literally means "to hold up [from beneath]." The abbreviation **SDGs** stands for "Sustainable Development Goals" (but to me "sustainable development" seems to be an **oxymoron**).

Why do we say "suffix" rather than "subfix," although the original prefix is *sub~*? The answer is that "suffix" is easier to pronounce. The way sounds in speech change to become the same as a neighboring sound is called **assimilation**. Assimilation makes pronunciation more efficient.

Q. How do I pronounce medical terminology?　（医学用語をどう発音する?）

I assume that everyone reading this book has a smartphone and/or access to a computer with an internet connection. If my assumption is correct, then the quickest way to check correct pronunciation is to use an online dictionary. For example, if you wanted to check how to pronounce "**ankylosing spondylitis**" (a type of arthritis that causes the bones in the spine to fuse), put "ankylosing spondylitis + pronunciation" into a search engine. You could also watch a few short online videos about ankylosing spondylitis and listen to how the term is pronounced by different people. Some medical words have silent letters or unusual pronunciation; for example, in **pneumonia**, the "p" is silent and the word starts with a "nu," and in **xenotransplantation**, the Greek root *xenos* (meaning "foreign") is pronounced with a "z" ("zeno"). With your smartphone, however, it's easy to check the correct pronunciation of such words.

Q. There are many thousands of medical words. How can I learn all of these by heart?　　　　　　　（医学用語は山ほどある。どうやったら全部覚えられるのだろう?）

No one is expecting you to memorize thousands of medical terms. However, once you grasp the basic rules on how medical terms are formed, it will become much easier to analyze and remember new medical vocabulary that you encounter. For example, imagine that you come across the term "**osteogenic sarcoma**" in a journal paper on cancer. With your knowledge of prefixes, suffixes, and roots, you could **deconstruct** (break down) this term to figure out its meaning. I know that *oste/o* means "bone," *genic* means "produce," *sarc/o* means "flesh," and *~oma* is a suffix meaning "tumor." So, I could guess that osteogenic sarcoma is "cancer of the flesh that develops in bones." Now, I check online (hopkinsmedicine.org) and find this: *"Osteogenic sarcoma is a cancer that starts in the bone. It often starts in the ends of the bones where new bone tissue forms as a young person grows."* I also learn online that **sarcoma** is a type of cancer that starts in tissues like bone, muscle, cartilage, and fat. Although there are thousands of medical terms, the WFEs that create these terms number "only" around 300. So, as you learn more WFEs, you will become more efficient at deconstructing a newly encountered medical term to get a rough idea of its meaning.

Q. What is the point of becoming familiar with English medical terminology?
　　　　　　　　　　（そもそも何のために医学用語を学ばなければいけないの?）

- It is estimated that over 90% of articles in medical journals are in English. If you are pharmacist, doctor, or other healthcare professional in Japan, then learning medical vocabulary will make it easier for you to find out about the latest research.

- English medical vocabulary is taught to trainee healthcare professionals throughout the world, so it serves as a universal language that helps global communication.

- Medical terminology also makes communication more efficient because, although some of the terms are long, they condense lots of information into one or two words. For example, in the sentence *the patient took medicine to treat dyslipidemia*," if the word "dyslipidemia" did not exist, you would need to explain it like this:

"The patient took medicine to treat a blood lipoprotein disorder that promotes the development of atherosclerosis, and which is characterized by increased low-density lipoprotein cholesterol, decreased high-density lipoprotein cholesterol, and increased serum triglycerides." (33 words)

Saying or writing "dyslipidemia" is much more efficient than repeating the above 33 words each time.

- If you get sick and become a patient, knowing medical terminology can improve communication with healthcare providers and enable you to become more knowledgeable about your condition. This in turn can help you to make important decisions about your treatment.

・ETYMOLOGY （語源）

Etymology is the study of the origins and historical development of words. It is very easy to check the etymology of a word with an online search. For example, if you wanted to find the etymology of "prognosis," you could do the following search: "prognosis + etymology." The entry of the *Online Etymology Dictionary* is shown below:

PROGNOSIS (n.) （予後（名詞））: 1650s, "forecast of the probable course and termination of a case of a disease," from Late Latin *prognosis*, from Greek *prognōsis* "foreknowledge," also, in medicine, "predicted course of a disease," from stem of *progignōskein* "come to know beforehand," from *pro-* "before" (see **pro-**) + *gignōskein* "come to know" (from PIE root **gno-** "to know"). (https://www.etymonline.com/word/prognosis)

If you then click on "**gno-**," you will be taken to a list of other words containing this root, which means "to know/knowledge." Other words with this root include **diagnosis**, **agnostic**, **ignorant**, **acknowledge**, and **recognize**. If, for example, you click on "diagnosis" you will jump to a new entry:

DIAGNOSIS (n.) （診断（名詞））: "scientific discrimination," especially in pathology, "the recognition of a disease from its symptoms," 1680s, medical Latin application of Greek *diagnōsis* "a discerning, distinguishing," from stem of *diagignōskein* "discern, distinguish," literally "to know thoroughly" or "know apart (from another)," from *dia* "between" (see **dia-**) + *gignōskein* "to learn, to come to know," from PIE root **gno-** "to know." (https://www.etymonline.com/word/diagnosis)

Learning medical terminology can seem like studying a foreign language. This is because more than 90% of roots used in medicine are originally from **Latin** (the language of the ancient Romans) and **Greek** (the language of ancient and modern Greece). Around 60% of words in everyday English are also from Latin and Greek, but many of the Latin and Greek roots used in medicine are not common in everyday English. Checking a word's etymology will give you a deeper understanding of that word, and learning more words with the same root can help you to expand your vocabulary. Etymology is also interesting, as the following random examples should illustrate:

- **Atrium**: The upper chambers of the heart are called the **left atrium** and **right atrium**. In ancient Roman houses, the *atrium* was the entrance-hall. In our body, the two **atria** are the entrance-halls to the heart.

- **Cancer**: It is said that it was Hippocrates who named cancerous tumors *karkinos*, which is the Greek word for "crab." It is not known why "the father of medicine" chose this name around 400 BCE, but here are a few possibilities: a crab's shell is hard and so is a cancerous tumor; both the pinch of crab's claw and cancer are painful; if a crab grabs you with its claw, it is tenacious and won't let go, and cancer too can be a relentless disease; and the swollen veins surrounding a tumor resemble the shape of a crab.

- SD（追記）: **Do you like cacti?　Yes, cactuses are really fascinating plants.**
  You will notice that the plural of *atrium* is *atria*. Because many medical terms originate from Greek and Latin, the rules for forming the singular and plural forms often follow the rules of the original language rather than English. Table 1 below shows some of the rules for forming plurals of Greek and Latin words. Some words have both a traditional (i.e., Greek and Latin) plural form and an English plural form. For example, "melanomas" is used more frequently than "melanomata," and in everyday writing and speech, most people would write "formulas" rather than "formulae." And, although "cacti" is the Latin plural of "cactus," the English plural (cactuses) is completely OK to use.

Table 1.

Some Singular and Plural Medical Words　（いくつかの単数形および複数形の医学用語）

Singular ending (単数末尾)	Singular （単数形）	Plural （複数形）
~a	vertebra, formula, pleura	vertebr**ae**, formulae, pleurae
~x	thorax	thora**ces**
~ix	appendix, cervix	appendic**es,** cervices
~is	metastasis, diagnosis, testis	metastas**es**, diagnoses, testes
~ma	sarcoma, melanoma	sarcoma**ta**, melanomata
~um	bacterium, ovum, atrium	bacteri**a**, ova, atria
~us	nucleus, glomerulus, bronchus	nucle**i**, glomeruli, bronchi,
~y	biopsy, deformity	biops**ies**, deformities

- **Muscle** comes from *mus*, the Latin word for "mouse." The movement of a muscle under the skin was thought to resemble the movement of a mouse under the skin.
- **Vaccine** is from the Latin word *vacca* meaning "cow." It was coined by the British doctor Edward Jenner (1749-1823) for the technique of making someone immune to **smallpox** by deliberately infecting a person with the **cowpox virus** (*variolae vaccinae*). Incidentally, the Spanish for "cow" is *vaca*.
- **Hippocampus** is a structure of the brain that has vital role in memory. We have two hippocampi, one in each cerebral hemisphere. The name *hippocampus* derives from a Greek word for sea horse because the shape of the hippocampus resembles a sea horse. The Greek word *hippos*, meaning "horse," is in other words such as **hippopotamus** (lit. "river horse") and **hippodrome**, a place in ancient Greece for horse racing. The root *drome* is from the Greek *dramein*, meaning "to run." A **syndrome** is a group of symptoms that tend to occur, or run, together.
- **Herpes** is a viral infection that often causes cold sores around the mouth. It comes from the Greek word *herpein*, meaning "to creep." The blisters of herpes *creep* slowly across the skin. **Herpetology** is a branch of zoology concerned with snakes and frogs, and other **reptiles** and **amphibians**. These animals creep along the ground (*herpeton* is Greek for "a thing that creeps").
- **Orthopedics** is a branch of medicine concerned with the study and treatment of the **musculoskeletal system** (i.e., bones and muscles). The WFE *ortho~* means "straight" and *paidios* means "child." The term orthopedics was coined in the 17th century by a French doctor (the French word is *orthopédie*). It began as a medical specialty to correct or straighten skeletal problems, including spinal deformities and broken bones, in children. A **pediatrician** is a doctor (*iatros* = "doctor") who specializes in the care of children. In the term "**pediatric orthopedics**," a branch of medicine devoted to treating children's musculoskeletal conditions, the root for "child" is used twice.

In writing this book, *Wikipedia*, a free online encyclopedia, was a useful resource.

The word **encyclopedia** is derived from the Greek *enkyklios paideia*, which literally means "learning in a circle" (*en~* = "in"; *kyklios* = "circle"), but can be translated as "all-round knowledge" or "general education." The root *pedia* (= "education/learning/knowledge") is derived from *paidios*, which in ancient Greece was the education of children.

Not all medical words are derived from Greek or Latin, some are **eponyms**. An eponym is a word derived from the name of a person, a place, or a thing. Here are some examples:

Diseases or conditions named after people: Parkinson's disease, Alzheimer's disease, Cushing's syndrome, Down's syndrome, Kawasaki disease, Hansen's disease (also known as leprosy).

Anatomical parts named after people: loop of Henle, Bowman's capsule, islets of Langerhans, Purkinje fibers, Bundle of His.

Medical tests named after a person: roentgenogram (named after Roentgen; now commonly called a radiograph or x-ray), Apgar score.

Diseases named after places: Lyme disease, Ebola, Marburg virus disease.

Diseases named after a thing: Takotsubo cardiomyopathy, named after a Japanese octopus fishing pot called a *takotsubo* (蛸壺).

There is a debate about the **merits and demerits of using eponyms** in the field of medicine. Some people say that using, for example, nephron loop, glomerular capsule, pancreatic islets, subendocardial branches, and atrioventricular bundle are easier to understand and more informative than loop of Henle, Bowman's capsule, islets of Langerhans, Purkinje fibers, and Bundle of His, respectively. If you are interested to learn more about this debate, just put the words "eponym debate medicine" into the search box of your web browser.

・ABBREVIATIONS　（略語）

An abbreviation is a shortened form of a word or phrase. Healthcare professionals use abbreviations to save time when communicating. In written communication, abbreviations also save space, which is why I have used quite a few in this book. Although abbreviations can be useful, they may not be understood by patients. They can also cause confusion. For example, **ED** could mean **erectile dysfunction**, **eating disorder**, **emergency department**, or **effective dose** (of course, context will usually make clear which meaning of ED is meant). Two main types of abbreviation are initialisms and acronyms:

- **Initialisms** are formed by combining the first (initial) letters of a phrase. In speech, you pronounce each letter of an initialism. Examples include: **HIV** (short for *human immunodeficiency virus*), **MRI** (an abbreviation of *magnetic resonance imaging*), and **IBD** (short for *inflammatory bowel disease*).

- **Acronyms** are usually made up of the initial letters of a phrase, but the initial letters are pronounced as a word. Examples include: **AIDS** (short for *acquired immunodeficiency syndrome*), **NSAIDs** (pronounced "en-saids"), is an abbreviation for *nonsteroidal anti-inflammatory drugs*, and **CRISPR** (pronounced "crisper"), a genetic engineering technique, stands for *clustered regularly interspaced short palindromic repeats*.

   Brevity is important when writing, so I will stop here and leave you to do a few practice exercises on medical terminology. (BTW, the words "abbreviation," "brevity," and "brief" are all derived from the Latin word *brevis*, meaning "short." In case you don't know, BTW is an initialism meaning "by the way.")

Well, what do you know?

（どのくらいわかるようになったか試してみよう）

1. Are the statements that follow each medical term true or false?

   a) lymphoma: This has 1 root and 1 suffix.

   b) cardiovascular: This has 1 prefix, 1 root, and 1 suffix.

   c) thrombocytopenia: This has 2 roots, 2 combining vowels, and 1 suffix.

   d) ischemia: This has 1 prefix and 1 suffix.

   e) pericardium: This has 1 prefix, 1 root, and 1 suffix.

   f) cryptorchidism: This has 2 prefixes and 1 suffix.

2. Circle the best answer.

a) *epi* in the word *epidemic* is a:	**a.** root	**b.** prefix	**c.** suffix
b) *pnea* in the term *dyspnea* is a:	**a.** root	**b.** prefix	**c.** suffix
c) *hepato* is a:	**a.** combining form	**b.** prefix	**c.** suffix
d) *anti* in *antihypertensive* is a:	**a.** prefix	**b.** root	**c.** suffix
e) *kinetics* in *pharmacokinetics* is a:	**a.** prefix	**b.** root	**c.** suffix
d) *gram* in *electrocardiogram* is a:	**a.** prefix	**b.** root	**c.** suffix

3. Use the WFEs (prefixes, roots, suffixes) below to form a term that fits with the definition. The number in parentheses is the number of WFEs required.

hypo · adeno · toxico · rrhea · arthr · neo · ic · hyper · oncho · ~~scope~~
logy · enter · carcin · natal · onco · galacto · algia · gene · ism
oma · derm · gastro · itis · pituitar · lysis · ~~colono~~

E.g., An instrument used to view the colon. (2) = colonoscope

   a) An illness caused by infection and inflammation of the gut. (3)

   b) The study of poisons. (2)

   c) Cancer that occurs in the glandular tissue. (3)

d) Relating to the region beneath the skin. (3)

e) Flow of milk from the breast unrelated to pregnancy or breastfeeding. (2)

f) Joint pain. (2)

g) Relating to newborn babies. (2)

h) A gene that has the potential to cause cancer. (2)

i) Over secretion of one or more pituitary hormones. (3)

j) The separation of a nail from the nail bed. (2)

4. This exercise is to practice deconstructing and interpreting medical terms. For the words below (1-5), do the following steps. An example is done for you with the term "hyperthermia." Use a separate piece of paper to do this exercise.

1. *phagocytosis*   **2.** *hyponatremia*   **3.** *polymyalgia*

4. *intravenous*   **5.** *osteoporosis*

Step 1: Split the term into its constituent WFEs: hyper**/**therm/ia.

Step 2: Write the meaning of each WFE: *hyper* = "above normal" + *therm* = "temperature" + *~ia* = "pathological condition."

Step 3: Combine the meaning of the WFEs to form a rough definition. It is often best to form the definition by first giving the meaning of the term's final WFE, then the meaning of the first WFE, and lastly the middle WFE.

Hyperthermia is a condition (*ia*) in which there is an above normal (*hyper*) temperature (*therm*).

Step 4: Check your rough definition online:

"Hyperthermia is an abnormally high body temperature."

(https://my.clevelandclinic.org/health/diseases/22111-hyperthermia)

5. What do the abbreviations in bold mean? Use context and the Japanese translation to help you. Check your answers on the internet.

a) HT (高血圧) is when blood pressure is consistently too high.

b) BUN (尿素窒素) is a test that measures the amount of urea nitrogen in the blood.

c) HD (血液透析) is a process of cleaning the blood when the kidneys are not working normally.

d) A **CPAP** (持続的気道陽圧(呼吸療法)) machine is used in the treatment of sleep apnea.

e) In combination with cardiopulmonary resuscitation (CPR), using an **AED** (自動体外式除細動器) can save the life of a person who has suffered cardiac arrest.

f) If a **HPAI** (高病原性鳥インフルエンザ) virus becomes able to transmit efficiently between humans, an influenza pandemic could result, potentially causing many more deaths than the COVID-19 pandemic.

Chapter 1 Diabetes mellitus
（糖尿病）

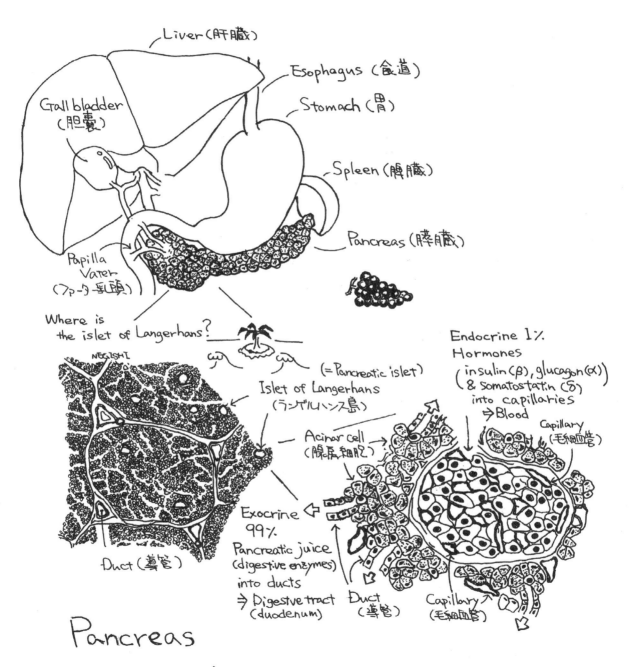

Liver（肝臓）
Esophagus（食道）
Stomach（胃）
Gall bladder（胆嚢）
Spleen（脾臓）
Pancreas（膵臓）
Papilla Vater（ファータ乳頭）

Where is the islet of Langerhans?

NEGISHI

(= Pancreatic islet)

Islet of Langerhans（ランゲルハンス島）

Acinar cell（腺房細胞）

Endocrine 1%.
Hormones
(insulin (β), glucagon (α)
& somatostatin (δ)
into capillaries
⇒ Blood

Capillary（毛細血管）

Exocrine 99%
Pancreatic juice
(digestive enzymes)
into ducts
⇒ Digestive tract
(duodenum)

Duct（導管）

Duct（導管）

Capillary（毛細血管）

Pancreas

The ingenious gland,
Secreting enzymes outward and hormones inward

NAVvocab 60 （案内役の単語 60）

1. adipocyte・脂肪細胞
2. ailment・軽いまたは慢性の病気
3. atherosclerosis・動脈硬化
4. autoimmune・自己免疫
5. bariatric surgery・肥満外科療法
6. contraindicated・禁忌の
7. deleterious・有害な
8. diabetes mellitus・糖尿病
9. diabetic retinopathy・糖尿病網膜症
10. diagnosis・診断
11. dialysis・透析
12. endocrine・内分泌
13. etiology・病気の原因
14. euglycemia・正常血糖
15. exocrine・外分泌の
16. exogenous・外因性の
17. facilitated diffusion・促進拡散
18. gangrenous・壊疽にかかった
19. gastrointestinal tract・消化管，胃腸管
20. glucosuria・糖尿
21. glycemic index・グリセミック指数
22. glycogenolysis・グリコーゲンの分解
23. hepatic gluconeogenesis・肝臓での糖新生
24. hyperglycemia・高血糖症
25. hypoglycemia・低血糖症
26. hypothalamus・視床下部
27. immunogenic・免疫原性
28. pathogenesis・病気の発症機序
29. inextricably linked・密接に関わっている
30. ingest・摂取する，飲み込む
31. insatiable appetite・飽くことのない食欲
32. islets of Langerhans・ランゲルハンス島
33. isolated・単離した
34. microvascular complications・細小血管合併症
35. monosaccharide・単糖
36. morbidity・病的状態，罹患率
37. mortality・死亡率
38. nocturia・夜間頻尿
39. normal range・検査の正常範囲
40. obesity・肥満
41. ophthalmologist・眼科医
42. osmotic diuresis・浸透圧利尿
43. pancreas・膵臓
44. pathophysiology・病態生理学
45. peripheral neuropathy・末梢神経障害
46. pharmacological intervention・薬理学的介入
47. polydipsia・多渇症，多飲症
48. polyphagia・多食症
49. polysaccharide・多糖
50. pre-prandial・食前の
51. prognosis・予後
52. retention・滞留
53. secrete・分泌する
54. skeletal muscle・骨格筋
55. stem cell therapy・幹細胞治療
56. synthetic・合成の
57. urinalysis・尿検査
58. visceral fat・内臓脂肪
59. well-tolerated・忍容性が良い
60. xenotransplantation・異種移植

1-1 Essay — Diabetes: A Mismatch Disease

（糖尿病：ミスマッチ病）

[1]Have you ever tasted urine? I have. When my son was small, he sometimes did a **pee**[E8] in a glass at night and left it by the kitchen sink because he was too lazy to go to the toilet. One morning, mistaking the yellow liquid for homemade *ume* (plum) juice, I took a sip of it. Apparently, until the 1800s doctors tasted a patient's **urine** as a way to detect **diabetes mellitus** (**DM**)[E3]. If the urine was sweet—*mellitus* is Latin for "as sweet as honey"—a positive **diagnosis** could be made. Urine tasting has long been replaced by more accurate testing methods such as the **HbA1c** blood test, but **urinalysis** for the presence of glucose is still used. But why could **glucosuria**, the presence of glucose in the urine, be a **sign**[E11] of diabetes? To answer this question, we need to understand the basics of DM.

[2]Most of the food we eat is **metabolized** into **glucose**, the form of sugar the body requires as a fuel. Let's say I eat a bowl of *udon* noodles (I pick this food because, having lived for three years in Kagawa Prefecture, I must have eaten hundreds of bowls of this prefecture's specialty, *sanuki udon*). The **starch**, a **polysaccharide**, in the noodles will be broken down in the **gastrointestinal** (**GI**) **tract** by physical and chemical digestion into glucose, a **monosaccharide**. The glucose will then be absorbed through the wall of the **small intestine** into the bloodstream. This causes a rise in blood glucose. However, shortly after this rise, blood glucose will fall again as glucose is taken up by body cells. These cells metabolize the glucose to produce energy, or they convert the glucose into a form that can be stored as **glycogen**[E5] or as fat.

[3]It is a **peptide hormone** called **insulin**[E5], released in response to **elevated** blood glucose, that enables glucose from the blood to enter the cells. Insulin is **secreted** from the **pancreas**, an organ around 15 cm long, that is located behind the stomach and shaped like a sweet potato. The pancreas has both **exocrine** and **endocrine**[E4] functions. It is the endocrine cells, named **islets of Langerhans** (also called **pancreatic islets**), that secrete insulin. Specifically, insulin is produced in **β** (**beta**) **cells** of the islets of Langerhans.

[4]An increase in blood glucose is detected by the β-cells, causing them to release more insulin. The islets of Langerhans also contain **α** (**alpha**) **cells** and **delta cells**, which secrete **glucagon** and **somatostatin**, respectively. When Insulin binds to receptors in the plasma membrane of **skeletal muscle** cells and **adipocytes** (fat cells), it acts like a key that unlocks the "doors" to the cell, thereby allowing the entry of glucose into the cell. Of course, this lock and key **analogy** is a simplification, and the take up of glucose is a much more complex process involving **facilitated diffusion** through a **glucose transporter**

called **GLUT4**[D4]. As glucose is transported into cells, blood glucose levels fall, and this fall suppresses further insulin secretion. This is a good example of **negative feedback**.

[5]While insulin acts to lower the level of blood glucose by moving glucose inside cells, glucagon acts to raise the level of blood glucose. You can see that insulin and glucagon are **antagonistic hormones**, a pair of hormones with the opposite effect. They are vital in the regulation of blood glucose, helping to maintain it within a **normal range** (or **reference range**). For non-diabetics, the normal range for blood glucose is approximately 4-6 mmol/L (**millimoles per liter**) before eating (known as **pre-prandial** blood glucose). A blood glucose level above the normal range is called **hyperglycemia,** below it is **hypoglycemia**, and within the normal range is termed **euglycemia**.

[6]As well as the crucial function of enabling the uptake of glucose into cells, insulin has various other important metabolic effects. The main effects of insulin are summarized in Table 1.1. From this table it can be seen that insulin has different actions in different tissues, and that insulin is an **anabolic** hormone, promoting the construction of complex molecules from smaller units, and inhibiting **catabolism** (the breakdown of complex molecules into smaller ones).

[7]Diabetes mellitus occurs when the pancreas cannot produce enough insulin (i.e., **hyposecretion**) and/or when the body does not respond properly to insulin (i.e., **insulin resistance**). Insulin hyposecretion and/or insulin resistance leads to hyperglycemia. Glucose is too important for the body to lose, so 100% of it is normally reabsorbed by the millions of **nephrons** in the kidneys. However, when blood glucose levels rise above a certain level (known as the **renal threshold**), the nephrons become unable to reabsorb all the glucose back into the bloodstream, causing glucose to be excreted in the urine. This is why the urine of a **diabetic**[E2] tastes sweet (and that of my son, who, fortunately, does not have the condition, did not).

[8]**There are several types of DM**[D12], but the main ones are **type 1 diabetes** (**T1D**) and **type 2 diabetes** (**T2D**). Table1.2 compares various aspects of TID and T2D. There are important differences between the **etiology and pathogenesis of T1D and T2D**[D2], but many of the symptoms and complications are the same. Three of the classic symptoms to watch out for in both types can be represented by 3 T's: feeling *Tired* (**fatigue**); going frequently to the *Toilet* to pass large amounts of dilute **urine** (**polyuria**); and increased *Thirst*, which has the medical name **polydipsia**[E10]. Polyuria occurs because the **retention** of glucose in the **tubules** of the nephrons pulls more water into the tubules by osmosis. This increase in the volume of urine excreted is called **osmotic diuresis**. The body responds to the loss of water in the urine by stimulating thirst. The feeling of thirst increases the urge to **ingest** fluids, thereby helping to **compensate** for the extra fluid lost in the urine.

[9]The suffix "poly" in polyuria and polydipsia means "many", and there is another key

"poly" symptom: **polyphagia**, or excessive hunger. In DM, this symptom can occur because glucose from the blood is unable to enter the cells, so glucose cannot be converted into energy. The lack of energy causes the **hypothalamus** in the brain to stimulate hunger, a sensation that motivates eating. After eating food, most non-diabetics no longer feel hungry; however, for some people with untreated DM, the hunger remains even after eating; they describe having an "**insatiable appetite**." Despite eating more, sudden and unintentional weight loss can occur, particularly in T1D. This happens because the body uses fat to produce energy instead of using glucose (which cannot enter muscle and fat cells without insulin). As you can see from the above explanation of symptoms, a knowledge of the **pathophysiology** of DM helps to understand why the different symptoms develop.

Table 1.1

Effect of Insulin in Main Insulin-Sensitive Tissues　（インスリン感受性組織の働き）

Organ/tissue （臓器/組織）	Effect of Insulin　（インスリンの作用） （↓suppression ↑promotion）	Meaning of terminology （用語の意味）
The liver[D10]	↓ **glycogenolysis**	Breakdown of glycogen
	↓ gluconeogenesis	Formation of glucose from non-carbs
	↓ ketogenesis	Production of ketone bodies
	↑ glycogenesis	Glycogen synthesis
	↑ lipogenesis	Formation of fatty acids from glucose
Muscle	↑ glucose uptake	
	↑ protein synthesis	
	↓ protein degradation	
	↑ glycolysis	Breakdown of glucose
	↑ glycogenesis	
	↓ glycogenolysis	
Fat	↑ glucose uptake	
	↑ lipogenesis	
	↓ Lipolysis	

[10]Adam, a family friend, has worked in advertising for many years. In the 1990s, when he was employed by a top advertising agency in London, Adam often went with colleagues or clients for business lunches. During these lunches, he enjoyed lots of good food and several glasses of wine (**alcohol** contains 7 calories per gram, almost as much as fat, which has 9 calories per gram). After the main course, Adam always had a room for a dessert, even if he was full (he, of course, is not the only one with a "**dessert stomach**"). Moreover, a busy work schedule left Adam with little time for exercise. As a result of a **sedentary** lifestyle and

overeating, Adam put on a lot of weight. **Obesity**[D8] is a key risk factor for T2D. When he was in his late 40s, Adam noticed that he was urinating more than usual. He often woke up several times at night to visit the toilet (frequent night-time peeing is called **nocturia**), but he just **attributed** this to stress. However, one morning Adam noticed that his toes felt numb. Concerned, he went to his doctor, and after some tests he was diagnosed with T2D. The numbness was a symptom of nerve damage called **peripheral neuropathy**[E9], one of the **complications** of chronic hyperglycemia.

Table 1.2

Differences Between Type 1 and Type 2 Diabetes （1 型糖尿病と 2 型糖尿病の違い）

	T1D （1 型糖尿病）	**T2D** （2 型糖尿病）
What is the pattern of onset?	Abrupt	Gradual
What is the age at onset?	Usually before age 20*	Usually after 35†
What is the cause?	**Autoimmune condition**: the immune system mistakenly attacks pancreatic β-cells. Sometimes triggered by an infection.	More likely to develop in people who are overweight. Genetic **predisposition** probably more important than in type 1 diabetes.
Is there a body type that is more likely to develop it?	Thin or normal	Often overweight or obese
How is it treated?	Treatment must include insulin. Without insulin the person will die.	**Oral antidiabetics.** Insulin may be needed as the disease progresses.
What is the state of the endogenous insulin?	Low or absent	Low, but sometimes increased‡
It is preventable?	No	Can often be prevented through exercise and diet.

* T2D in adolescents was almost unheard of before the 1990s, but it is now becoming common. The decrease in the age of onset is due mainly to childhood obesity and a lack of physical activity.
†T1D diabetes can begin at any age as was shown when Theresa May, the second female prime minister of the UK (from 2016 to 2019), was diagnosed with T1D at the age of 56.
‡Hyperinsulinemia, the presence of excess insulin in the blood, can result from insulin resistance. The pancreas attempts to compensate for insulin resistance by secreting more insulin. Hyperinsulinemia can be an early indicator of T2D.

[11]Adam needs to have a regular checkup at a local hospital, where his feet are checked by a **podiatrist**, a medical specialist who treats problems with people's feet. The podiatrist carefully examines Adam's feet for nerve damage, termed **diabetic neuropathy**. This check is important because nerve damage can cause people to become insensitive to pain, leading to small injuries on the foot to go unnoticed. This nerve damage, together with the **slow healing of wounds**[D9] means diabetics are **susceptible** to **foot ulcers**. If not treated, ulcers can become **gangrenous**, leading in serious cases to foot **amputation**.

[12]During his regular checkup, Adam's kidney function is tested for **diabetic nephropathy,** also called **diabetic kidney disease**, a condition that can lead to kidney failure and dependence on **dialysis.** Adam's eyes are also examined by an **ophthalmologist** in order to check for early signs of **diabetic retinopathy**, the most common cause of blindness in adults in the UK and the second leading cause in Japan.

[13]The complications described above are caused, either directly or indirectly, by the **deleterious** effect of long-term hyperglycemia on blood vessels. And it is these **vascular** complications that are primarily responsible for the **morbidity** and **mortality** in DM. The complications can be categorized into two groups, according to the size of blood vessels affected: **microvascular complications**, which occur in small blood vessels (e.g., neuropathy, diabetic nephropathy, and retinopathy); and **macrovascular complications,** which affect larger blood vessels (e.g., **coronary artery disease**, **stroke** and **peripheral artery disease**). Diabetics are also prone to **dyslipidemia** (abnormal levels of blood lipoproteins), which is an important risk factor for **atherosclerosis** (hardening and narrowing of the arteries).

[14]**World Diabetes Day** is marked every year on November 14, the birthday of Frederick Banting. He was a Canadian doctor who, in 1921, successfully **isolated** insulin from the pancreatic extracts of dogs. The co-discover with Banting was Charles Best, who was still a medical student at the time. The following year, a 14-year-old Canadian boy with T1D became the first person to receive an injection of insulin from the pancreas of cows. Prior to that day, T1D was always fatal, and most people died within a year of diagnosis (the boy went on to live for another thirteen years, dying of pneumonia at the age 27 in 1935).

[15]For decades, the only source of insulin was from animals, namely cows (**bovine** insulin) or pigs (**porcine** insulin). The main problem with animal-derived insulin was that it could trigger an allergic reaction in some people. Bovine insulin was more **allergenic** than porcine insulin because, compared to human insulin, the insulin from cows is structurally more different than that from pigs (porcine insulin differs from human insulin by only one amino acid, while bovine insulin differs from human insulin by three amino acids). However, from the early 1980s, **synthetic human insulins** became widely available. Because synthetic human insulin is identical in structure to endogenous human insulin, it is much less **immunogenic** than animal-derived insulin (immunogenicity is the ability of a foreign substance to **induce** an immune response). Synthetic human insulin is made using **genetic engineering**. This technology involves the human gene for insulin being incorporated into an *E. coli* bacterium, which then reads the insulin gene, causing it to manufacture insulin.

[16]In 1996, the first insulin **analog** was approved by the **Food and Drug Administration (FDA)** in the USA. Insulin analogues are synthetically made human insulin that have small structural or other changes that give them certain beneficial characteristics. For example, the addition of zinc ions to the insulin results in a drug that has a more gradual **onset** and a longer duration. **Hypoglycemia**[D5], an abnormally low blood glucose level, is the most serious complication of insulin treatment.

[17]Insulin injections replace the insulin the pancreas does not produce. Although these injections can enable a person with T1D to live a relatively normal life, the average life expectancy of people with T1D is still shorter than the general population. Insulin injections are not a **panacea**[E7] for T1D because they do not cure the underlying problem. In the future, treatments such as **islet xenotransplantation** and **stem cell therapy** may mean that insulin injections will no longer be needed.

[18]In T1D, beta cells in the pancreas make no insulin, so people with T1D must inject insulin to control blood glucose levels. On the other hand, in people with T2D, the pancreas still makes some insulin, meaning that insulin injections are often not necessary. However, T2D is a progressive disease, and in a **significant minority** of patients the secretion of endogenous insulin declines so much that **exogenous** insulin, in the form of insulin injections, becomes necessary.

[19]Many people with T2D are prescribed orally administered drugs, called oral antidiabetic drugs, to help control blood sugar levels. **There are several classes of oral antidiabetics**[D11]. In the UK, the most commonly prescribed oral antidiabetic is **metformin**[D7]. Metformin has been approved for diabetes treatment since the late 1950s, but its history is much older. Its active ingredient is **derived** from a plant that was used in Europe for hundreds of years to treat various **ailments**. Metformin lowers blood sugar levels primarily by suppressing **hepatic gluconeogenesis** (i.e., decreasing the production of glucose in the liver). It also increases **insulin sensitivity** in the liver and skeletal muscle. Metformin is generally **well-tolerated**, but it can have **side effects**, including **loss of appetite** and stomach upset. Some people with diabetes also have **chronic heart failure** (CHF), but for several decades, metformin was **contraindicated**[D1] in people with this heart condition. However, evidence from more recent studies suggest metformin can be taken by people with CHF, if the **benefits outweigh the risks**.

[20]Adam has lived with T2D for many years, and, so far, he has not had any serious complications. This is likely due to him following a healthy **diet** (e.g., he cut out most foods with a high **glycemic index**), losing weight, and becoming more physically active. In addition to these lifestyle changes, **pharmacological interventions** have also been important: Adam takes metformin, **antihypertensive medication**, and **statins** (to lower blood cholesterol levels). His successful management of his condition is also because he

takes medication as directed—good **drug adherence** improves the **prognosis** of people with T2D.

[21]It used to be thought that T2D could not be reversed, but research has shown that people with T2D can reduce their blood sugar glucose level to a normal range without medication. How can this reversal be achieved? It's simple: by losing weight. Actually, it's not so simple because, to achieve such a reversal, a person must lose a lot of weight in a short period of time by following a very low-calorie diet. **Calorie restriction** is combined with physical activity, partly because regular **exercise enhances insulin sensitivity**[D3].

[22]It is thought that reversal of T2D through diet occurs because rapid weight loss causes a big reduction in **visceral fat**, which is fat stored around the liver, intestines and other organs in the abdomen. There is increasing evidence that excess visceral fat leads to chronic low-grade inflammation and that this inflammation is involved in the pathogenesis of T2D. Reversal of diabetes is not a cure; instead, doctors talk of diabetes **remission**. Remission is not possible for everyone, but losing extra weight will benefit nearly all people with T2D. Very-low-calorie diets are extreme diets and should be undertaken under the supervision of a medical team, including a **dietician**.

[23]Another way to lose a lot of weight is by weight-loss surgery, also called **bariatric surgery**[E1]. There is a large **body of research** showing that bariatric surgery can often bring about diabetes remission, but it is major surgery that has risks. It would be much better if T2D could be prevented—after all, **prevention is better than cure**. Diabetes is the world's fastest growing chronic condition, and although it is not infectious in the same way as COVID-19, the global rise in T2D has been described as a "pandemic." The diabetes pandemic is becoming a **grave problem** for many healthcare systems around the world.

[24]To understand how DM could be prevented, we need to know the factors that are driving the global increase in T2D. While genes can **predispose** a person to developing T2D, lifestyle factors such as an unhealthy diet and lack of physical activity are extremely important. The global increase in T2D is **inextricably linked** to the increase in obesity. In the UK, around 32% of people are obese (defined as having a **BMI** of over 30%). Whenever I visit London, I am always **taken aback** by the number of very big people walking around. Although **Japan has a relatively low obesity rate**[D6] of around 4%, T2D is a serious and growing problem in this country too.

[25]There are still a few societies in the world that remain relatively untouched by the modern world. In such societies T2D is very rare or absent. One such society is the **Hadza people** of Tanzania. The Hadza are **hunter-gatherers**, relying on hunting animals and **foraging** for roots, nuts and fruit. The ancestors of modern humans were also

hunter-gatherers. Over millions of years our bodies adapted to the hunter-gatherer lifestyle, a lifestyle of being physically active for much of the day and eating a varied, high-fiber diet.

[26]Compare that to the world in which you live—a world with cars, elevators, escalators, smart phones, mostly sedentary jobs, and convenience stores crammed with **ultra-processed food** that is **calorically dense**, and yet nutrient-poor. We can say that T2D is a classic example of what **evolutionary anthropologists** call a "**mismatch disease**," or diseases that are a consequence of our hunter-gatherer bodies being poorly adapted to the modern world. Although we can't press a time-machine app on our smartphones and return to being **Paleolithic** hunter gathers, we can take lessons from the hunter-gatherer way of life to help reduce the risk of T2D and other lifestyle diseases.

1-2　Eleven Etymologies (E)　（11 の単語を詳しく）

1) ***Bariatric surgery* is weight loss surgery that is sometimes used to treat people who are obese.** There are several types of weight loss surgery; one type, called a **gastric bypass**, involves the top part of the stomach being attached to the small intestine. A person who has undergone a gastric bypass will have a smaller stomach, so the amount of food that he or she can eat will be greatly reduced. Weight loss after this surgery happens rapidly, and within one year after surgery a person can lose 60 to 80% of excess body weight. Studies have shown that soon after surgery, often within 24 hours, the blood glucose level of people with T2D returns to normal levels (i.e., it becomes **euglycemic**). In other words, bariatric surgery can actually reverse T2D. The fact that the reversal of T2D often occurs before any significant weight loss has occurred means that it cannot be explained only by weight loss. It is thought that changing the **anatomy** of the digestive tract with gastric bypass surgery affects the secretion of **gut hormones**, which in turn improves glucose metabolism and resolves the T2D. Incidentally, drugs for the treatment of T2D have been developed that mimic gut hormones. These drugs, called **incretin mimetics**, were first discovered in the saliva of a lizard called the **Gila monster**, the only **venomous** lizard in the USA.

WFE: In bariatric *bar* means "weight/pressure" and *iatric* means "medical treatment/doctor."
*& There are **baroreceptors** in certain arteries that sense changes in blood pressure.*
*& A **pediatric psychiatrist** is a doctor who diagnoses and treats children with mental health conditions. (ped~ = "child"; psych = "mind")*

Although rare, there are cases of healthcare workers infecting patients with an infectious disease. For example, around 20 years ago, a doctor in Israel who had hepatitis C infected several patients with the hepatitis C virus. This is an example of **iatrogenic** infection (*genic* = "to cause"; so, iatrogenic means "caused by a doctor or medical treatment"). **Iatrogenic harm** is unintended harm caused by a doctor or other healthcare professional. A pharmacist that **dispenses** the incorrect medication to a patient and causes that patient to have a serious adverse reaction is an example of iatrogenic harm. A more everyday term with a similar meaning is **medical error**.

SD 1A: I've got a very painful corn on my foot, who should I see?

Podiatry is a medical specialism that deals with the prevention, diagnosis, and treatment of problems affecting the foot. People often visit a **podiatrist** if they have a **foot corn** (hard layers of thickened skin caused by friction), or some other problem with the foot. Podiatrists help people with diabetes look after their feet by screening for peripheral nerve damage, and by checking for ulcers and other foot injuries. They help to prevent foot damage by trimming toenails, removing hard skin on the foot, and recommending special diabetic shoes that protect against foot ulcers. In the UK, to become a podiatrist you usually need to do an **undergraduate** or a **Master's degree** in podiatry. Studying full time, it takes two to three years to become a **qualified** podiatrist. In Japan, however, podiatry is not a recognized **medical specialty** and there is no podiatry course available. The word "podiatry" is made up of *pod*, the Greek for "foot," and *iatros*, meaning "doctor/treatment." Other words with *pod* are **tripod**, **podium**, and **cephalopod**. Cephalopods are animals that have their feet (tentacles) directly attached to their head (*cephalo* = "head"). One example of a cephalopod is an **octopus** ("eight feet"). Incidentally, in Japanese, the word *tako* (たこ) means both "octopus" and "corn" (hard skin). This is an example of a **homonym**, two words that have the same spelling and pronunciation but have different meanings (*homo* = "same" + *nym* = "name"). The WFE *pus* is the Latin for "foot." It is found in many words, including the verb **impede**, and the nouns **pedal**, **pedestrian**, **expedition**, **biped**, **centipede**, and **pedigree**.

2) *Diabetic* is an adjective that means "a person with diabetes." However, nowadays, many people do not consider it acceptable to refer to a person by the disease they have. Instead of saying "Adam is a diabetic" it would probably be better to say, "Adam has diabetes" or "Adam is living with diabetes." Saying "Adam is diabetic" makes it sound as if Adam and the disease are the same, rather than diabetes being just one part of his life. Here are three more examples. Rather than "she is **schizophrenic**", consider using, "she has **schizophrenia**"; rather than "he is **epileptic**," consider saying, "he has **epilepsy**"; and rather than referring to someone as "**blind**," perhaps use the phrase "someone living with sight loss."

The British Psychological Society has suggested that the phrase "obese person" should be avoided because it is **stigmatizing** and offensive. It calls for the phrase "a person with obesity" or "person living with obesity" to be used instead. As people's views change over time, language changes too. In the past, the word "**retarded**" or "mentally retarded" was the normal way to describe people with limitations in mental functioning. However, "retarded" is now judged to be **offensive**. In the 2020s, terms such as **"intellectual disability"** and **"cognitive disability"** are usually used instead.

*People with Down syndrome will be **mentally retarded** to some degree. (?)*

*People with Down syndrome will have some degree of **cognitive disability**.*

3) ***Diabetes mellitus*** **is a chronic metabolic disorder characterized by high blood glucose.**

WFE: The word "mellitus" comes from the Latin root for "honey"; "diabetes" is from a Greek word meaning "siphon." So, lots of sweet urine passes through the body as if it were a siphon. The prefix *dia~* has several meanings, but in the word diabetes it means "through." Other words with this prefix are: **diarrhea** (*dia~* = "through" + *rrhea* = "flow"); **diameter** (*dia* = "across"; *meter* = "measure"); **dialysis** (*dia~* = "apart"; *lysis* = "separation"). In **diagnosis**, the WFE *~gnosis* means "to know/ knowledge." Diagnosis can be thought of as a judgement [on what is wrong with someone] that comes *through knowledge*." Another important medical word containing *~gnosis* is **prognosis** (lit. "know before"), which is the likely outcome or course of a disease.

SD 1B: "Japanese Diet Member Diagnosed with Diabetes on Calorie-Cutting Diet"

This title of this Box is a fictional headline from a newspaper. Two characteristics of newspaper headlines are **ellipsis** and **alliteration**. Ellipsis is the **omission** of one or more words that can be understood from context. To make the headline grammatically complete, you would need to add several words:

ᴬJapanese Diet member ᵂʰᵒ ʷᵃˢ diagnosed with diabetes ʰᵃˢ ᵍᵒⁿᵉ on ᵃ calorie-cutting diet

Let's focus on three words in the headline: Diet, diet, and calorie. The first **"Diet"** in the headline refers to the **National Diet**, or Japan's parliament. In Japanese, the Diet is called *Kokkai* (国会). The second "diet" in the headline is related to food intake. The word "diet" is derived from the Greek word *diaita*, which means "daily work/way of life." Over time, "diet" came to mean a way of eating that is advised by a doctor. The etymology of "Diet" is somewhat unclear, but it may also be derived from *diaita*. This could be the connection: In the same way that a person on a diet follows a set of rules about which foods to eat and which foods to restrict, the National Diet follows a schedule to pass laws.

The word **calorie** is a French word that comes from the Latin *calor* meaning "heat." A calorie is a unit of energy. A calorie written with a lower case "c" is the amount of energy it takes to raise the temperature of 1 gram of water by 1°C (degree Celsius). A **C**alorie, with an upper case "C," is short for kilocalorie (kCal), which is the amount of energy it takes to raise the temperature of 1 kilogram of water by 1°C. When you check the calorie content on the back of a food package, it is kilocalories (Calories with a big "C") that is being referred to.

Scientists measure the calorie content in food by burning the food in device called a **bomb calorimeter**. The heat that is given off by the **combustion** of the food is used to calculate the calorie content of a particular food. However, if you are trying to watch your weight, just comparing the calories contained in different food items is of limited value. This is because foods will have a different **caloric availability**. Professor Giles Yeo, an obesity geneticist at

Cambridge University, defines this important concept in his book "Gene Eating" (2018):
"Caloric availability is the amount of calories that can actually be extracted during the digestive process, as opposed to the total calories that are locked up in the food." (p. 62)

Unlike a bomb calorimeter, the human digestive system cannot extract all the calories from a particular food. The proportion of calories that can be extracted will depend on various factors, including genetics, sex, age, gut microbes, the time of day we are eating, and how active or sedentary a person is. But most important is the type of food. For example, compare sugar, sweet corn, and tortillas. If we go to the supermarket to buy granulated sugar to make a cake, the sugar you will buy is **sucrose**, which is made up of one fructose molecule and one glucose molecule joined together. If you ate 100 calories of sucrose, it is likely that the process of digestion would extract more than 95 calories. This is because enzymes in the small intestine only have to split sucrose into fructose and glucose. And glucose can be used immediately as fuel. On the other hand, if you ate 100 calories of canned sweet corn, the digestive system would absorb many fewer calories than the 100 calories that are contained in it. Many of the calories are locked in the **cellulose** shell of the sweet corn, and this cannot be digested (so it passes out of the body—take a look in the toilet the morning after you have eaten sweet corn for dinner). The caloric availability of sweet corn is much lower than sucrose. Corn flour is made by drying sweet corn kernels and grinding them up very finely. This flour can be used to make **tortilla**, a thin pancake that is a **staple** of Mexican cooking. Compared to sweet corn, the highly processed tortilla will have a much higher caloric availability. Grinding the corn kernels breaks down the cellulose and makes more of the calories accessible to the body. So, just looking at calories does not tell you how many calories your body can take from a certain food.

Another example that Professor Yeo gives is celery. One medium-sized stick of celery is only 6 calories, but if it is cooked, for example, in a soup, the caloric availability increases to 30 calories. This is because most of celery's calories are stored in **cellulose,** and cooking breaks down the cellulose, allowing the digestive tract to extract more calories. As with cooking, **fermentation** also improves digestibility by breaking down substances such as starch and fiber. For example, the caloric availability of *Kkakdugi* (カクテキ), a type of kimchi made from diced radish, would be higher than the same amount of raw radish. Using fire (cooking) and fermentation are ways to partly digest foods *before* we eat them. This **predigestion** reduces the amount of energy required for digestion and increases caloric availability.

Finally, which would you choose if you were on a diet? Three and a half squares of milk chocolate or one medium-sized apple? Both contain 100 calories, but when you make your choice, remember that milk chocolate has a much higher caloric availability than an apple. Milk chocolate is also high in **fat**, and fat is the most efficient fuel to digest. Fat provides 9 calories per gram but it only requires around 3% of consumed calories to digest. To digest food costs the body energy, which is sometimes called the **thermal effect of food**, and fat takes the least energy to digest. (Because protein is the most chemically complex of the **macronutrients**, it takes the most energy to digest, with nearly 30% of the calories consumed from protein being required to digest it. Carbohydrates take between 5-10% of consumed calories to digest). In case you're still tempted to choose the milk chocolate, consider that the apple contains many more vitamins and minerals.

4) *Endocrine* refers to hormones and the glands that produce and secrete these hormones. A **gland** is an organ or specialized cells that synthesizes one or more substances for use in the body. The **endocrine system** is made of **endocrine glands,** which are also called **ductless glands** because they secrete hormones directly into the bloodstream, and not through a **duct** (a small tube). Hormones are chemical messengers that are carried in the blood to target cells. Hormones alter the activity in cells and tissues causing various changes (the word "hormone" is derived from a Greek word meaning "to excite into activity"). Hormones produce their effects in tiny amounts, being measured in the body in parts per trillion (ppt); 1ppt is equivalent to a quarter of a teaspoon of sugar dissolved in an Olympic-sized swimming pool. In school biology lessons, I learnt about the **primary endocrine glands**, whose main function is hormone secretion. Such glands include the **hypothalamus, pineal**, and the **pituitary** in the brain; the **thyroid** and **parathyroids** in the throat; the **islets of Langerhans** in the pancreas; the **adrenal glands**, on top of the kidneys; and the **ovaries** and **testes,** which are the **gonads** (reproductive glands). However, I did not learn that many other organs secrete hormones in addition to their primary function. Examples of such **secondary endocrine glands** and their hormones include the heart (**atrial natriuretic peptide**), kidney (e.g., **erythropoietin**), and the **gastrointestinal tract** (e.g., gastrin, ghrelin). **Adipose tissue**, commonly called fat tissue, used to be considered just a store for energy, but now it is known to be one of the body's largest endocrine organs, secreting a number of hormones called **adipokines**.

Whereas endocrine glands release hormones directly into the bloodstream, another type of gland, **exocrine glands**, release substances via ducts onto a surface or into a cavity. For example, sweat glands secrete sweat onto the surface of the skin, **salivary glands** secrete **saliva** into the mouth, and **mammary glands** produce and secrete milk. One type of exocrine gland (called **parietal cells**) in the stomach secretes **hydrochloric acid** (HCl) onto the lining (**epithelium**) of the stomach. More than 95% of the pancreas is comprised of exocrine tissue, while only between 2% to 5% consists of endocrine cells that secrete insulin and other hormones. The exocrine part of the pancreas produces **pancreatic juice**, which contains enzymes to digest food (the enzymes include **lipase, trypsin**, and **amylase**, which break down fat, protein, and carbohydrates, respectively). Pancreatic juice is secreted via ducts into the **duodenum**, the first part of the small intestine.

WFE: The prefix *endo~* of **endocrine** means "within" and *crin,* from the Greek *krinein,* means to "to separate." An **endoscope** (*scope* = "look") is medical device used to examine the hollow organs of the body such as the colon, stomach, and bladder. The word **endogenous** means "to be produced internally"; *genous* is from the WFE *gen* (= "birth/origin/ produce").

*& Around 25% of cholesterol in the body comes from the diet; the rest is **endogenous** cholesterol produced in the liver.*

Other words in this essay with this suffix are **allergenic** and **immunogenic**.

The prefix *exo~* in exocrine means "outside/external."

*& Fire is an <u>**exothermic**</u> reaction, in other words, one that produces heat.*

*& There is concern that the trade in <u>**exotic**</u> pets will spread zoonotic diseases and spark another pandemic.*

*& Two characteristics of arthropods, which include insects and spiders, are having an <u>**exoskeleton**</u> and jointed limbs.*

The word "duct" is from the Latin *ducere* meaning "to lead." **Air ducts** are pipes that carry (or "lead") air between two points, and in the human body the **common bile duct** is a tube that carries ("leads") bile from the liver and gallbladder into the small intestine. The meaning of "lead" is in the following words: <u>**conduct**</u>, <u>**introduce**</u> (*intro~* = "inside"), <u>**reduce**</u> (*re~* = "back"), <u>**educate**</u> (*e~* → ex~ = "out"; so, "lead out"). Note that *duc* is a variant of *duct*.

5) *Glycogen* is a polysaccharide composed of thousands of glucose units joined together. Stored mainly in the liver and muscles, glycogen is converted into glucose when energy is needed.

WFE: *Glyco* means "sweet," and *~gen* means "to produce/to cause"; *gluco~* has the same meaning. In this essay, we have met a number of words with *glyco/gluco*:

- <u>**glucose**</u>: the suffix *~ose* is used to name sugars. Glucose is a simple sugar or **monosaccharide** (*mono~* = "one"). Sucrose is a **disaccharide** (*di~* = "two") composed of glucose and fructose.

- <u>**glucosuria**</u>: glucose in the urine (*uria* = "urine").

- <u>**HbA1c test**</u>: a blood test used to diagnose DM and to monitor blood glucose levels in people with DM. The test indicates blood glucose levels over the last 2 to 3 months by measuring how much glucose is bound to red blood cells. The higher the blood glucose levels and the longer the duration of the hyperglycemia, the more glucose attaches to hemoglobin. HbA1c is short for **glycated hemoglobin**. Glycated hemoglobin has undergone **glycation**, a chemical process in which a sugar molecule joins to a protein or fat molecule.

- <u>**hypoglycemia**</u>: *hypo~* (= "low") + *glyc~* (= "sugar") + *~emia* (= "blood").

- <u>**hyperglycemia**</u>: *hyper~* (= "high").

- <u>**neuroglycopenic**</u>: *neuro~* (= "nerves/nervous system") + *glyco* (= "sugar") + *pen* (*penia* = "lack of") + *~ic* (suffix forming an adjective).

- <u>**glucagon**</u>: a hormone that raises the level of blood glucose.

- <u>**euglycemia**</u>: a normal level of sugar in the blood; *eu~* = "good/normal."

- <u>**glycogenolysis**</u>: the breakdown of glycogen into glucose; *lysis* = "breakdown/separation/loosen." Other words with *~lysis* include **dialysis**, **analysis**, **autolysis**, **paralysis**. **Lysis** is the breakdown of a cell caused by damage to its outer membrane.

  *Ɛ Some types of snake venom cause **lysis** of red blood cells. This is called **hemolysis**.*

  The noun **catalyst** contains a variation of "lysis" (*cata* = "down"):

  *Ɛ For a chemical reaction to take place, a certain minimum amount of energy, called the activation energy, is required. A **catalyst** is a substance, such as an enzyme, that can lower the activation energy without being changed or destroyed during the reaction.*

- **gluconeogenesis**: *gluco* (= "sugar") + *neo* (= "new") + *genesis* (= "produce"). The synthesis of new glucose from noncarbohydrate sources such as protein and fat. Other words with the suffix ~*genesis* include **carcinogenesis**, **pathogenesis**. When used alone **genesis** means "the beginning":

  *Ɛ The **genesis** of agriculture can be traced back to around 11,000 BCE.*

SD 1C: Genmai GI vs white rice GI

The **glycemic index** (GI) is an important concept that all diabetics should be aware of. Even if you do not have DM, being aware of it can help you to choose healthier foods. Do you like riding the rollercoaster at an amusement park? I would pay *not* to ride on a rollercoaster, but some people love the thrill of soaring sharply and then dropping almost vertically. Lots of **peaks and troughs** may be great for rollercoaster rides, but when it comes to blood glucose levels, such ups and downs should be avoided. The GI is a value given to foods based on how quickly a certain food causes an increase in blood glucose levels. It measures how much a certain food raises blood sugar compared to pure glucose. A food with a GI of 30 raises blood sugar only 30% as much as pure glucose, whereas one with a GI of 100 acts just like pure glucose. Orange juice has a high GI (around 70), but that of a whole orange is much lower GI (around 40). The main reason for this is that in the whole fruit much of the sugar (fructose) is contained within the cells, surrounded by the **cell wall**. Dietary fiber is in many parts of a plant, but the cell wall is the main fiber-containing structure. Because the digestive system cannot completely breakdown the cellulose-containing cell wall, the amount of sugar absorbed into the bloodstream is reduced and the absorption takes a relatively long time. (The fiber in an orange not only lowers the GI, but it also plays an important role in gut health because fiber improves **gut motility** and has a beneficial impact on the gut microbiome). On the other hand, when oranges are made into commercial orange juice, most of the fiber in the fruit is removed, and the sugar becomes **free sugar**. Free sugar is easily absorbed and reaches the bloodstream very quickly. White rice also has a high GI (around 73), meaning it causes spikes in blood sugar. The high prevalence of T2D in high in Japan is partly related to the high consumption of white rice and other **refined carbohydrates**. The GI of brown rice, called *genmai* (玄米) in Japanese, is about 50.

  Soft drinks are full of free sugar that causes sharp spikes in blood glucose, and they are an important factor in the increased incidence of obesity and T2D. In 2018, the UK introduced a **levy** on sugary drinks (the "**sugar tax**") as a way to encourage **beverage** manufacturers to reduce the sugar content of the drinks they produce. People concerned about their health should avoid soft drinks. However, because sugary soft drinks raise blood sugar levels quickly, they are an effective treatment for **hypoglycemia**, a potentially serious complication of insulin therapy.

6) *Insulin* **is a hormone that regulates the amount of glucose in the blood. It is produced in the pancreas by groups of cells called islets of Langerhans**. In 1867, while in his early 20s and still in medical school, a German pathologist called **Paul Langerhans**, discovered some cells in the pancreas. He reported that under the microscope these cells looked like tiny islands scattered around the exocrine tissue of the pancreas. Langerhans died in 1888, aged 41, but after his death, a French researcher named the cells that Langerhans had identified as *islets de Langerhans* ("**islets of Langerhans**"). The word "insulin" was first introduced in 1909.

It is remarkable to think that in 1838, over a decade before Paul Langerhans was born, a pig's **cornea** was transplanted into a human for the first time. Transplantation of an organ, tissue, or cells between two different species is called **xenotransplantation**. In theory, T1D could be cured with a transplant of a pig's pancreas (pigs are the most suitable animal because their organs are about the same size as that of humans). I mention xenotransplantation because on January 7, 2022, the first pig-to-human heart transplant was announced by doctors at the University of Maryland Medical Center. Prior to the Maryland transplant, organ transplants from animals had failed, mainly because the immune system of patients rapidly **rejected** the animal organ. The Maryland transplant, however, used a heart from a pig that had been genetically engineered to avoid immune rejection. (The patient, a man called David Bennett, died two months after the transplant of heart failure, but the pig's heart showed no signs of rejection by David's body.) There is a shortage of human donors, so genetically engineered pigs could one day provide new pancreases for people with DM. However, xenotransplantation has been condemned as being unethical—Why should animals be killed to save humans? In addition, people worry that xenotransplantation of a pig's organ could transmit a microbe to the human recipient and cause the emergence of a new **zoonotic disease**.

WFE: The suffix *~in* indicates a protein, and *insula* means "island." So, the term "insulin" means "a protein [hormone] secreted by isolated and scattered cells that resemble islands." In general English, **insular** is used to describe people who are closed-minded and only know about their own country or group:

*℮ Travelling and living abroad helps people to learn about other cultures and become more open-minded. As a result of the COVID-19 pandemic and other factors, fewer young Japanese people are going abroad to study. There is concern that this will make Japan more **insular**.*

I suspect that the average North Korean citizen is quite insular. Where is North Korea? It is on the **Korean Peninsula** (*pene~* = "almost"; lit. "almost an island"). In the word **xenotransplantation**, *xeno~* means "foreign/different in origin." Two words to remember with this WFE are **xenophobia** (*phobia* = "fear of") and **xenobiotic** (*~bios* = "life").

*℮ Some British people voted for Brexit in 2016 because they did not like foreigners. But most Brexit voters were not **xenophobic** and wanted to leave the **EU** for other reasons.*

℮ Microplastics are small pieces of plastic (<5 mm) that come from plastic pollution. They

*have been found in fish and in the feces of human babies. There is concern that this **xenobiotic** (i.e., a substance that is foreign to an organism) can harm the health of people and animals.*

SD 1D: Could stem-cell therapy be a cure for T1D?

With **stem-cell biology** it is possible for insulin-producing cells to be produced in the laboratory and then **infused** into a patient. The infused cells can then start producing insulin. In 2021, it was reported that an American man named Brian Shelton had been cured of T1D using this kind of stem cell therapy. In the future, this therapy may become widely available for people with T1D. Recent advances in stem-cell therapy owe a lot to the work of Dr Shinya Yamanaka (山中 伸弥), who first succeeded in generating **iPSC** in 2006 (for which he was awarded the 2012 **Nobel Prize in Physiology or Medicine**, jointly with Sir John Gurdon, a British biologist).

The abbreviation iPSC stands for **induced pluripotent stem cells**. These cells are derived from **somatic cells** (i.e., any cell of the body except sperm and egg cells) that have been reprogrammed to become stem cells. Stem cells have the capability to then develop into almost any type of cell. Dr Yamanaka and his team discovered a way to reprogram cells to an **embryonic**-like state that can give rise to different types of cells. Until the about 14 days after **conception**, the human **embryo** is composed of undifferentiated cells. It is only in the third week that these cells start to **differentiate** (specialize) to become the heart, liver, eyes, hair, and all the other different cells, tissues and organs in the body. Dr Yamanaka's iPSC technology provided a way to take, for example, a normal skin cell, and reprogram it to how it was as a week-old embryo, when it had the potential to become almost any cell in the body. The word "induce" means to "cause something to happen" (*duce* = "to lead, to guide"). The prefix *pluri~* in "pluripotent" means "many", and "potent" means "power/potential." So, an iPSC has been *induced* to return to a stem cell that has the *potential* to differentiate into *many* cell types.

7) ***Panacea* is a solution for all problems.** In Greek mythology, *Panaceia* is the goddess of healing.

WFE: Panacea is from the Greek word *panakeia,* meaning "cure-all" (*pan* = "all"; *akos* is derived from *~iatric* = "to heal").

*& During the COVID-19 **pandemic**, vaccines helped save many lives. However, they were not a **panacea**.* (*demos* = "people"; so, a pandemic affects all people)

*& Pancreatic cancer is cancer that starts in the **pancreas**.* (*kreas* means "flesh"; so pancreas literally means "all flesh," perhaps because it has homogenous, fleshy appearance).

SD 1E: Insulin is a lifesaver but not a panacea

The advent of insulin injections in 1922 changed T1D from a fatal disease to a chronic condition that people could live with for many years. However, for several reasons insulin injections are not a panacea for DM. Until the late 1970s, all insulin came from animals. But animal-sourced insulin sometimes triggered an allergic reaction in patients because the structure of animal insulin is slightly different from human insulin. In 1978, the first **synthetic human insulin** became available. Synthetic insulin works better than animal insulin, it does not trigger allergies, and it avoids ethical concerns. However, synthetic insulin is very expensive, so many people living with DM in lower-income countries, and even in the USA, cannot afford it.

Another reason that insulin is not a panacea is related to the route of administration: Insulin can only be taken by **non-oral** means, most often by **subcutaneous injection** (although **insulin pumps** are increasingly used). The medical term for non-oral ways to get a drug into the body is **parenteral administration** (*enteron*= "intestine" +*para~*= "beside/beyond"; think of "parenteral" as meaning "avoiding the intestine"). Taking insulin orally would be more convenient, but because insulin is a peptide hormone it would quickly be **degraded** in the stomach by gastric acid and digestive enzymes. There is another way to administer insulin: through the lungs by **inhalation**. In 2014, the Food and Drug Administration (FDA) approved an inhaled human insulin, with the brand name Afrezza. Inhaling insulin means it is absorbed through the lungs into the bloodstream, which is a very rapid method of drug delivery. However, there are concerns about the possible **deleterious** effects of inhaled insulin on the respiratory system. These concerns may explain why Afrezza has not been **authorized** for use in Japan, the UK, and other counties. Finally, while an insulin injection can replace endogenous insulin, it cannot make the pancreas start making insulin again. This is the main reason insulin is not a panacea for TID.

8) *Pee* **is an informal word for "urine."** (As a verb, "pee" is an informal way to say "urinate"). "Pee" is most often used informally, while "urine" is more formal and medical sounding. In asking for a sample from a patient, a doctor may say to a child, "We need a little bit of your pee in this cup." In making the same request to an adult, a doctor would probably say, "Please use this cup to provide a urine sample." The way language is used in different situations is called **register**.

9) *Peripheral neuropathy* **is damage to nerves outside of the central nervous system (the brain and spinal cord), which often affects the hands and feet**.

WFE: The prefix *peri~* means "around" (a submarine has a **periscope** for looking around the surrounding area), and *neuro~* means "nerve." The WFE *pathos* has several meanings. For example, in "**pathologist**" it means "disease," while in "**sympathy**" it means "feel/suffer" (lit. "feel/suffer together"). An important word for healthcare professionals is **empathy**.

*€ Having been raised by a single mother in a one-room apartment in a poor neighborhood of Osaka, Dr Tanaka could feel **empathy** for patients in financial hardship.* (em~ → en~ = "in"; so, empathy is the "ability to share another person's feelings or suffering.")

Apathy, which literally means "an absence of feeling" (*a~* = "not"), is a lack of enthusiasm and concern for things around you. Apathy can be a symptom of mental health problems.

€ Cannabis is the world's most widely used illicit drug, and some studies show that long-term

*use of cannabis is associated with a lack of motivation and **apathy**.*

*& Many younger voters in Japan are not interested in politics and think that even if they do vote, nothing will change. Such **voter apathy** leads to a low election turnout, which is not good for democracy.*

10) *Polydipsia* is excessive thirst, accompanied by drinking excessive amounts of fluid. The prefix *poly~* is very common in medical English. For example, insulin is a **polypeptide** hormone that is composed of many peptides (strings of amino acids). **Polyphagia** is the medical term used to describe "excessive hunger or increased appetite." The WFE *phagia* means "eat." A type of white blood cells is a **macrophage**, which literally means "big eater." **Polypharmacy** is the regular use of several, often at least five, medicines. More common in older people, polypharmacy increases the risk of drug interactions and side effects. A **polypill** is a medicine that contains multiple medications. It is also known as **fixed-dose combination therapy**. It has been proposed, for example, that people at risk of cardiovascular disease should be offered a polypill containing a combination of blood pressure lowering medicine, a statin for dyslipidemia, and low-dose aspirin to prevent the formation of potentially deadly blood clots.

Outside of medicine, you can find *poly~* in some difficult words:

*& Japan's Shinto is an example of a **polytheistic** religion which worships many kami (神) or gods.*

*& Professor Rose is a leading expert in pharmacology, but he also writes about politics, philosophy, and history. In addition, he speaks five languages fluently, and he is an expert on Chinese and Japanese food. He is a true **polymath**. (~math = "learning")*

11) *Sign*: The words "sign" and "symptom" are often used **interchangeably**. However, in medicine there is a difference between the two words. A sign can be identified by the patient and also by other people. For example, a cough can be heard, and the **radial pulse** (on the wrist) can be **palpated** (felt with the fingers). Some signs need to be identified by medical professionals using various tests (e.g., a chest X-ray can help identify a **tumor** in the lung, which could lead to a diagnosis of lung cancer). **Vital signs** are measurements of the body's most basic functions. Vital signs are the heart rate (pulse), breathing rate (or respiration rate), body temperature, and blood pressure. A sign is **objective** evidence of a disease. A **symptom**, on the other hand, is **subjective**, which is identifiable only by the person experiencing it. For example, loss of smell (**anosmia**) is a symptom of COVID-19, while fever is a sign; feeling thirsty all the time can be a symptom of DM, while slow wound healing is a sign; and stomach cramps are a symptom of ulcerative colitis, while blood in the feces is a sign. Doctors cannot identify or test for thirst, loss of smell, or stomach cramps, which is why they need to ask questions of patients to help reach a diagnosis.

WFE: The word "symptom" contains *sym~*, a common prefix, which means "together/at the same time." It is usually spelt *syn~*, but is changed to *sym~* before the letters "b," "m," and "p," and is changed to *sy~* before "s" (e.g., **system**). The prefix *a~* means "not/without," so **asymptomatic** means "showing no symptoms of a particular disease."

ℰ *For the first 10-20 years of chronic hepatitis C infection, many people are* **asymptomatic** *or have non-specific symptoms such as chronic fatigue and depression.*

The prefix *a~* usually becomes *an~* before a vowel. For example, **anemia** (*~emia* = "blood"), **anoxia** (*~oxia* = "oxygen"); and **anorexia,** meaning "without appetite" (*orexis* = "appetite"). Anorexia, the medical term for "loss of appetite" is a symptom of many conditions. **Anorexia nervosa** is a serious eating disorder (*nervosa* = "obsession"). An **agnostic** is a person who is unsure whether or not God exists (*~gnos* = "to know" e.g., **di<u>agnos</u>is, pro<u>gnos</u>is**). On the other hand, an **atheist** does not believe in the existence of God (*a~* = "not"; *theism* = "God").

Let's return to *syn~* and *sym~*. **Synthesis** means to "make something by combining different materials" (*~thesis* = "to put"). Plants obtain energy by **photosynthesis**, a process that makes ("puts together") sugar using sunlight (*photo~*), carbon dioxide, and water. You may have watched **synchronized swimming** (*chron* = "time"; e.g., chronic). During the COVID-19 pandemic, many university teachers were required to pre-record their lessons. Rather than all students learning from the teacher at the same time, each student could study at a time they wanted. The is termed **asynchronous learning**.

1-3   Dozen in Detail (D)   （12 の話題を詳しく）

1) *Contraindicated* is the adjective form of the noun **contraindication**. The prefix *contra~* means "against," and a contraindication is a reason (e.g., a medical condition, age, being pregnant) *against* using a medical treatment or procedure because it may cause harm. A contraindication may be absolute or relative. An **absolute contraindication** is when a particular treatment or procedure is absolutely inadvisable. For example, **thalidomide** is effective as a treatment for **leprosy** and certain types of cancer; however, it is a potent **teratogen**, infamous for causing severe and living-threatening **birth defects**. Therefore, thalidomide must never be used—it is absolutely contraindicated—in women who are pregnant or by women who could become pregnant. A **relative contraindication** means the drug should be avoided, but it may be used if the benefits outweigh the risks.

In medicine, an **indication** for a drug is the reason the drug is used; for example, DM is an indication for insulin treatment. Many drugs have more than one indication; for example, aspirin is indicated for reducing inflammation in conditions such as rheumatoid arthritis and also as a **prophylaxis** against **ischemic stroke** and **myocardial infarction**. When a drug is **approved** by a **regulatory authority** (e.g., the **FDA** in the USA), it will be approved for one or more specific indications. Sometimes a drug is used to treat an illness other than the authorized indication. This is called an **off-label** use of a drug. For example, beta-blockers are a class of drug indicated for hypertension and heart conditions, but in the USA, they are also widely used off-label to treat **migraine** and **anxiety**. The FDA has not approved beta blockers for these conditions, but there is data to show that they are effective in treating them.

2) *Etiology and pathogenesis of T1D and T2D*: <u>T1D</u> is an **autoimmune disease** that results when a person's own immune system destroys the β-cells of the pancreas. However, what causes this autoimmune destruction has not yet been fully **elucidated**. Genetic factors play a role, suggested by the fact that if one parent has TID, their children have up to a 9% chance of developing it (the lifetime risk for the general population is about 1%). Also, the rates of T1D are highest in Northern Europe; for example, in Finland, the country with the world's highest incidence of T1D, the **incidence** of T1D per 100,000 children aged 0 to 14 is around 58. In contrast, in Japan the incidence is around 2. This suggests a **genetic susceptibility** of **Caucasians** to T1D compared to Japanese (and other East Asians). Indeed, research has identified genetic mutations in the **genome** of people in Scandinavia that may increase the risk of diabetes. On the other hand, there has been a rapid increase in T1D across Europe since the 1950s. For example, the incidence TID in Finnish children under 15 years of age doubled between 1980 and 2005. Such an increase cannot only be due to genes because evolutionary processes that alter our genes generally happen over generations. Therefore, environmental factors have to explain most of this increase. In short, it appears that autoimmune destruction of β-cells is triggered by an unknown environmental factor(s), probably in people who are **genetically susceptible**.

T1D is usually diagnosed when hyperglycemia causes symptoms such as polydipsia, polyuria, and weight loss. This usually occurs when between 80-90% of β-cells have been destroyed. Before the availability of insulin injections in 1922, the complete lack of endogenous insulin due to β cell destruction resulted in people with T1D usually dying within a month or a few years at most. Often the cause of death was **diabetic ketoacidosis**. This is a life-threatening complication that occurs when cells are unable obtain glucose (remember that insulin is the key that "unlocks" the cell and allows glucose to enter it). Instead, the liver metabolizes fat into molecules called **ketone bodies**, which can be used as a source of energy by muscle and other tissues. However, the over production of ketones, as happens in diabetic ketoacidosis, causes the blood to become too acidic. (Blood is normally slightly basic, with a normal pH range of 7.35 to 7.45; a pH below 7.35 is considered to be in acidosis.) Acidosis due to the ketone bodies is called **ketoacidosis**. Ketoacidosis causes symptoms such as **nausea**, shortness of breath, **arrhythmia**, and **confusion**. Untreated, it can lead to **coma** and death.

Although a person with a family history of <u>**T2D**</u> is **predisposed** to developing T2D, for the disease to actually develop usually depends a lot on the influence of the environment. In other words, T2D is a **multifactorial disease** that results from a combination of genetic and environmental factors. The two key environmental factors that can lead to T2D are overeating and physical inactivity. The human body responds to the consumption of excess calories by storing the extra calories as fat in **adipose tissue**. Excess energy is converted into lipids and stored in **adipocytes**. As more and more lipids fill the adipocytes, they get bigger, like balloons being inflated. This increase in cell size, called **hypertrophy**, is mostly responsible for "putting on weight." (**Hyperplasia**, an increase in adipocyte number, also contributes to weight gain, but to a lesser extent). Some people store a lot of energy in **subcutaneous adipose tissue** (fat under the skin), but still maintain a normal blood glucose. But other people, due to genetic factors, have a lower capacity to store excess calories in subcutaneous adipose tissue, and fat accumulates around their internal organs. It is such **visceral fat** (also called **abdominal obesity**) that is a key cause of insulin resistance.

While insulin resistance is most often caused by abdominal obesity, it is also associated with other factors such as a sedentary lifestyle, stress, and certain medications. There are also several hormones that work against the action of insulin, particularly adrenaline, glucagon, growth hormone, and cortisol. Any condition or medication that increases these insulin **counterregulatory hormones** can increase the risk of developing insulin resistance. Whatever the cause of the insulin resistance, the β-cells in the pancreas will compensate by secreting more insulin. However, the β-cells cannot increase insulin production indefinitely, and after a period of time—usually several years—the β-cells become exhausted and begin to fail. With less insulin being secreted, the concentration of glucose in the blood rises. The elevated blood glucose leads to β-cells secreting even less insulin because of the toxic effect of glucose on those β-cells. With a further reduction in insulin, the hyperglycemia will worsen, which will **impair** the β-cells even more.

SD 1F: Why do more men get T2D?

Men tend to have more visceral fat, which is one reason for the higher prevalence of T2D in men, who are almost twice as likely to develop it compared to women. Women tend to store fat under the skin (subcutaneously) in their hips, thighs, and bottom. The main reason visceral fat is more dangerous than subcutaneous fat is because visceral fat is more **metabolically active**, producing hormones and **proinflammatory cytokines**.

SD 1G: What could be the mystery environmental factor for TID?

One hypothesis is that some factor of modern life is causing changes in the **gut microbiome**, which is important in regulation of the immune system. Another is related to **vitamin D**

deficiency. Research has shown that children in Europe who develop T1D are most often diagnosed in the winter months. What could explain this? Here are two possible reasons: firstly, people who develop T1D often have in their blood a certain type of **autoantibody** (called islet cell autoantibody) that attacks the β-cells of the pancreas. These autoantibodies most often first appear in autumn and winter, when there is little sunlight—and sunlight is necessary for the skin to **synthesize** vitamin D (although it can also be obtained from the diet). Vitamin D is thought to be important for regulating the immune system. So, vitamin D deficiency could be contributing to the development of autoantibodies. Secondly, infections with viruses are most common in winter, and T1D often develops after a **viral infection**. It is hypothesized that certain viruses directly destroy pancreatic β-cells, or they trigger the immune system to attack the β-cells.

SD 1H: Why sugar isn't always sweet

My eldest son is a bad-tempered teenager now, but when he was a little boy, he was really sweet. "Sweet" in this context means "cute" or "nice." However, sweet blood, or more precisely, chronic hyperglycemia, is far from nice for the body. One reason elevated blood glucose is damaging is that the glucose becomes bound to fats and proteins in a process called **glycation**, resulting in the formation **advanced glycation end products** (**AGEs**). These AGEs impair the function of β-cells, damage blood vessels, and induce the release of pro-inflammatory cytokines (inflammation has an important role in the pathophysiology of T2D).

3) Exercise enhances insulin sensitivity: Exercise is an activity that requires physical effort and is done to maintain or improve health and fitness. There are different types of exercise, including **aerobic** exercise and strength training. My daily run around the local park, followed by bodyweight exercises such as push-ups and pull-ups, helps me to keep fit, and it reduces stress and anxiety, improves sleep, and gives me a feeling of well-being. Because of the great physical and mental health benefits of physical activity, it is often said that if exercise could be made into a pill, it would become the most prescribed medicine in the world. For people with DM the importance of exercise cannot be overstated.

- Regular exercise helps with weight loss, and losing excess body fat, especially visceral fat, makes the body respond more effectively to insulin.
- Weight loss also reduces the risk of cardiovascular disease by helping to lower both blood pressure and blood cholesterol. In particular, exercise reduces the amount of LDL (low-density lipoprotein), which is also called "bad cholesterol" because it contributes to atherosclerosis formation.
- Regular aerobic exercise can help to lower blood glucose levels even without weight loss. One reason for this is that exercise makes skeletal muscle cells more sensitive to insulin and increases the uptake of insulin into muscle cells. Exercise does this by inducing an increase in the **expression** of **GLUT4** in the plasma membrane of muscle cells (GLUT4

is a glucose transporter protein that is necessary for glucose to enter muscle cells).

- Another effect of exercise is its anti-inflammatory one: exercise promotes the secretion of **anti-inflammatory cytokines** (cytokines that reduce inflammation).

SD 1I: Sumo wrestlers are "fat and fit"

Sumo wrestlers are notable because, although they have a very large calorie intake and put on a lot of weight, they do not generally develop T2D. The intense training that sumo wrestlers do for hours each day is thought to prevent the accumulation of **visceral fat**. Sumo wrestlers may look fat, but most of this fat is **subcutaneous** (under the skin). However, when sumo wrestlers retire, they usually cannot maintain the level of physical activity they did when competing. Unless they drastically reduce their calorie intake, excess calories become stored as dangerous visceral fat. Retired sumo wrestlers often develop T2D and other lifestyle illnesses, resulting in a **life-expectancy** that is around two decades shorter than the average Japanese male.

4) *GLUT4* **stands for glucose transporter type 4.** Glucose is transformed into energy in the process of **cellular respiration**. As the name suggests, cellular respiration takes place within the cell, mostly in organelles called **mitochondria**. But how does glucose get into the cell? The cell membrane is composed of a **lipid bilayer**, which is **hydrophobic** (i.e., it tends to repel water). On the other hand, glucose, because of its chemical structure, is highly **hydrophilic** (i.e., it has a strong **affinity** for water and mixes well with it). So, it is clear glucose would be unable to just passively diffuse across the cell membrane into the cell. What is needed to transfer glucose across the plasma membrane is a glucose transporter. Glucose transporters are proteins in the cell membrane that facilitate the transport of glucose across the plasma membrane (this process is called **facilitated diffusion**). There are two main groups of glucose transporters, the first being GLUT. So far, 14 types of GLUTs have been identified. GLUT1, GLUT2, GLUT3, GLUT4 and GLUT5 appear to have the most important role in humans. The different GLUTs differ in their location; for example, GLUT1 is found in red blood cells, while GLUT2 is found in the liver, pancreas, and small intestine. They also differ in their properties; for example, GLUT3, found in the brain, neurons, sperm, and other tissues has a very high affinity for glucose, while GLUT2 has a low affinity for it. GLUT4 is found mostly in skeletal muscle and adipose tissue. It has a high affinity for glucose. The key difference between GLUT4 and the other GLUTs is this: **GLUT4 is insulin-dependent,** while the others are insulin independent. In other words, without insulin, glucose cannot enter skeletal muscle and fat cells, but in other tissues glucose uptake does not depend on insulin.

In addition to GLUT, there is another group of glucose transporters called **SGLT** (sodium-dependent glucose transporter). SGLT1s are found in **enterocytes** (cells in the intestine) and serve an important role in glucose absorption. SGLT2s, located in the nephrons of the kidney, are responsible for the reabsorption of glucose from the nephron back into the bloodstream, preventing the loss of glucose in the urine. Both types of SGLT are insulin-independent. In DM, when blood glucose levels are abnormally high, SGLT2s become saturated and unable to reabsorb all the glucose, resulting in some glucose being lost in the urine (**glucosuria**). A class of oral antidiabetic drugs called **SGLT2 inhibitors** work by inhibiting SGLT2. Drugs that inhibit SGLT1 have also been developed. **SGLT1 inhibitors** lower blood glucose mainly by reducing the absorption of glucose from the intestine.

SD 1J: How GLUT4 allows glucose into the cell

Let's focus on how glucose enters skeletal muscle and other insulin-sensitive cells. When insulin concentrations in the blood are low, GLUT4 remains in **vesicles** (storage sacs) in the **cytoplasm** of cells. After a meal, glucose that is absorbed from the digestive system enters the bloodstream. The raised blood glucose stimulates the release of insulin from the pancreas. When this insulin binds to receptors on the membrane of insulin-sensitive cells, it causes the vesicles to change location, or **translocate**, from the cytoplasm to the plasma membrane, and then fuse with it. Inserting GLUT4 into the plasma membrane enables the cells to easily take up glucose. In liver and other cells that do not require insulin for glucose uptake, the glucose transporters are located permanently in the plasma membrane (i.e., they do not have to translocate from the cytoplasm).

5) *Hypoglycemia* is a condition in which blood glucose level is abnormally low. It is the most serious side effect that can result from insulin injections (it can also be caused by taking certain oral antidiabetics). Hypoglycemia most commonly occurs when a person with DM unintentionally injects too much insulin, but it can also occur due to skipping a meal. In addition, although exercise is important for the management of diabetes, it can also cause hypoglycemia. This is because when we exercise our muscles require more energy. At the onset of exercise, the muscles use stored glycogen to obtain energy, but as exercise continues, they rely more on glucose in the blood. This causes blood glucose levels to drop. The risk of **exercise hypoglycemia** can be reduced by eating a snack before exercising or by decreasing the pre-exercise insulin dose. When blood glucose levels drop too low, the secretion of **adrenaline** is triggered. This leads to various symptoms such as weakness, feeling hungry, **nausea**, **tachycardia**, and **anxiety**. A further drop in blood glucose deprives the brain of enough glucose to function properly (the brain cannot synthesize glucose or store it as glycogen, so it requires a continuous supply of glucose from the blood circulation).

Hypoglycemia can cause the brain to dysfunction, leading to various symptoms, including dizziness and confusion. Symptoms caused by the brain being deprived of glucose are called **neuroglycopenic** symptoms. If not treated, severe hypoglycemia can result in **coma** (called a **hypoglycemic coma**), and death. The **take-home message** is that insulin injections are a life-saver, but if the dose is too high, exogenous insulin can kill. Insulin users must take care to use the correct dose because insulin has a **narrow therapeutic index** (i.e., there is only a small difference between a dose that maintains blood glucose within normal levels and a dose that causes blood glucose to drop too much, causing hypoglycemia).

SD 1K: An antidote for insulin overdose

The immediate treatment for hypoglycemia is to eat or drink something sugary. If hypoglycemia causes a person to lose consciousness, people around must call an ambulance. In hospital, treatment for an insulin overdose includes giving **IV** glucose treatment and/or an injection of **synthetic glucagon**. Glucagon is a hormone that raises blood glucose levels by stimulating glycogen stored in the liver to be converted to glucose, which then enters the bloodstream. In this way, synthetic glycogen can counteract the effect of insulin; in other words, it is an **antidote** to insulin overdose.

6) Japan has a relatively low obesity rate compared to other high-income countries. Despite this, the number of people with T2D in Japan is rapidly increasing. Japan's increase in T2D is due to several reasons, including an aging population (middle-aged and older adults have the highest risk of developing T2D), and an increase in the number of people being diagnosed since new checkups for metabolic syndrome were introduced in Japan in 2008. But the main factors underlying the rise in T2D relate to eating habits and lack of exercise. The traditional Japanese diet is not perfect (it is high in salt), but it is generally considered to be very healthy. Included in the traditional Japanese diet are raw fish, pickled vegetables, fermented soybeans (*natto*), and dried seaweed. While traditional Japanese food is still widely eaten, Japanese people now eat much more high-calorie, highly-processed foods than they used to. An unhealthy diet, little exercise, and other factors (e.g., a tendency for Japanese people, especially men of working age, to eat their food fast and to eat late at night) are leading to more obesity. And obesity is a key risk factor for T2D. The link between obesity and T2D is complex, but it is related to obesity leading to chronic, systemic inflammation that causes insulin resistance, the dysfunction of β-cells, and ultimately T2D.

But wait a second! I wrote above that Japan has a "relatively low obesity rate." It is true that compared to the USA, and the UK, there are many fewer people who are obviously obese in Japan. But studies have shown that the onset of T2D occurs at a lower BMI in Japanese compared to Caucasians. While Caucasians can often put on a lot of weight before the onset of T2D, Japanese people tend to have a lower safe fat-carrying capacity. So, many Japanese people diagnosed with T2D appear to be only slightly overweight or are even of normal weight. Japanese people tend to more readily accumulate visceral fat, and they also have less muscle mass (the more muscle mass, the lower the risk for insulin resistance). Studies also suggest that β-cells of Japanese people tend to have a lower capacity to secrete insulin after a meal.

7) *Metformin* **is probably the most widely prescribed drug for the treatment of T2D**. Like aspirin and morphine and many other drugs, metformin was originally derived from a natural source. It is a **synthetic derivative** of a plant called French lilac (*Galega officinalis*), which was used for hundreds of years in Europe to treat many conditions. As a drug to treat T2D, metformin works in several ways to control blood sugar, including by suppressing **hepatic gluconeogenesis**, the synthesis in the liver of glucose from non-carbohydrates such as amino acids and fatty acids. In diabetics, hepatic gluconeogenesis occurs at a faster rate than in non-diabetics, and this contributes to hyperglycemia. This is why metformin's suppression of hepatic gluconeogenesis is so important. An advantage of metformin is that it does not increase insulin secretion by the pancreas, so there is minimal risk of it causing hypoglycemia. Some people taking metformin get side effects such as stomach upset and **flatulence**, but it is generally **well-tolerated**.

Metformin appears to have other therapeutic effects apart from lowering blood sugar; for example, there is evidence that metformin is **cardioprotective**, and taking metformin is associated with a reduced risk of **dementia**. During the COVID-19 pandemic, there were reports that people taking metformin had a reduced mortality from COVID-19. A pharmacologist would say that metformin is a drug with **pleiotropic effects**, meaning that it has other actions, usually beneficial ones, apart from the one(s) for which it was originally developed. An **indication** for a drug is the reason it is used, and metformin is indicated to treat T2D. However, it is also prescribed **off-label** for several other conditions. An example of metformin's off-label use is the treatment of weight gain caused by taking certain **antipsychotics**.

SD 1L: Drug repurposing

Do the following Google search and see how many hits (search engine results) you get: "metformin + repurposing." My search results included articles on "*Repurposing Metformin for Cancer Treatment...*", "*Metformin Repurposing for Parkinson Disease Therapy...*", "*Drug repurposing of metformin for Alzheimer's disease...*", and many more. But what is repurposing of metformin? Well, **repurposing** means to find a new you use for something; for example, turning a school that has closed into a sports center. And **drug repurposing** means exploring how existing drugs can be used to treat new medical conditions. Metformin has been a treatment for T2D for over 60 years, but researchers are testing whether it can be used for new indications, including certain types of cancer, and Alzheimer's disease.

The advantage of drug repurposing is that an existing drug has already been studied for safety during its original clinical trials; therefore, compared to developing a completely new drug, repurposing an existing one should need less time and money to bring it to market for a new indication. Another advantage of repurposing existing drugs is that many of them are older drugs whose **patents** have expired. **Off-patent generic drugs** are much cheaper and have fewer restrictions on their use than **originator drugs** (i.e., drugs developed and patented by the original pharmaceutical company). An example of drug repurposing is **thalidomide**, which was once used for morning sickness, but found a new life as a treatment for **multiple myeloma**, a type of blood cancer, and also as a treatment for a serious complication of **leprosy**. (If you're a pharmacy student and you don't know about the **thalidomide scandal** [サリドマイドの薬害], then you have **a gap in your knowledge** that needs to be filled.)

8) *Obesity* **and being overweight are, according to the WHO, an "abnormal or excessive fat accumulation that presents a risk to health." A body mass index (BMI)** of over 25 is usually considered as overweight, while a BMI of over 30 is obese. Being overweight or obese is a risk factor for developing T2D. Research from the UK suggests there is a seven times greater risk of T2D for obese people compared to people with a healthy weight. However, obesity is not the only risk factor for T2D—genetics, ethnicity, and age are others—and it is important to say that not all people who are obese will get T2D, and not all people with T2D are obese. Moreover, distribution of fat in the body is more important than just looking at BMI. People with **abdominal obesity** (or **visceral fat**) are at a much great risk of diabetes than people whose fat is mostly under the skin (**subcutaneous fat**) and located around the lower body. During the annual medical checkup at Meijo University, where I presently work, one of the measurements the nurse takes is **waist circumference**. This is a measure of abdominal obesity. In Japan, a weight circumference of 85cm or over in a man, and 90cm or over in a woman indicates an excess of abdominal fat. Why people with central obesity are more **prone** to developing T2D has not been completely **elucidated**, and what is known is rather complicated. But, **in a nutshell**, it appears that excess abdominal fat promotes the release of **pro-inflammatory cytokines** from fat cells. These cytokines lead to chronic inflammation in the body, and this inflammation appears to induce insulin resistance. It is important to appreciate that adipose tissue is not just an **inert** store of fat, like a block of butter. Rather, adipose tissue is a highly active endocrine organ that secretes various hormones, collectively known as **adipokines**, that effect the metabolism. Abdominal obesity increases the secretion of **pro-inflammatory adipokines**, contributing to insulin resistance.

SD 1M: The modern world is making us fat

What goes through your head when you see someone who is obese? Do you think that they are greedy, with no self-control, who eat too much junk food, and are too lazy to exercise regularly or cook healthy food? While **personal responsibility** needs to be considered when talking about obesity, we should not ignore other factors. Some people put on lots of weight because of a medical condition (e.g., **hypothyroidism**, **Cushing syndrome**, **polycystic ovary syndrome**), drugs (e.g., **corticosteroids**, **oral contraceptives**, **antidepressants**), and certain genes that affect things like appetite, **satiety**, and metabolism. Most importantly, we live in an environment in which it is very easy to put on too much weight. Think about all the fast-food restaurants near your university and all the high-calorie foods that fill the shelves of supermarkets. Companies use clever advertising to tempt people, especially young people, to buy sugar-loaded soft drinks and ultra-processed foods. When I went to Alabama in the USA, I visited urban areas in which there were no shops selling fresh fruit or vegetables. In these areas, known as "**food deserts**," death rates from DM and other chronic illnesses are much higher than in areas with easy access to shops selling healthy foods. We also live in a world in which we hardly have to move our bodies. Online shopping means we don't even have to walk to the shops. In short, we are living in an environment that makes us fat—an **obesogenic environment**.

9) **Slow healing of wounds**: People with DM are **prone** to getting chronic wounds (i.e., wounds that do not heal well), especially on the feet. In around 15% of people with DM, impaired wound healing will cause a **foot ulcer** to develop. If not treated in time, the tissue around a foot ulcer dies and may become infected. In some cases, a foot ulcer does so much damage that the foot will need to be **amputated**. The pathophysiology of impaired healing in DM is complex, but here are some of the causes.

- DM increases the risk of developing **peripheral artery disease** (**PAD**). This condition results from plaques composed of cholesterol and other substances forming in the walls of peripheral arteries. This plaque build-up, called **atherosclerosis**, can cause narrowing of arteries, leading to a reduction in blood flow. **Impeded blood flow** results in less oxygen and nutrients reaching the wound.
- Hyperglycemia in DM is thought to cause **dysfunction** of the immune system**,** making wounds vulnerable to infections and impeding healing.
- An important process in wound healing is **angiogenesis** (the formation of new blood vessels). High blood glucose in DM impairs angiogenesis.
- **Peripheral neuropathy** is a complication of DM. It occurs because chronically high blood sugar levels can directly damage the nerves, and also due to the effect of DM on reducing blood flow to the nerves. This can cause decreased sensation in the feet and toes, making it more difficult for a person with DM to notice a wound until it has become infected.

10) *The liver* **is the largest internal organ and acts as the body's glucose reservoir**. When the blood glucose level becomes too high, **hepatocytes** (liver cells) can take in glucose and store it, and when the level of blood glucose drops too low, hepatocytes release glucose into the blood. The liver stores glucose in the form of **glycogen**, a polysaccharide (made up of many connected glucose molecules). When needed (e.g., when we are sleeping or between meals), the liver releases glucose into the blood by turning glycogen into glucose, a process called **glycogenolysis**. The liver is the only organ that can directly release glucose into the bloodstream. This glucose is taken up by neurons in the brain and by other cells to produce energy. Muscle tissue is also a major glycogen store, but when glycogen is converted back to

glucose in the muscle, it is used only by muscle cells themselves and is not released into the blood. Incidentally, the main reason a typical man's body contains more water (60%) compared to that of a typical adult women's (55%) is related to glycogen: each gram of glycogen is bound to 3-4 g of water, and skeletal muscle stores much more glycogen than adipose tissue; therefore, because men are generally more muscular than women (who have more fat tissue), men's bodies contain more water.

Insulin stimulates the synthesis of glycogen in the liver. But there is a limit to how much glycogen the liver can store: when the liver's glycogen storage is **saturated** (at around 5% of the liver's mass), further synthesis is inhibited and excess glucose is converted into fatty acids. Fatty acids are not soluble in water—oil and water don't mix—so in order to be carried in the blood, fatty acids are combined in the liver with proteins to form **lipoproteins**. Lipoproteins are then transported in the bloodstream to various tissues, including fat tissue.

11) There are several classes of oral antidiabetics, drugs which help to control blood glucose. This essay described one oral antidiabetic drug, metformin. Let's look at one more example. Approved in Japan in 2014, **SGLT2 inhibitors** are a relatively new class of antidiabetic. If we consider that a key sign of diabetes is **glycosuria** (the presence of glucose into the urine), then the way SGLT2 inhibitors work may at first seem **counterintuitive**. What they do is *increase* the amount of glucose excreted in the urine, which in turn leads to a lowering of blood glucose levels. After all, it is chronic hyperglycemia (not glycosuria) that causes the dangerous complications of diabetes. The abbreviation SGLT2 stands for **sodium-glucose co-transporter-2**. The capacity of the kidney to reabsorb glucose back into the blood is due to SGLT 2 in the nephrons of the kidney. Inhibiting SGLT2 prevents glucose reabsorption, leading to glycosuria and the lowering of blood glucose. SGLT2 prevents valuable glucose from being lost in the urine, which was advantageous for survival for most of human evolution when food was scarce. But now that consuming too many calories is a bigger problem for many people, this glucose conservation mechanism could be said to be disadvantageous. SGLT2 inhibitors prevent the body from holding onto glucose that is not needed. Some studies have found that SGLT-2 inhibitors are associated with an increased risk of developing **urinary tract infections**. This may be because the excess glucose in the urine provides a **conducive environment** for the growth of microorganisms.

There are many examples of drugs developed for a certain purpose that are later found to have other therapeutic effects. SGLT2 inhibitors are one such example. They were originally developed to lower blood glucose levels in T2D, but research shows that they also greatly improve outcomes in people with **chronic kidney disease** (CKD) and in heart failure. It is not exactly known why SGLT2 inhibitors protect the kidney and the heart, but it is thought to be partly related to the fact that, because SGLT2 reabsorbs sodium along with glucose, SGLT2 inhibitors promote **natriuresis** (i.e., the excretion of sodium in the urine). This increase in sodium excretion helps to lower blood pressure.

SD 1N: Has tirzepatide been approved to treat obesity?

Tirzepatide is the generic name of a drug that was approved by the FDA in 2022 to treat T2D. This drug stimulates the release of GIP (glucose-dependent insulinotropic polypeptide) and GLP-1 (glucagon-like peptide-1). Both GIP and GLP-1 are hormones released from the intestine after eating, and they act to stimulate the secretion of insulin from the pancreas. These hormones also promote **satiety** (i.e., help people feel full after eating). Recent studies have found that tirzepatide, which is administered as a weekly injection, can also bring about a substantial weight reduction in obese people who don't have diabetes. By the time you read this, it is possible that tirzepatide will have been approved as a treatment for obesity by the **regulatory authority for drug approval in Japan**. Why not check the internet to find out?

12) There are several types of DM, with one kind, **gestational diabetes**, only affecting women. Gestational diabetes is DM that occurs during pregnancy in women who didn't have DM before getting pregnant. During pregnancy, a woman's body undergoes hormonal and physiological changes that increase insulin resistance and make it difficult for the pancreas to produce enough insulin. Gaining weight during pregnancy, and the secretion from the **placenta** of certain hormones with a **contra-insulin effect** are thought to be involved in the pathogenesis of gestational diabetes. This type of diabetes usually develops in the second or third **trimester** of pregnancy (i.e., between 3 to 9 months). After a woman with gestational diabetes gives birth, her blood glucose levels usually return to normal. However, women who have experienced gestational diabetes have a higher risk of developing T2D in the future.

When DM occurs due to another medical condition or a medication it is called **secondary diabetes**. For example, **chronic pancreatitis** (inflammation of the pancreas) can lead to diabetes. An adverse side effect of **oral corticosteroids** is that they raise blood sugar levels by stimulating glucose production in the liver, and they increase insulin resistance by inhibiting glucose uptake in muscle and fat tissue. When taken for long periods, the hyperglycemic effect of corticosteroids can sometimes lead to T2D.

Another drug class that can cause DM is **immune checkpoint inhibitors.** Treatment of some types of cancer has been revolutionized by immune checkpoint inhibitors, the first of which was approved by the FDA in 2011. These drugs block checkpoint proteins on certain immune cells. Checkpoints act like a brake on the immune system, preventing an over-aggressive immune response. But by holding back the immune system, checkpoints sometimes prevent the immune system from killing cancer cells. Blocking checkpoints with immune checkpoint inhibitors **unleashes** the immune system to attack cancer cells. Unfortunately, unleashing the immune system sometimes leads to an autoimmune reaction, with the immune system attacking healthy tissue in the body. If the pancreas is attacked, T1D can result. Although T1D induced by immune checkpoint inhibitors is a rare adverse effect, it is irreversible, and, if not treated properly, can result in life-threatening diabetic ketoacidosis.

1-4　Well, what do you know?

（どのくらいわかるようになったか試してみよう）

Are the following statements true (T) or false (F)?

1. The sole function of insulin is to enable glucose to enter cells.
2. Insulin is secreted by specialized exocrine cells in the pancreas.
3. The onset of T1D is always in childhood.
4. Visceral fat is associated with the development of T2D.
5. People with T2D will always require insulin injections.

What is the meaning of the underlined WFE?

1. Although it is not usually serious for most patients, **diarrhea** can cause serious dehydration in children and can be fatal.
2. Rubber condoms were first made in 1855, and now they are the most widely used **contra**ceptive product in the world.
3. Polio, or poliomyelitis, is an infectious disease caused by the poliovirus. The virus affects the brain and spinal cord, causing **paralysis** and sometimes death.
4. People who say that they "don't know" if God exists are **agnostics**.
5. The relationship between blood testosterone levels and health in men is controversial. Even so, it is increasingly common for elder men to supplement **endogenous** testosterone with injections of this hormone.
6. Ecstasy (MDMA) is an example of an **empathogen**, a drug that increase a person's feelings of empathy and friendliness towards others.
7. An estimated 10% of all adults in China currently live with T2D. In the late 1980s, it affected only 2.5% of the population. The increase in T2D is associated with the rising prevalence of obesity in China, which in turn is driven by various **obesogenic** environmental factors.

Choose a word from below to replace the underlined word(s)

a) glycosuria   **b)** sedentary   **c)** hypersecretion   **d)** pathology

e) systemic   **f)** hypoglycemia   **g)** physiology

1. People on insulin need to monitor their blood sugar levels because administering too much insulin can cause <u>abnormally low blood sugar</u>.

2. A tumor in the pituitary gland can lead to <u>excessive release</u> of growth hormone, causing gigantism (a condition characterized by excessive growth and height significantly above average).

3. If you use steroid eye drops correctly, there is little danger of the drug entering <u>general</u> circulation.

4. Leading <u>a low physical-activity</u> lifestyle raises the risk of developing DM.

5. Paul Langerhans discovered the cells that secrete insulin. His main field of expertise was <u>the study of disease</u>.

1-5   May Jo's Health-Podcast

(メイ・ジョーの健康ポッドキャスト)

Podcast presenter May Jo (MJ) and Dr Janet Kwon (Dr) are talking about the high incidence of T2D in indigenous Australians.

MJ: We have a question from a listener. Sam in Sydney has texted to say that five of his friends or colleagues have been diagnosed with type 2 diabetes just in the last year. Sam's question is this: "Is type 2 diabetes increasing in Australia, and if it is, why?". To answer this question is Dr Janet Kwon, an endocrinologist at Sydney's Newtown Hospital.

Dr: Well Sam, the answer to the first part of your question is straightforward. The prevalence of type 2 diabetes is increasing in Australia. In fact, diabetes is the fastest growing chronic condition in Australia. But it's not just Australia; type 2 diabetes is increasing globally.

MJ: What's the cause of this increase?

Dr: There are various interrelated factors such as the ageing population, dietary changes, and a more sedentary lifestyle, but the main reason is that there are so many more people who are obese or overweight.

MJ: Are you saying that if everyone was of normal weight, there'd be no more type 2 diabetes?

Dr: No, people whose weight is normal can develop it, perhaps because they have a genetic predisposition. But it's estimated that if obesity was eliminated from the Australian population, the incidence of type 2 diabetes would drop by nearly 50%.

MJ: What's the situation like with Aboriginal Australians *?

Dr: The situation is really serious. Indigenous Australians are around three times more likely to have T2D compared to the non-indigenous population. In some remote rural communities up to 40% of the population has type 2 diabetes. And type 2 diabetes is having a terrible impact on the health of Aboriginal peoples and leading to many premature deaths.

MJ: Why are indigenous Australians at greater risk of type 2 diabetes than non-indigenous Australians?

Dr: It's partly because the factors that increase the risk of type 2 diabetes are even worse in Aboriginal communities. They tend to eat more processed foods and engage in more risky behavior such as heavy drinking and cigarette smoking. Poor living conditions and social breakdown underlie the worse health outcomes in aboriginal communities.

MJ: Is the westernized lifestyle a cause of the increase in type 2 diabetes in indigenous Australians?

Dr: I would say that the western lifestyle is not just a cause, it is *the* cause.

MJ: Really?

Dr: Yes. When the aboriginal peoples lived a traditional hunter-gather lifestyle, type 2 diabetes just did not exist. The way they lived before the British settled—or as some people would say "invaded"—Australia in 1788, was how humans lived in the Paleolithic era before the development of agriculture. Type 2 diabetes in indigenous Australians is a mismatch disease.

MJ: What do you mean?

Dr: Well, aboriginal peoples lived for thousands of years in an environment where food was often scarce, and they developed a metabolism that was efficient at conserving energy.

MJ: But the westernized lifestyle is so different from the hunter-gatherer one.

Dr: That's right. Now indigenous Australians tend to eat too much calorie-dense food and have a sedentary lifestyle. The energy-conserving metabolism that was advantageous when they were hunter-gatherers is now disadvantageous.

MJ: So, genetic traits that once helped indigenous Australians to survive have now become maladaptive.

Dr: Exactly.

MJ: Can the concept of mismatch diseases explain the dramatic increase in type 2 diabetes worldwide?

Dr: Yes, to some extent. Have you thought about why we crave sweet foods?

MJ: No, why do we?

Dr: Well, since *Homo Sapiens* emerged around 200,000 years ago, until the dawn of agriculture around 11,000 years ago, humans were hunter-gatherers. Eating fruit from trees or honey collected from the nests of wild bees was the most efficient way for them to obtain the sugar that could be converted into fat. The early humans who could store most fat had the best chance to survive periods of famine and pass on their genes.

MJ: But in the modern age, high-calorie foods are plentiful and easy to obtain. You don't have to climb a tree to get a chocolate cake or a sugar-loaded soft drink!

Dr: That's right. The environment has changed completely, but modern humans remain genetically wired to crave sugary foods.

MJ: Perhaps in another 1000 years, human physiology will have evolved to be perfectly healthy on a 100% junk-food diet and a couch potato lifestyle.

Dr: I suppose it could happen, but it would take a lot longer than 1000 years. For people alive today, the best way to prevent type 2 diabetes is by maintaining a healthy body weight, eating a balanced with lots of fruit and vegetables, taking regular exercise, drinking alcohol only moderately or not at all, and not smoking.

MJ: It's advice that we all know, but too few of us follow. That's all we have time for today. Thank you, Dr Kwon.

Dr: My pleasure, thanks for having me.

* The people who had been in Australia for at least 65,000 years before the British arrived in 1770 used to be called "Aborigines". However, this word is now considered inappropriate by many people. More appropriate terms are Aboriginal Australians, indigenous Australians, and First Nations Australians.

51

Chapter 2　Chronic kidney disease
（慢性腎臓病）

Kidneys

The strainer of blood and the tap of urine
as the guardian of the body fluid

Proximal tubule
（近位尿細管）

Renal corpuscle
（腎小体）
=
Gromerulus
（糸球体）
+
Bowman's
capsule
（ボーマン嚢）

Distal
tubule
（遠位尿細管）

Mesangial cell
（メサンギウム細胞）

Capillary
（毛細血管）

Renal corpuscle（腎小体）

Renal corpuscle
（腎小体）

Proximal
tubule
（近位）

Distal
tubule
（遠位）

Henle's
loop
（ヘンレ
ループ）

Nephron
（腎単位）

Collecting
duct
（集合管）

Renal corpuscle（腎小体）

Cortex
（皮質）

Medulla
（髄質）

Renal
column
（腎柱）

Liver
（肝臓）

Adrenal
gland
（副腎）

Beans?
Kidney
（腎臓）

Ureter
（尿管）

Urinary bladder
（膀胱）

Cortex
（皮質）

Medulla
（髄質）

Renal vein
（腎静脈）

Renal artery
（腎動脈）

Renal pelvis
（腎盂）

Renal
papilla
（腎乳頭）

Renal pyramid
（腎錐体）

NAVvocab 60 （案内役の単語 60）

1. acute kidney injury・急性腎障害
2. acute tubular necrosis・急性尿細管壊死
3. active transport・能動輸送
4. afferent arteriole・輸入細動脈
5. albuminuria・アルブミン尿
6. anachronistic・時代錯誤
7. anthropomorphize・擬人格化する
8. antidiuretic hormone・抗利尿ホルモン
9. anuria・無尿（症）
10. arrhythmia・不整脈
11. asymptomatic・無症状
12. benign prostatic hyperplasia・前立腺肥大症
13. bicarbonate ion・炭酸系イオン
14. comorbidity・併存症
15. contaminated・汚染された
16. crush injury・圧挫損傷
17. debilitating・衰弱させる
18. dietician・栄養士
19. endothelium・内皮
20. erythropoiesis・赤血球産生
21. erythropoietin・エリスロポエチン
22. euthanize・安楽死させる
23. extracellular fluid・細胞外液
24. genetic susceptibility・遺伝的感受性
25. glomerulonephritis・糸球体腎炎
26. glomerulus・糸球体
27. hematuria・血尿
28. hemodialysis・血液透析
29. hydrostatic pressure・静水圧
30. intractable disease・難病
31. multifactorial・多因子
32. mycotoxin・マイコトキシン (カビ毒, 真菌毒)
33. myocyte・筋細胞
34. nephrolithiasis・腎結石症
35. nephrosclerosis・腎硬化症
36. nephrotoxin・腎毒素
37. oliguria・乏尿
38. osmosis・浸透圧
39. Paleolithic diet・旧石器時代の食事方法を手本にしたダイエット
40. palliative care・緩和ケア
41. palpate・触診する
42. peripheral edema・末梢性浮腫
43. peritoneal dialysis・腹膜透析
44. peritubular capillary・傍尿細管毛細血管
45. pleiotropic effects・多面的効果
46. polycystic kidney disease・多発性嚢胞腎
47. predisposed (to)・〔病気〕にかかりやすい素因を持っている
48. prevalence・有病率
49. proteinuria・タンパク尿
50. redundancy・余剰性
51. renal cortex・腎皮質
52. renal ischemia・腎虚血
53. renal medulla・腎髄質
54. rhabdomyolysis・横紋筋融解症
55. sepsis・敗血症
56. striated muscle・横紋筋
57. ultrafiltration・限外濾過
58. uremia・尿毒症
59. urinary system・泌尿器系
60. vascular calcification・血管石灰化

2-1 Essay — CKD: A Gradual Loss of Kidney Function
（慢性腎臓病：腎機能が少しずつ失われていく病気）

[1]We suspected something was wrong when she **lost her appetite**. She hardly ate anything, and even refused smoked salmon, her favorite treat. She started to drink a lot and would spend hours in the empty bathtub, licking up any water that dripped from the tap. Her once shiny coat became dull and dry, and, as she lost weight, her ribs started to stick out. One spring day in 1985, I put her in a cardboard box and together with my dad took her to a **vet**[E11] near our house in north London. The "her" that I am writing about was Tootsie, the family cat. She was 18 years old at the time and I was 17. In the **veterinary clinic's** waiting area, Tootsie lay on my lap, and sitting next to us was a man with a big Labrador. The dog was friendly and sniffed Tootsie's face. When young and **healthy**, Tootsie would have run away at the sight of a dog, but the sick Tootsie in that waiting room did not even blink. I may be **anthropomorphizing**[E2], but she seemed to have a **look of resignation** on her face. Perhaps she sensed she was dying, so even a big dog could not scare her.

[2]My dad and I entered the veterinary exam room, and I put Tootsie on a table. The vet asked us about Tootsie's symptoms and then she **palpated** her abdomen. After a few minutes the vet said, "Your cat has **kidney**[E6] failure." I asked the vet, "Is it serious?" "Yes, I'm afraid it is," she replied. "You can either take her home and she will probably die in a week or so, or I can **put her to sleep**[E8] now." At that point, I started crying and walked out of the room. A few minutes later, my father followed with tears in his eyes. I don't know what the vet did with Tootsie's body after she was **euthanized**, but animals **put down** at veterinary clinics are usually **cremated**. Even now, I regret we did not take Tootsie's body home to be buried in the garden that she had played and hunted in all her life.

[3]**Chronic kidney disease (CKD)**, the condition from which Tootsie died, is the number one cause of death in older cats. It is also a leading cause of **morbidity** and **mortality** in *Homo sapiens*. And the **prevalence** of CKD in people is increasing around the world. In Japan, where it is estimated that one in eight adults suffer from CKD, the condition has been called a "new national disease" (新たな国民病). Chronic kidney disease is a gradual loss of kidney function that happens over months or years. Kidney function can also decline more rapidly, a condition called **acute kidney injury (AKI)**. Before looking in detail at CKD and AKI, we will review the functions of the kidney.

[4]When I was at school in the 1970s and 1980s, one dish that was regularly served for school lunch was **steak and kidney pie** (**offal** is a common ingredient in traditional British food). In **primary school**, I enjoyed this dish and often had a second helping, but

after entering **secondary school** I went off eating it. This was because biology lessons started in secondary school, and in one biology lesson I learnt that the kidneys make **urine**. Learning this **put me off** eating kidney.

[5]Biology lessons in secondary school were taught by Mr. Pond, a **short-tempered** but **engaging** teacher. (Mr. Pond, was a World War II **veteran**, who would often **digress** from the topic of the lesson and tell stories of fighting against the Imperial Japanese Army in the jungles of Burma.) In his lesson about the **urinary system**, Mr. Pond taught us that the kidneys are shaped like kidney beans (although the **legume** is named after the body organ, not the other way round), and that people have two kidneys, each one about the size of an adult fist, located at the back of the abdomen on both sides of the spine.

[6]Mr. Pond drew a simplified diagram of a kidney on the blackboard (there was no PowerPoint in the early 1980s), showing how it is formed of two layers: the inner part, called the **renal medulla**, and an outer layer, called the **renal cortex**, which he shaded in with a darker color (because the cortex receives 90% of the blood supply to the kidney, it has a darker red color than the underlying medulla). The renal cortex and medulla are composed of **nephrons**, the **functional units** of the kidney that filter the blood and produce urine. Mr. Pond emphasized that the kidneys are very important in maintaining **homeostasis**, a state of internal stability, by regulating the body's salt and water concentration, and by filtering waste products from the blood, which are **excreted** from the body in the urine.

[7]Mr. Pond's biology lesson when I was 12 years old was very interesting, but it only touched on a few of the kidney's many functions. Other functions include: regulating the composition of the **extracellular fluid**[D9]; secreting **erythropoietin**, a hormone that stimulates **erythropoiesis** (the production of red blood cells); producing **renin,** an enzyme important in blood pressure regulation; and converting vitamin D obtained from the sun or from the diet into a form that is usable by the body. A Japanese word for "crucial" is *kanjin* (肝心). Although this word is usually written with the Chinese characters for liver (肝) and heart (心), it can also be represented as "肝腎," using the character for kidney (腎) instead of heart. After reading Table 2.1, which summarizes the kidney's functions, it should become clear why "腎" is well-suited for a word meaning "crucial" or "essential."

[8]The kidneys make up only 0.5% of the body's total body weight, but they are highly **vascularized** and receive around 20% of the total cardiac output. This large **renal blood flow** reflects the fact that, to be effective filters, the kidneys require a plentiful blood supply. To understand the filtering and waste production roles of the renal system, we need to understand the basic structure of the kidney.

[9]Each kidney is made up of around one million microscopic filtering units called **nephrons**, and each nephron can be divided into two parts: a **glomerulus**[E4]—a bundle of

tightly packed blood capillaries that filter the blood (a process called **filtration**)—and a **tubule** ("little tube"). The fluid filtered by the glomerulus, called the **filtrate**, moves along the tubule. However, a nephron tubule is nothing like a plastic hose pipe that just carries water from one point to another. Rather, through a process of **reabsorption** and **secretion**, the filtrate is changed as it moves along the tubule. The importance of reabsorption is shown by the fact that although the glomeruli filter about 200 liters of blood every 24 hours, a person's average urine output is only about 1.5 liters. Blood is around 90% water, so if all the water contained in the filtered blood was excreted rather than being reabsorbed, the daily urine output would be around 180 liters a day!

Table 2.1

Functions of the Kidney　（腎臓の働き）

Function　（働き）	Explanation　（説明）
Excretion of waste products of metabolism	Urea and creatinine and other substances are filtered into nephron tubules and not reabsorbed. The kidneys are important in **drug excretion**[D8].
Maintains balance of electrolytes	Excess electrolytes in the blood are excreted by nephrons. Fine-tuning of electrolyte regulation is under hormonal control.
Maintains acid-base balance	Nephrons reabsorb **bicarbonate ions** from urine into the blood and secrete **hydrogen ions** into the urine.
Regulates extracellular fluid	Regulates the volume and osmolality of the plasma by excreting more or less water.
Regulates blood volume	Blood volume must be maintained to ensure adequate blood pressure for circulation. **RAAS**[D12] is a hormone system vital in blood pressure regulation.
Production of renin	Renin is an enzyme involved in the regulation of blood pressure.
Production of active vitamin D (calcitriol)	Calcitriol, secreted by cells in the nephron, has a vital role in calcium absorption from the intestines and the maintenance of healthy bones.
Secretion of **erythropoietin**[E3] (EPO)	EPO stimulates **erythrocyte** (red blood cell) production in bone marrow.

[10]Let's look more closely at the process of filtration, reabsorption, and secretion. Each kidney receives oxygenated blood from the heart through a **renal artery**, which branches into increasingly smaller blood vessels to become **afferent arterioles**. The afferent arterioles deliver blood to the many **glomeruli**. Because the pressure of blood in the glomerulus (called the **hydrostatic pressure**) is very high, water and solutes from the blood plasma are forced through the wall of the glomerulus and into a cup-like structure called the **Bowman's capsule**. The filtrate that has collected in the Bowman's capsule then enters the first part of the tubule called the **proximal convoluted tubule**[E7] (PCT).

[11]Because the wall of the glomerular capillary acts like a very fine-meshed **sieve**, large

molecules cannot pass through. So, after **ultrafiltration** in the glomerulus, the filtrate at the start of its journey through the nephron does not contain large molecules such as **albumin**, a type of blood protein, nor blood cells. The filtrate does, however, contain various dissolved substances that are small enough to pass through the tiny pores in the **endothelium** (wall) of the glomerulus. These dissolved substances include glucose, amino acids, ions, urea, and **creatinine** (a waste product produced by muscles). In the PCT a lot of the dissolved substances that the body does not want to lose, such as glucose and amino acids, are reabsorbed back into the body. Cells in the PCT contain many **mitochondria**, an energy-producing **organelle**. Energy is needed since much reabsorption in the PCT occurs by **active transport** processes.

[12]More reabsorption occurs in the PCT than in any other part of the nephron tubule. The PCT reabsorbs about 65% of water, sodium, potassium, and chloride; 100% of glucose; 100% of amino acids; and 85% of bicarbonate. After the PCT, the filtrate, which is by now much more concentrated, flows into a U-shaped part of the nephron called the **loop of Henle** (named after the German anatomist who first described it in the 19th century), where more water and ions are reabsorbed. The loop of Henle leads into the **distal convoluted tubule**. The final section of the nephron is called the **collecting duct**.

[13]All along the nephron substances are reabsorbed back into the blood via the **peritubular capillaries**, or secreted from the peritubular capillaries into the **lumen** of the nephron tubule. Secreted substances include hydrogen ions, creatinine, ions, and other types of waste products, including drugs. To describe the process of secretion and reabsorption in detail is beyond the scope of this essay, but here are three key points to remember. Firstly, there are various mechanisms by which substances are reabsorbed and secreted, including **active transport**, **diffusion**, **facilitated diffusion**, and **osmosis**. A quick glance at a **<u>comparison of the composition of blood, filtrate, and urine</u>**[D4] will show the amazing effect of these mechanisms. Secondly, different portions of the nephron vary in their reabsorption capacity. For example, the **thick ascending limb** of the loop of Henle is impermeable to water. Thirdly, certain **<u>hormones are intimately involved in renal function</u>**[D10]. For example, **antidiuretic hormone** (ADH), secreted by the **pituitary gland** in the brain, is of great importance in regulating water excretion.

[14]Having undergone reabsorption and secretion, the filtrate that reaches the end of the collecting duct has become urine. In a person with normally functioning kidneys, urine largely consists of what the body does not need. The urine leaves the collecting ducts, collects in the **renal pelvis**, a funnel-shaped structure, and then flows into one of the two **<u>ureters</u>**[E10]. Each ureter is a muscular tube that carries urine to the **urinary bladder**, a muscular sac that stores the urine until **urination**. When a person urinates, urine is released from the bladder through the **urethra** to the outside of the body.

¹⁵"The Horse Whisperer" (邦題:モンタナの風に抱かれて) is a movie starring Robert Redford that was released in 1998. The movie is based on a 1995 novel by an English author called Nicholas Evans (1950-2022). In August 2008, Nicholas and his wife were on holiday in Scotland with two other family members. As well as being a world-famous author, Nick was also a keen cook and he enjoyed searching the countryside for edible plants and mushrooms to use in his dishes. One evening during the holiday, Nicholas went to a nearby forest to pick some mushrooms for dinner. After picking a basketful of what he thought were porcini mushrooms, Nicholas returned to the holiday cottage and fried the delicious-looking mushrooms. These butter-fried mushrooms, sprinkled with parsley, were enjoyed by the four family members with some wine.

¹⁶The following morning all four woke up feeling unwell. Worried that they may have food poisoning, Nicholas looked in a mushroom identification book that happened to be in the kitchen. To his horror, he saw that the mushrooms he had picked were not porcini, but a highly poisonous fungi called *Cortinarius speciosissimus*, commonly known as the deadly webcap. This mushroom contains orellanine, a highly potent **nephrotoxin** (a substance that damages the kidneys). Of the many kinds of **mycotoxins**, or toxic compounds naturally produced by some types of fungi, orellanine is **notorious** for selectively targeting the kidney and severely damaging the nephrons.

¹⁷By lunchtime, Nicholas and the other three people were suffering from severe nausea, vomiting and other horrible symptoms. They were rushed to hospital. By the morning of August 9, Nicholas was not urinating at all, a condition called **anuria**, and the other three people were only producing a few drops of urine. They had all suffered **AKI**, an abrupt decrease in kidney function. All four were put on **hemodialysis**, a procedure that removes waste products and excess fluid from the blood when the kidneys stop working properly. AKI can be reversible, and one of the family members regained enough kidney function to be taken off dialysis. But for the other three, their kidney function did not recover. In 2011, after three years on dialysis, Nicholas had a **kidney transplant operation** with a kidney that was donated by his daughter, who was 29 at the time (this is a **living-donor transplant**). The other two family members continued with dialysis until they received kidney transplants in 2012. By mistaking a deadly poisonous mushroom for an edible one, Nicholas almost killed himself and three other people. In the media, he described the "horrible guilt" he felt about the event.

¹⁸The Japanese archipelago lies along the **Pacific Ring of Fire** and is situated in an area where four **tectonic plates** converge. This is relevant to our discussion on AKI because Japan's geographical location makes it one of the world's most active earthquake zones, and earthquakes can result in people suffering **crush injuries**. The Hanshin-Awaji earthquake that hit the city of Kobe on January 17, 1995 caused many buildings to

collapse. The earthquake occurred when many people were still in bed, so hundreds became trapped alive under rubble, with their legs or other body parts crushed by heavy objects. The compression of skeletal muscle by heavy rubble for several hours damages the membrane of muscle cells, causing the muscle cells, or **myocytes**, to break down. This breakdown of myocytes allows various substances, including potassium and **myoglobin**, a muscle protein, to leak out of the myocytes. The name for this rapid breakdown of damaged skeletal muscle is **rhabdomyolysis**—*rhabdomyo* means "stripped muscle" (or **striated muscle**) and *lysis* means "breakdown."

[19]When a trapped person is pulled from the rubble by a rescuer, the pressure on the crushed muscles is suddenly released and blood can start flowing through the muscle again. This renewed blood flow sounds like good news, but it can cause dangerous complications because it quickly circulates the potassium and myoglobin, and various other substances, from the damaged myocytes. The excess potassium can disrupt the conductivity of the heart, causing **arrhythmias** or even cardiac arrest, but it is the massive release of myoglobin due to rhabdomyolysis that can quickly lead to AKI. Myoglobin is freely filtered across the glomeruli and becomes deposited within nephron tubules, causing obstruction of the tubules and damage to the cells of the proximal tubule. As if this were not bad enough for the kidney, myoglobin molecules further damage the kidney by constricting renal arterioles, thereby reducing renal blood flow. The combined effect of intratubular blockage, the direct toxic effect of myoglobin on tubule cells, and **renal ischemia** can lead to <u>**acute tubular necrosis**</u>[E1] , which is the death of tubular cells.

[20]We have seen above that AKI can be caused by eating mushrooms containing nephrotoxic mycotoxins and by crush injuries. But these two causes of AKI are quite rare. There are many more common causes of AKI, a few of which are **sepsis**, **chronic heart failure**[D3], and **kidney stones**, hard deposits of minerals that form inside the kidneys. Acute kidney injury is also a rare complication of **benign prostatic hyperplasia (BPH)**, an enlarged prostate gland that is common in older men. Various medications can increase the risk of AKI, including **NSAIDs** and **ACE inhibitors**. There have also been cases of AKI after taking **contaminated** medicine (e.g., in 2022, the death of over 60 children from AKI in Gambia, West Africa, was linked to cough and syrups contaminated with diethylene glycol and ethylene glycol). Some **Chinese herbal medicines** are also known to cause nephrotoxicity, despite the general belief that herbal medicines are **innocuous**. The etiology of AKI is often **multifactorial**, but the different causes can be divided into the three groups: <u>**prerenal, intrarenal, and postrenal**</u> [D11].

[21]While AKI happens within a short time period, from a few hours to a few days, **CKD** is the **progressive** loss of kidney over months or years (CKD is often defined as the presence of either kidney damage or decreased kidney function for three months or more). Some of the key differences between AKI and CKD are summarized in Table 2.2.

Table 2.2

Key Differences Between AKI and CKD　（急性腎障害と慢性腎臓病のおもな違い）

	AKI　（急性腎障害）	CKD　（慢性腎臓病）
Onset（発症）	Rapidly over hours to days. Onset of symptoms is sudden.	Gradually over months to years. Often asymptomatic until advanced.
Reversible（腎機能は元の状態に戻れるか？）	Often reversible if the underlying cause is quickly treated, but it can leave permanent kidney damage.	Irreversible, although progression can be slowed.
Causes（原因）	Often due to renal hypoperfusion or toxic **insult**[E5] to the kidney.	Most often due to diabetes mellitus and hypertension.
Urine output（尿排出量）	**Oliguria** or **anuria** (i.e., little or no urine output).	**Nocturnal polyuria** is a common symptom.
Dialysis（透析）	If required, usually temporary.	If required, is permanent.

[22]My wife's father, let's call him Mr. Y, who is now in his early 80s, has CKD. After graduating from a **prestigious** national university, Mr. Y spent his working life in a Japanese corporation, one of the millions of workers who contributed to Japan's post-war economic miracle. I would have liked to have asked Mr. Y about his experience of living with CKD, but, unfortunately, we are not really on speaking terms. At first, I thought he was upset because his daughter had married a foreigner, but he is not the type of man to hold such **anachronistic** views. No, I think the reason he is unfriendly towards me is that he **does not suffer fools gladly**. He has no time for **incompetent** people, and, in the eyes of Mr. Y, I am incompetent beyond help (and, to some extent, he is right). So, unable to talk directly with Mr. Y, I asked his daughter about the **chronology** of her father's CKD.

[23]After Mr. Y was diagnosed with CKD when he was in his mid-60s, his doctor prescribed **antihypertensives** and helped him to make lifestyle and dietary changes. These measures may have helped to slow down the **deterioration** of Mr. Y's kidneys, but after a few years, the decline in his renal function had progressed to a stage at which less than 15% of normal kidney function remained. Because Mr. Y's kidneys could no longer filter enough waste from the blood and remove excess fluid, **renal replacement therapy** became necessary to keep him alive. So, at age 70, Mr. Y began **peritoneal dialysis**, a type of dialysis treatment in which a person's own **peritoneum**, the lining of the abdominal cavity, is used as a filter to remove waste products from the blood. An advantage of peritoneal dialysis is that it can be carried out at home, meaning regular visits to a hospital's dialysis unit are not required. On the other hand, a major disadvantage is the risk of getting **peritonitis**, a potentially life-threatening inflammation of the peritoneum.

[24]After four years on peritoneal dialysis, Mr. Y needed to be switched to the other type of dialysis, **hemodialysis**. During hemodialysis, the patient's blood passes through a filter,

called a **dialyzer** (an "artificial kidney"). Mr. Y is driven by his wife to the dialysis center at the local hospital for his hemodialysis (hemodialysis can be done at home, but it requires the patient and the patient's family to have extensive training). While going to hospital 3 days a week, for around 4 hours each time, is a physical and mental burden for both Mr. and Mrs. Y, it does give them 4 days a week that are dialysis-free.

[25]Since the first person was successfully treated with dialysis in the Netherlands in 1945, the lives of millions of people with kidney disease have been extended. But dialysis is by no means a perfect replacement for real kidneys. Dialysis replaces the kidney's filtering function, but the kidney also has important **endocrine** functions, which dialysis cannot replace. In addition, dialysis can cause **complications** such as infection, depression, and itchy skin. The life expectancy of someone on dialysis is shorter than for a healthy person of the same age. For example, a Japanese person in their 40s on dialysis will live on average for 20 years fewer than a **healthy peer**. And a man who starts dialysis at age 70 in Japan can expect to live for another 6 years, compared to another 12 years for a healthy person of the same age. Of course, life expectancy on dialysis varies between people depending on the presence of **comorbidities** and other factors. According to statistics, Mr. Y would have been expected to die at around 76 years old, but he is now in his 80s and still enjoys a regular game of golf and a weekly lunch at his local *sushiya*.

[26]Mr. Y was diagnosed with hypertension when he was in his early 30s. **Hypertension** is one of the two main risk factors of CKD, the other one being **diabetes**. Persistently raised blood pressure causes **nephrosclerosis**, or hardening of the walls of the small arteries and arterioles in the kidney, and it also damages the nephrons themselves. Not only does hypertension damage the kidneys, but damage to the kidneys can also cause hypertension. My wife also told me that her father's mother (i.e., my wife's **paternal grandmother**) also suffered from kidney disease for many years. Kidney disease can run in families, so perhaps Mr. Y has a **genetic susceptibility**.

[27]One more factor that **predisposed** Mr. Y to developing CKD was his age. All vital organs lose some function as we get older, but the kidneys are particularly susceptible to the effects of aging. If you are reading this book, it is likely that you are between the ages of 18 and 25 years of age. If this is so, then by the time you are 70 years old, your kidneys will probably have lost around 50% of their nephrons. It is such a loss in nephron number that results in a decline in kidney function with increasing age. This age-related decline is the main reason CKD is more common in people aged 65 years or older. This age-related renal decline also leaves elderly people more vulnerable to kidney damage from infection or from the use of certain medications such as NSAIDs and **lithium**.

[28]Apart from hypertension and diabetes, there are several other common conditions that increase a person's susceptibility to CKD. These include **chronic heart failure**, **gout**,

nephrolithiasis[E9] (more commonly known as **kidney stones**), and **urinary tract infections** (**UTIs**). There are also rarer conditions that can lead to CKD, including **systemic lupus erythematosus** (**SLE**), **polycystic kidney disease** (**PKD**), and **IgA nephropathy**. In Japan, these three conditions are classified as **intractable diseases** by the **Ministry of Health, Labor, and Welfare**. (To qualify as an intractable disease, it must be relatively rare, with the number of patients fewer than around 0.1% of the population of Japan, difficult and expensive to treat, and usually incurable. A person with one of the 338 designated intractable diseases can apply for financial assistance from the government.) The most common of these three conditions is SLE, an autoimmune disease in which the body's immune system attacks healthy tissues by mistake. In some people with SLE, the immune system attacks the glomeruli, causing them to become inflamed. Kidney damage due to SLE is known as **lupus nephritis**. In PKD, an **inherited disease**, many fluid-filled sacs, called **cysts**, develop in the kidneys. These cysts cause the kidneys to enlarge, and they interfere with the kidney's ability to filter waste products. There are around 30,000 people with PKD in Japan, of whom around 50% will go on to develop kidney failure by the age of 60. The last of these three intractable diseases, IgA nephropathy, is caused by the accumulation of IgA, an antibody, inside the glomeruli. This accumulation causes inflammation and damage to the glomeruli.

[29]**CKD can be divided into 5 stages**[D5] depending on the remaining level of kidney function. Because the kidneys have a considerable **redundancy**, or extra capacity, the early stages of CKD are often asymptomatic. This is why CKD is often called a "silent disease." In fact, it is possible to lose up to 90% of kidney function before experiencing any symptoms. In people who are **asymptomatic**, CKD is usually only diagnosed if a blood or urine test that is carried out as part of a routine health check happens to detect a kidney problem (this is called an **incidental medical finding**). Although humans are born with a big surplus of nephrons, at some stage in the progression of CKD, the loss of nephrons becomes so great that various signs and symptoms begin to appear. These include **extreme fatigue,** which occurs due to **uremia,** a buildup of toxins in the blood, and due to a deficiency of red blood cells (**anemia**); persistent itching (**uremic pruritus**); swelling in the ankles and feet (**peripheral edema**) due to fluid overload; and **muscle cramping** due to **electrolyte imbalances**. Changes in urine volume and frequency often occur, such as **oliguria** (producing abnormally small amounts of urine) and **nocturia** (excessive urination at night). Blood in the urine (**hematuria**) is a sign of CKD, although it can also indicate a UTI or kidney cancer. People may also notice **foamy urine,** a sign of **proteinuria** (protein in the urine). The symptoms of advanced CKD can be extremely **debilitating** and cause a significant decline in a person's quality of life.

[30]There are various tests and procedures used in the diagnosis, evaluation, and monitoring of CKD. Blood and urine tests are commonly used. Urinalysis checks for things that the urine should not contain, particularly blood, glucose (glucose in the urea is called **glycosuria**), and **albumin** (albumin in the urine is known as **albuminuria**). The presence of such substances in the urine may indicate damage to the glomerular filter. Blood tests measure the level of waste products such as <u>**blood urea nitrogen (BUN) and creatinine**</u>[D2]. Determining the level of creatinine is particularly important because it is used to calculate the **estimated glomerular filtration rate (eGFR)**, which is a measure of how much blood passes through the glomeruli each minute. The eGFR is the most accurate way to measure kidney function and it used to determine a person's stage of kidney disease. **Nephrologists**, doctors who specialize in diagnosing and treating kidney disease, may also use **imaging techniques** (e.g., ultrasound, MRI, or CT) and **biopsy** to get more information (e.g., an ultrasound scan can assess kidney size—in CKD the kidneys usually shrink; and a kidney biopsy is used to determine the presence of **glomerulonephritis**, an autoimmune disease in which the glomeruli become inflamed).

[31]Because the kidneys are important for so many body functions, CKD can cause various **complications,** including **anemia**, a reduction of the total number of circulating red blood cells. Anemia in CKD is complex, but the main cause is decreased renal production of **erythropoietin (EPO)**, a hormone that stimulates bone marrow to make red blood cells. Some of the complications of CKD are related to <u>**disturbances of acid-base balance** and **electrolyte disorders**</u>[D7]. Abnormally high levels of potassium, known as **hyperkalemia,** is a common electrolyte disorder in CKD. In healthy kidneys, potassium is secreted from the blood into the nephron tubule and then excreted (approximately 90% of potassium is excreted in urine); however, in CKD potassium excretion declines, causing it to build up in the blood. Because potassium is important for nerves and muscles to function properly, and for maintaining cardiac rhythm, hyperkalemia can lead to muscle weakness and cramps, and heart **arrhythmia**. A deterioration in mineral homeostasis due to poor kidney function can also lead to <u>**CKD-MBD**</u> [D6] (**chronic kidney disease-mineral and bone disorder**). One possible consequence of CKD-MBD is **vascular calcification**, the deposition of minerals on the wall of blood vessels. This accelerates **atherosclerosis** and increases the risk of a heart attack.

[32]The word "heart" appeared twice in the previous paragraph, suggesting that CKD can have negative effects on cardiac health. In fact, cardiovascular disease is the leading cause of mortality in people with CKD. In the UK, over 45% of people with CKD die of cardiovascular diseases. The **pathogenesis** of heart problems in people with CKD is complex, but the key message is that renal dysfunction can induce or worsen heart problems, while cardiac dysfunction can induce or worsen kidney problems.

[33]Although the kidneys can repair themselves to a limited extent, they lack the liver's ability of regeneration. For this reason, lost kidney function is generally considered to be irreversible. However, if diagnosed in the early stages, the progression of CKD can be slowed or even stopped with appropriate lifestyle changes and drug treatment. Exercise benefits people with CKD in many ways; for example, it helps to lower blood pressure, maintain bone and muscle strength, improve appetite, and improve physiological well-being. Diet also has an important role in protecting the kidneys from further damage. People with CKD may be given advice by a **dietician** on consuming a kidney-friendly diet. Often, dietary changes are made to restrict the consumption of salt, potassium, phosphorus, and protein. For example, bananas and avocados are very nutritious, but due to their high potassium content they may need to be avoided by some people with CKD. Especially in the USA, some people have advocated a **Paleolithic diet** for CKD patients. This is a modern version of the diet our hunter-gatherer ancestors are thought to have eaten during the Old Stone Age, before humans began farming around 11,000 years ago.

[34]It is important for people with CKD who have diabetes mellitus and/or hypertension to have good adherence to **antidiabetic and antihypertensive pharmacotherapy**[D1]. One class of drugs, called **SGLT2 inhibitors**, were originally developed as an oral antidiabetic, but they have been found to be effective at slowing the progression of kidney disease, even in CKD patients who do not have diabetes mellitus. SGLT2 inhibitors provide an example of a drug with **pleiotropic effects**, or having actions other than those for which it was originally developed. There are many drugs to treat the various symptoms and complications of CKD. For example, **edema** caused by water retention can be treated with **diuretics**; anemia can be treated with **erythropoiesis-stimulating agents**; and bone disease can be treated with **phosphate binders** (drugs that reduce the amount of phosphorus that is absorbed into the blood) and with **calcitriol analogs** (synthetic forms of calcitriol, the active form of vitamin D).

[35]It was mentioned earlier that CKD can be divided into five stages. Stage 5 kidney disease is also called **end stage renal disease (ESRD)**, and it usually occurs when the eGFR is 15 or lower. Such an eGFR indicates that the kidneys have lost around 85% of their function. At this stage, the kidneys are close to failing or have already failed, and there are only two treatments remaining that can prolong life by years: dialysis or **kidney transplant**. Without dialysis to take over some of the functions of the failed kidneys, or a new kidney from a donor, toxins and fluid will build up in the body and death from renal failure will usually come within days or weeks. Not everyone with ESRD chooses dialysis. Some people will decide against this treatment because they feel it will have too great an impact on the remainder of their life. Such people are offered **palliative care**, the primary goal of which is to optimize the quality of life for people with **terminal illnesses** (i.e.,

illnesses that cannot be cured and are likely to lead to death).

[36]In June 2019, I returned to the UK from Japan to visit my father, then aged 90, in hospital. I remember sitting with my mother and sister discussing my father's medical care with a doctor. The doctor told us that my father, who at the time had an eGFR of 25 (CKD stage 4), would not qualify for dialysis, even if his kidneys failed completely, because of his age and the fact he had chronic heart failure. In August 2019, my father died of **pneumonia**, an infection of the lungs. The risk of pneumonia is higher in patients with CKD, but I have no idea if my father's failing kidneys contributed to his death.

[37]It was in school that I first learnt about the urinary system from Mr. Pond, my biology teacher. A few years later, I saw firsthand with Tootsie, the family cat, how kidney failure is **incompatible** with life. However, with renal replacement therapy, the lives of people whose kidneys have failed can be extended. Thanks to dialysis, Mr. Y, my father-in-law, has lived for over a decade without functioning kidneys. The kidneys work away quietly at the back of the abdomen, filtering the blood and making urine. When healthy, it is easy to forget about them. But after my experiences with Tootsie, Mr. Y, and my father, I know that healthy kidneys should not be taken for granted.

2-2 Eleven Etymologies (E) （11 の単語を詳しく）

1) *Acute tubular necrosis* **(ATN) is a kidney disorder in which the tubule cells in the nephron of the kidneys are damaged**. This can lead to acute kidney failure. Common causes of ATN are low renal blood flow, drugs that damage the kidneys, and severe systemic infections. The word *necrosis* means "the localized death of body cells." Necrosis can have various causes including interruption of blood supply, infection, and venom (e.g., from a venomous snake bite). Someone who is exposed to extreme cold can get **frostbite**, which is when tissue becomes frozen and the cells die. Dead tissue in certain parts of the body, often the nose, fingers, or toes, turn black. Necrosis is caused by factors external to the cell and it is always **pathological** (i.e., relating to, or caused by, a disease). Another form of cell death is **apoptosis**, which is programmed and can be part of an organism's normal physiology.

WFE: The Greek word *nekrosis* means "a state of death." The suffix *~osis* indicates an abnormal state, and the root *nek*, means "death." **Nectar**, the "drink of the gods" in ancient Greece, literally means "to overcome death." It was said that a person who drank nectar would become **immortal** (*im~* → *in~* = "not" + *mortal* = "to die"; so, "to live forever"). The meaning of nectar extended to mean a sweet juice, usually made from fruit, and the sweet liquid produced by flowers:

& *Butterflies use a proboscis, a long tongue-like structure, to reach* **nectar** *inside flowers.*

Have you ever eaten a **nectarine**? This fruit developed from a peach by a natural genetic mutation and differs from a peach in that it has smooth skin (i.e., it has no fuzz, or tiny hairs, on its skin). The name "nectarine" means "[to taste] like nectar." The Greek root *nek* is also the origin of the Latin *nocere* meaning "to harm, injure." If by accident you touch a very hot frying pan, you will quickly withdraw your hand and feel pain. This response is due to receptors in your skin that respond to harmful stimuli and send a signal to the brain. These pain receptors are called **nociceptors**. Some other words containing *nocere* (or variations of it) are underlined in this sentence:

& *The man in the café was reading a book and drinking a cup of coffee. Although he looked* ___**innocuous**___, *he was really a dangerous terrorist. In his bag was a bottle containing a liquid that produced a* ___**noxious**___ *gas. He planned to kill many* ___**innocent**___ *people.*

Finally, a Latin phrase that every doctor knows is ***primum non nocere***, meaning "first, do no harm [to your patients]." This phrase is a statement of the principle of **non-maleficence** (*mal~* = "bad/harm" + *fic* = "do"; so, **maleficence** is to "do harm" and non-maleficence is "do no harm"). That doctors should not harm their patients sounds obvious, but doctors do sometimes have to inflict harm. For example, the surgeon who operated on my brain (see Chapter 4) caused me a lot of post-operative pain and left me with a big scar on my scalp. But the benefit of the operation far outweighed its *nocere* (harm). One doctor who went completely against the principal of *primum non nocere* was Harold Shipman, a British doctor who killed over 200 of his patients by administering lethal doses of diamorphine (pharmaceutical heroin). Shipman killed himself in his prison cell in 2004.

2) Anthropomorphizing: *Anthropomorphize* **means to give human characteristics to non-human animals, plants, or inanimate objects such as a rock or a car** ("inanimate" means non-living; the Japanese word *anime* is derived from the Latin *anima* meaning "living/breathing"). For example, in the fairy story "Little Red Riding Hood," the wolf is given the human characteristic of being bad and devious.

WFE: The root *anthropo* means "human being," and *morphe* is the Greek for "shape/form" (e.g., **metamorphosis**; *meta* = change). So, anthropomorphize literally means to "become the form of a human." The suffix *~ize* means to "make" (e.g., **globalization** = "to make the world become more global or connected"). Words that contain *anthropo* include **anthropology** (the study of human societies and cultures) and **misanthrope** (a person who dislikes people). **Philanthropist** literally means "a person who loves humans" (*phil* = "like/love"), but this word is used to describe people, usually very rich people, who use their money for the benefit of others. A famous philanthropist is Bill Gates, the cofounder of Microsoft.

Anthropogenic means "caused by humans," and **anthropogenic climate change** is global warming that is caused by human activity, such as the burning of fossil fuels. The impact of humans on the Earth is huge, and we are now in an age in which humans are affecting the climate, ecology, geology, and other systems of this planet. This most recent geologic period has been named the **Anthropocene** (~*cene* = "recent/new"). **Anthropocentrism** is the idea that humans are the most important or *central* entity on Earth.

3) *Erythropoietin* (EPO) is a peptide hormone that is essential to the production of erythrocytes or red blood cells (RBCs). EPO is synthesized in the kidney by specialized cells called **renal interstitial fibroblasts**. The production of EPO is regulated by oxygen levels in the renal blood, with low oxygen levels triggering a greater production of EPO production. The secreted EPO is carried in the blood to the **bone marrow**, where it stimulates the production of RBCs. Found in the center of most bones, bone marrow is a soft, spongy tissue that is rich in blood vessels. There are two types of bone marrow: red and yellow. It is **red bone marrow** that produces RBCs. Red marrow is found mainly in the **flat bones**, such as the hip bone, **sternum**, and ribs. In CKD, kidney cells produce less EPO, which can lead to **anemia**. A decline in the synthesis of EPO impairs **erythropoiesis** (the process which produces RBCs), and can result in anemia. Around 90 percent of people with CKD develop anemia, the symptoms of which include tiredness and breathlessness. The secretion of EPO is regulated by the amount of oxygen in the blood that is flowing to the kidney. When the blood oxygen concentration is normal, EPO is made by only a few cells in the kidney, but when blood oxygen is too low (**hypoxia**), many more interstitial cells begin to make it. In environments where blood oxygen levels drop, for example at **high altitudes**, the production of EPO by the kidneys can increase by more than 100 times greater than normal.

EPO was one of the first drugs produced through **recombinant DNA technology**, which involves cloning the gene for erythropoietin. The first **recombinant human EPO** was approved for use by the FDA in 1989 to treat anemia and renal failure. Recombinant erythropoietin drugs are known as **erythropoietin-stimulating agents** (ESAs), or **synthetic EPO**. Synthetic EPO is not only used in the treatment of amenia caused by kidney disease, but also for anemia resulting from certain medical treatments such as chemotherapy. It has also been administered as an alternative to a blood transfusion; for example, because of religious beliefs, a person who is a **Jehovah's Witness** will refuse a blood transfusion, but he or she may accept treatment with a synthetic EPO.

In sport, doping with synthetic EPO is a big problem. Synthetic EPO was banned by the **World Anti-Doping Agency** in the early 1990s, but some endurance athletes continue to inject this drug to increase RBC levels and, consequently, aerobic capacity. In 2012, a famous US cyclist called **Lance Armstrong** admitted he used synthetic EPO all seven times that he won the Tour de France (a famous bicycle touring race). Because it can lead to the bone marrow making more RBCs, EPO can cause the blood to become excessively **viscous**, increasing the risk of blood clots.

WFE: The WFE *erythro* means "red" (e.g., **erythroderma** is abnormal skin redness); *poiet* means "to make," and *in~* means "protein." So, erythropoietin is literally "protein for making erythrocytes." The Greek WFE *poieo*, "to make," can also be found in the other medical terms such as **hematopoiesis** (the formation of blood cells) and **myelopoiesis** (the production of bone marrow; *myelo* = "bone marrow"). The word **poem** is also derived from this WFE (a poem is something that is made or created).

SD 2A: An alternative to synthetic EPO

The 2019 Nobel Prize in Physiology or Medicine was awarded to three scientists for discovering how cells sense and adapt to oxygen availability. The scientists showed that when oxygen levels are low (hypoxia), a protein called **hypoxia-inducible factor** (HIF) builds up in body cells. The rise in HIF stimulates the production of EPO. This Nobel-winning discovery led to the development of a drug called **roxadustat**, a type of drug called a hypoxia-inducible factor prolyl hydroxylase inhibitor (HIF-PH). By inhibiting the breakdown of HIF, roxadustat promotes erythropoiesis, thereby increasing the oxygen-carrying capacity of the blood. While synthetic EPO must be injected, roxadustat is in tablet form and is taken orally. The oral route of administration makes it more convenient to take compared to an injection. In the future, it may replace synthetic EPO as the main treatment for anemia in people with CKD. The development of roxadustat is just one example of how a breakthrough in **basic research** has been key in creating a new medicine.

4) *Glomerulus* **is a network of capillaries at the beginning of a nephron.** Glomeruli filter blood into the Bowman's capsule in a process called **ultrafiltration**, in which fluid is "pushed" across a semipermeable membrane by a driving force called **hydrostatic pressure**. If the glomeruli are damaged, it can have serious consequences. In fact, **glomerulonephritis**, a condition in which glomeruli are injured, is the third most common cause of CKD.

WFE: The Latin word *glomus* means "a ball of yarn." The Italian anatomist who named this structure in the 17th century must have thought that the ball of capillaries comprising the glomerulus resembled a ball of yarn. The term "glomerulonephritis" literally means "inflammation (*~itis*) of glomeruli in the nephron." Most English words are made plural by adding an "s," but because many medical terms are derived from Latin and Greek, they often follow different **pluralization** rules. For example, one rule is that when a singular form of the word ends with "*~us*," you drop the "*~us*" and add "*~i*" (e.g., glomerulus/glomeruli; thrombus/thrombi; embolus/emboli; alveolus/alveoli). Another rule is when a singular form ends with "*~um*," replace the "*~um*" with an "*~a*" (e.g., bacterium/bacteria; atrium/atria). The glomerulus is supplied with blood by the **afferent arterioles**, and blood leaves the glomerulus through the **efferent arterioles**. The efferent arterioles feed the peritubular capillaries that surround the nephron tubule. In the word *afferent*, the prefix *a~* is a simplified form of *ad~*, which means "towards," and *ferre* means "to carry." So, afferent means to "carry toward." On the other hand, the prefix *e~* in *efferent* is from *ex~* (before "f" the "x" is dropped), meaning "out" (as in the word "exit"). Other words containing *ferre* include **transfer**, **ferry**, and **suffer** (*su~* is from the prefix *sub~*, meaning "under").

5) Insult: If you insult someone you say or do something that offends him or her. However, in the essay, insult is used to mean "an injury or trauma to the body." For example, a blocked blood vessel in the brain that deprives a part of the brain of blood could be described as a **cerebral insult**. This is an example of a word whose meaning in medicine is different from its meaning in everyday English.

WFE: Insult literally means "to leap (jump) on." The *sult* WFE is from the Latin *salire*, meaning to "leap, jump." Words containing this WFE include **assault**, **somersault**, and **salmon**, a fish that often leaps out of the water. If you studied biology at high school, you may know the phrase **saltatory conduction**, describing how an electrical impulse moves along a **myelinated nerve axon** by skipping from one **node of Ranvier** to the next node of Ranvier.

6) Kidney: There are five organs in the human body that are considered vital for survival: the heart, brain, kidneys, liver, and lungs. If you check the etymology of these words, you will find that they do not come from Greek or Latin, but from Old English. However, as Table 2.3 shows, many medical words concerned with these organs use Greek or Latin WFEs.

Table 2.3

Latin and Greek Roots for the Vital Organs

（なくてはならない臓器のラテン語とギリシア語の語根）

Old English （古い英語）	L/G root （ラテン語とギリシア語の語根）	Examples　（例）
brain	*cerebro*	intracerebral hemorrhage
heart	*cardio*	cardiac arrest, myocardium
kidney	*ren(L)*	renal failure, adrenaline, renin
	nephros(G)	nephritis, epinephrine
liver	*hepatos*	heparin, hepatitis
lung	*pulmo*	pulmonary artery
	pneum	pneumonia

L = Latin　　*G* = Greek

You can see from the table that the kidney has two roots: *ren* is the Latin root and *nephros* is the Greek root. The branch of medicine that is concerned with the kidney is called **renal medicine** or **nephrology**, and a doctor who specializes in this branch is called a **nephrologist**. Sitting on the top of the kidneys are triangle-shaped **adrenal glands**. The prefix *ad~* means "near," so the word "adrenal" literally means "near the kidneys." A less commonly used alternative name is **suprarenal gland** (*supra~* is from the Latin *super* meaning "above"). The adrenal glands produce many important hormones, including **adrenaline**, **cortisol**, and **aldosterone**. In **Addison's disease**, also called **adrenal insufficiency**, the adrenal glands produce too little cortisol and aldosterone. John F. Kennedy, the 35th President of the United States who was assassinated in 1963, suffered from this autoimmune condition. The suffix *~ine* forms the name of chemical substances, so adrenaline is "a chemical substance made near the kidney." Adrenaline was first isolated in 1900 by a Japanese chemist called **Jokichi Takamine** (高峰 譲吉; 1854-1922). For various historical reasons, in the USA the term **epinephrine** is used instead of adrenaline. The prefix *epi~* means "on," so epinephrine is a "chemical substance made on top of the kidneys."

SD 2B: When does a condition become chronic?

When used to describe an illness, the word "chronic" means lasting for a long period of time, usually more than three months. For example, on the UK's National Health Service (NHS) website, chronic pain is defined as pain that "carries on for longer than 12 weeks despite medication or treatment." Although a dictionary defines a chronic illness as one that persists for a long duration, many British people tend to associate the word chronic with "bad" or "serious." This illustrates an interesting point about words: in addition to the literal main meaning of a word, words often have an implied meaning. For example, the word "beach" **denotes**, or literally means, an area of sand or small stones along a sea or lake, but for many people it also **connotes** (i.e., suggests or implies) a place to relax, eat ice cream, and get a suntan. The **denotation** of *sakura* (桜) is a "flowering cherry tree," but in Japan, this word evokes various feelings and images. Some of the **connotations** of *sakura* are spring, new life, enjoying *hanami* (花見; "flower viewing"), and transient beauty. The root *chrono* is from the Greek *khronos*, meaning "time." Two other words in the essay with this root are **anachronistic** ("out of date/old fashioned"; *ana~* = "against"), and **chronology** (adj. **chronological**).

⅋ One study found that the biological age of men who smoked tobacco was 1.5 times older than their actual **chronological age**, while the biological age of female smokers was almost double that of their chronological age. In other words, smoking makes you age more quickly.

In contrast to a chronic medical condition that is long-lasting, an **acute** condition generally develops suddenly and lasts a short time. The origin of "acute" is the Latin *acutus* meaning "sharp, pointed." Other words derived from *acutus* are **acupuncture**, **acne**, **acid**, and **acumen**. Acumen means sharp in the **figurative sense**. For example, if a woman has great **business acumen**, she is probably very good at making correct decisions and judgments when making business deals. In Japanese, too, *surudoi* (鋭い), the adjective for "sharp," can also be used figuratively to mean a person with quick judgement or deep insight.

SD 2C: How many kidneys do you have?

Why do humans *usually* have two kidneys when we only need one to survive? Experts are not completely sure, but the most obvious answer is this: renal function is so important for survival that we evolved to have two kidneys, just in case one of them is damaged due to injury or disease. On the other hand, the heart and liver are also essential for survival, but we don't have two hearts or two livers. Having two kidneys could just be because of **bilateral symmetry**. Most multicellular organisms are the same on both sides ("lateral" means "side"), and humans have two arms, two legs, two eyes, two ears, two lungs, and two kidneys. In the first line of this section, I wrote "usually" because not all people have two kidneys. Read on to find out more.

- **Renal agenesis** is a **congenital** abnormality of the kidney (congenital means "existing from birth or during fetal development"; *con~* = "with" + *gen* = "born"). Agenesis is when an organ or body part is absent or not completely developed (*a~* = "without" + *genesis* = "origin/production"). **Bilateral renal agenesis** is being born with no kidneys. This occurs in around 1 in 3000 births. This disorder is **incompatible** with **postnatal** life—a **fetus** with this condition will be born dead (a **stillbirth**), or will die shortly after being born. One sign during pregnancy that the fetus could have this condition is **oligohydramnios** (i.e., a low amount of **amniotic fluid**). Normally, a proportion of the amniotic fluid is made up of the baby's urine, but a fetus with bilateral renal agenesis will not make any urine, hence the oligohydramnios. **Unilateral renal agenesis** is a complete absence of one kidney. This is quite a common condition, occurring in around 1 in 800 births. Unilateral renal agenesis is sometimes caused by a genetic mutation. The solitary kidney usually undergoes **compensatory hypertrophy** (i.e., it grows larger to help do the work of two kidneys). Many children with unilateral renal agenesis will have no long-term complications, but others will experience hypertension, proteinuria, increased susceptibility to kidney infections, and other problems.

- Some people have only one kidney because the other one had to be removed by a **nephrectomy**, the surgical removal of a kidney (*~ectomy* = "removal"). A nephrectomy may be done because of **traumatic injury** (e.g., a traffic accident) or disease. The most common reason for a **radical nephrectomy** (i.e., removal of an entire kidney) is kidney cancer. The most common type of kidney cancer is **renal cell carcinoma**, which starts in the lining of nephron tubules. In Japan, around 6 in 100,000 people get this type of cancer.

- A nephrectomy is also done to remove a healthy kidney from a living donor for a **kidney transplant**. A person who has voluntarily donated a kidney for transplantation into another person will only have one kidney. The donor's remaining kidney will **pick up the slack** for the kidney that has been removed. Would you donate one of your kidneys to someone? Who? A family member? There are people who donate a kidney to a complete stranger, an act that is called "non-directed **altruistic** kidney donation." **Altruism** means being selfless, and being willing to help others, even if it brings you no benefit. The meaning of the Latin *alter* is "other" (e.g., <u>alter</u>native). Following a kidney transplant, the recipient will need to take **immunosuppressants**, medications that suppress the immune system, to help prevent rejection of the transplanted kidney. Immunosuppression therapy is often not required if the transplant is between identical (**monozygotic**) twins.

In such cases, the donor of the kidney is genetically identical to the recipient, so there is little risk of **organ rejection** (*re~* = "back" + *ject* = "throw"; so, **reject** means "to throw back"; **inject** = "to throw in").

- When the transplant **recipient** receives a kidney from a donor, the transplanted kidney is placed in the anterior (front) part of the lower abdomen. The recipient's own kidneys that have failed are usually not removed, but are left in place. So, the recipient of a kidney donation will have three kidneys, one from the donor, and two original non-working kidneys. There are even cases of a recipient getting two kidneys from a deceased donor, meaning there are people with four kidneys!

SD 2D: Organ donation in different countries

I studied French at school, but I didn't learn much. In fact, I picked up more Japanese in my first week living in Japan than I learnt from five years of school French lessons. One of the few things that I do remember from my school days is that the French verb for "to give" is *donner*. This verb is from the Latin *donare*, meaning to "to give as a gift." The English word **donor** is derived from *donare*. A few other words with the same etymology are **dose** (one "giving" [of medicine]); **antidote** "give against"; and **pardon** (*par~* → *per~* = "completely"; lit. "give completely" → "to forgive"). An **organ donor** is "a person who gives permission for a part of their body to be taken, while they are alive (**living donation**) or after they are dead (**deceased donation**), and put into someone else's body to replace an organ that is not working correctly" (Cambridge Dictionary). A living donation of a kidney is possible because most people can lead a normal life with just one kidney. On average, a person has around 1 million nephrons in each kidney, although there is a lot of variation, with some people only having fewer than 300,000. With such a high nephron number, each nephron does not need to work at maximum capacity. When a living person donates a kidney, the nephrons in the remaining kidney work harder to compensate for the 50% reduction in the total number of nephrons. Studies have shown that soon after a living donation, there is a compensatory increase in blood flow to the remaining kidney. The remaining kidney also undergoes **hypertrophy** that enables it to compensate for loss of the donated kidney.

The world's first successful kidney transplant, which was in 1954, was from a living donor. Richard and Ronald Herrick were identical twins, but Richard had suffered double kidney failure. Joseph Murray, the doctor who transplanted Ronald's healthy kidney into Richard, was awarded the Nobel Prize for Physiology or Medicine in 1990. (Murray's 1954 operation, was not only the first successful kidney transplant, it was also the first time ever that a human organ had been transplanted successfully). Receiving a kidney from a living donor has several advantages over a kidney donation from a deceased person, but deceased kidney donation is the most common type. In the UK, for example, around 70% of kidney transplants are with organs from a deceased donor. Around the world, there are different approaches to deceased organ donation. In an **opt-in system**, a person must actively register to donate their organs after death. In Japan, for example, people can indicate their willingness to be a donor by signing in the consent space on the back of a driving license. In an **opt-out system**, people are **presumed** to have **consented** to be an organ donor when they die unless they registered online a decision not to donate when they were still alive. Since 2020, England has had an opt out system. Organ transplantation in Israel includes a priority system. For example, a person who is a registered donor will be given priority for an organ transplant over a person who has not registered. Top priority for organ transplantation is given to a living donor and his or her family members. This system is nicknamed "**Don't give; Don't get.**"

The number of kidney donors, both living and deceased, is not enough to meet the demand for people who are on dialysis waiting for a kidney. For this reason, many people with end-stage kidney disease die while waiting for a transplant. There is an urgent need for a new source of organs. Using animal organs could be one option. In 2021, surgeons in the USA successfully transplanted a kidney from a pig into a brain-dead human patient. **Xenotransplantation** *(xeno~* = "other/foreign"), the transferring of cells, tissues, and organs between species, could potentially solve the shortage of donor kidneys. However, xenotransplantation raises issues such as the risk of **zoonosis** and ethical concerns around the animal exploitation. Because of advances in stem cell technology, there is now the **tantalizing prospect** of kidney transplants using organs that have been grown *de novo* in the laboratory.

7) *Proximal convoluted tubule* **(PCT) is the first segment of the nephron and it is also the longest segment** (the complete nephron is around 30 mm long, and the PCT is about 14 mm in length). A large amount of **reabsorption** occurs in the PCT. Reabsorption is when water and **solutes**, substances dissolved in the water, move from the PCT into the capillaries that wrap around the nephron. These capillaries are called **peritubular capillaries**. From the peritubular capillaries, blood flows into the **renal vein** and is returned to the heart via a large vein called the **inferior vena cava**. Remember how important reabsorption is: each day the glomeruli in the kidney filter around 180 liters of filtrate into the nephrons, but an average person will urinate less than 2 liters of urine a day. This means that each day around 178 liters of water, together with solutes, is reabsorbed from the nephron tubules and returned to the circulatory system. The **distal convoluted tubule** (DCT) is the between the Loop of Henle and the collecting duct. Despite being only 5 mm long, and the shortest segment of the nephron, the DCT is very important in sodium reabsorption, potassium secretion, and in other homeostatic processes.

WFE: The convoluted tubule is so called because it is many loops and twists. Two things that have a **convoluted** surface are **walnuts** and human brains. I'm not sure why a walnut has many folds on its surface, but the convolutions on the brain give it a large surface area. By the way, walnuts not only look like a brain, but they contain a lot of **omega-3 fatty acids**, which have an important role in brain functioning and growth. The word **convoluted** is often used to describe communication that is complicated and not easy to follow.

& Good teachers avoid **convoluted** *explanations and make even difficult concepts easy to understand.*

"Convoluted" is composed of the prefix *con~* (= "together") and the Latin root *volvere*, meaning to "to roll." Two other words with this root are **evolution** (*e* = "out"; lit. "roll out") and **involve** (lit. "roll into").

Proximal and **distal** are words used in anatomy to describe the location of structures that have a beginning and an end. Proximal means "closer to its origin."

*℮ The arm begins at the shoulder and ends at the wrist joint, so the elbow is **proximal** to the wrist.*

The Latin *proximus* means "near/close." A word used in everyday English is **proximity**, meaning "close to":

*℮ One thing I like about the location of this university campus is its **proximity** to AEON, a big department store.*

Another related word is **proximate**. The phrase "**proximate cause**" is the direct cause of an accident or other event.

*℮ The underlying cause of the 2011 Fukushima nuclear plant accident was an earthquake and tsunami, but the **proximate cause** was a power failure at the plant.*

In "distal," the prefix *dis~* means "away from" (e.g., "distant" is literally to "stand away").

*℮ The wrist is **distal** to the elbow because it is farther away from the shoulder, the point at which the arm attaches to the body.*

In the word "peritubular," the prefix *peri~* means "around/surrounding." For example, the **pericardium** is the membrane that that surrounds and protects the heart. Other words with this prefix are **periscope** (lit. "instrument for viewing all around"), and **perinatal** ("the period immediately before, during, and soon after birth"). The membrane lining the abdominal cavity is called the **peritoneum** (*peri~* + *teinein* = "to stretch"; the peritoneum is the membrane that is "stretched around [the abdominal wall]"). In **peritoneal dialysis**, the peritoneum acts as a filter to remove waste products from the blood. The kidney is surrounded by a thick layer of adipose tissue, called **perirenal fat**, which helps to protect it. Our bladders fill even when lying down because urine is propelled from the kidneys to the bladder by **peristalsis**, waves of contraction and relaxation generated by smooth muscle in the walls of the ureters. Peristalsis is from the Greek *peristaltikos*, meaning "contracting around."

8) Put her to sleep: The **phrasal verb** (PV) "put to sleep" means "make a sick or injured animal die without pain." Another PV with a similar meaning is "to put down."

℮ The race horse suffered a serious injury, and it had to be put down by a vet.

One difficult point about learning PVs is that one PV can have multiple meanings. For example, in the sentence, *"His wife is always putting him down in front of other people,"* "to put down" means to criticize a person in a way that makes that person feel stupid. Native speakers of English frequently use PVs, and they are an important part of speaking and writing natural English. In this chapter's essay, a single-word verb, **euthanize**, is also use to describe "ending the life of a living being in order to end suffering." The noun form of this verb is

euthanasia. The difference between the phrasal verbs "put down" and "put to sleep" and "euthanize" is that the single-word verb can also be used for humans. Euthanasia is legal in some countries, but in many other countries, including Japan and the UK, it is illegal. Some people think it is wrong that a lethal injection by a vet can give a suffering animal a peaceful death, but a doctor cannot do the same for a dying human who is suffering.

WFE: The prefix *eu~* means "good" and *thanatos* means "death," so euthanasia means a "good death." Some animals (e.g., cockroaches, guinea pigs) pretend to be dead in order to escape, a behavior that biologists call **thanatosis**. In the following sentences, words that contain the prefix *eu~* are in bold.

*& One reason that people worry about legalizing **euthanasia** is because of the history of the word. In Nazi Germany "euthanasia" was a **euphemistic** way to describe killing people, such as disabled people, under the Nazi's **eugenics**-based social policies.*

*& One reason opioid drugs such as morphine and fentanyl are very addictive is because they produce a sense of **euphoria**, a feeling of intense excitement and happiness.*

*& **Eukaryotes** are organisms whose cells have a nucleus enclosed within a nuclear membrane. The cells of eukaryotes are much more complicated than those of prokaryotes.*

SD 2E: Is "palliative" a euphemism for "dying"?

The word "palliative" is from the Latin *pallium*, meaning "a cloak." Palliative care can be thought of as care that cloaks (or covers) a person from the symptoms and stresses of serious illnesses. Palliative care takes a **holistic approach**. This means that it considers not only physical care, including the **alleviation** of pain, but also the psychological, social, and spiritual well-being of the patient and patient's family. Palliative care does not focus on curing a disease, but on improving a person's quality of life. As this exchange shows, "palliative" is sometimes used as a euphemism for "dying":

A: *I heard your father was in hospital. How is he?*

B: *Actually, **he's palliative**. We're trying to find a place for him in a hospice.*

However, it is a **misconception** that palliative care is only for people who are dying. Although palliative care does include **end-of-life care** (care for people who only have a short time left to live), it can be used at any time during treatment. Some people spend years receiving palliative care. On the other hand, **hospice care** is short-term (often less than 6 months) for people who are nearing the end of life. Another common misconception about palliative care is that it is only for people with cancer. In fact, it is for any **life-limiting illness** (i.e., an illness that cannot be cured and will significantly shorten a person's life), including CKD.

9) *Nephrolithiasis*, **more commonly known as kidney stones, are solid masses made of minerals and salts that form inside the kidneys**. Urine contains dissolved substances such as calcium, **oxalate** (also known as **oxalic acid**) and **uric acid**. If a person's urine becomes too concentrated, these substances can come out of solution to form solid crystals. This process is known as **precipitation**. (You may have seen white crystals at the edge of shallow rock pools at the beach. Sea salt precipitates when around 90% of the sea water has evaporated). The crystals can **aggregate** (stick together) to form stones that can range from the size of a grain of sand to bigger than a golf ball. Kidney stones most often form in the **renal pelvis**, an area at the center of the kidney. A stone that remains in the kidney may not cause symptoms, but a stone often becomes symptomatic if it enters one of the ureters, the narrow tubes (only 3-4 mm in diameter) connecting the kidneys and the bladder. A stone that has become lodged in a ureter is called a **ureteral stone**. Symptoms of kidney stones include intense pain, nausea, fever, abnormal urine color, and hematuria (blood in the urine). Here is some more information about kidney stones:

- **Composition**: A kidney stone can be classified according to its biochemical composition. Calcium-based stones are the commonest. Most calcium stones are a mixture of calcium and oxalate (**calcium oxalate** stones make up around 75% of all kidney stones). Another common type of stone is composed of uric acid. **Hyperuricosuria**, the presence of excessive amounts of uric acid in the urine, is a key risk factor for uric acid stones. Another type of kidney stone, called a **struvite stone**, containing calcium, magnesium, and ammonium phosphate, is associated with bacterial infection.

- **Lifetime risk**: Kidney stones are quite common. In Japan, around 1 in 7 men and 1 in 15 women will get kidney stones during their lifetime. The incidence of kidney stones has been increasing in Japan in recent decades. Women are less likely to develop kidney stones, which is partly due to estrogen inhibiting **bone resorption** (the process by which bone tissue is broken down, releasing calcium and other minerals into the blood). However, the incidence of kidney stones in women rises after **menopause**.

- **Risk factors**: Not drinking enough water or sweating a lot causes a low urine volume, making the urine more concentrated (such urine will have a dark yellow color). In concentrated urine there is less fluid to keep the minerals and salts dissolved. Kidney stones are more likely to occur in summer when people lose a lot of water through **perspiration** (sweating), causing the kidneys to make the urine more concentrated. Apart from a **negative fluid balance** (i.e., fluid output is greater than fluid intake), there are several other risk factors for kidney stones. One of these is diet; for example, consuming too much salt increases the amount of calcium in the urine, making it more likely that kidney stones will form. **Hypercalciuria**, or high calcium in the urine, is present in 80% of kidney stone patients. It seems **counterintuitive**, but a diet low in calcium increases the risk of kidney stones. This is because calcium binds to oxalate in the digestive tract, and is removed from the body in the feces. But if there is too little calcium in the diet, more oxalate is absorbed from the digestive tract into the bloodstream, leading to more oxalate being carried to the kidneys and ending up in the urine. Foods rich in calcium include dairy products, canned fish with bones, and almonds. Certain conditions also increase the risk of kidney stones. For example, people with **Crohn's disease** are susceptible to kidney stones due to poor intestinal absorption of fats.

- **Complications**: One complication is kidney infection. Untreated infections can cause permanent renal damage and can also lead to **sepsis**, an extreme immune response to an infection that can be fatal. Kidney stones can also cause a **urinary tract obstruction** at different sites in the urinary system. For example, a kidney stone can block a ureter (**ureteral obstruction**) or pass into the bladder but get stuck in the urethra. If the flow of urine is obstructed, urine will back up behind the point of blockage. For example, a blockage by a stone in the left ureter will act like a dam. Unable to flow beyond the stone, urine will flow the "wrong way" and return to the left kidney. The build-up of urine in the left kidney increases pressure in this kidney, causing it to swell, a condition called **hydronephrosis**. Severe hydronephrosis can lead to permanent kidney damage.

- **Treatment**: Small kidney stones may not need treatment because they just pass through the urinary tract and leave the body in the urine. To help kidney stones leave the body it is important to drink lots of fluid. If the kidney stone is large, or if it is blocking the urinary tract, active medical treatment is required. A common type of treatment is **extracorporeal shock wave lithotripsy**. This noninvasive procedure uses shock waves from outside the body to break a kidney stone into smaller pieces. These smaller pieces will later pass out of the body in the urine.

WFE: The word **nephrolithiasis** is composed of *nephron* (= "kidney") + *lith* (= "stone") + *~iasis* (= a suffix indicating a disease). Let's focus on the Greek word *lithos* meaning "stone."

The medical treatment **extracorporeal shock wave lithotripsy** literally means "crushing stones from outside of the body with shock waves" (*extra~* = "outside" + *corpus* = "body" + *lithotripsy* = "crush stones").

I am writing this sentence on a computer powered by **lithium-ion batteries**. Lithium is a soft, white, alkali metal. It is the lightest of all the solid elements in the **periodic table** and has the chemical symbol Li. The suffix *~ium* is often used to indicate a metallic element (e.g., calcium, barium). Most people know that lithium is used in rechargeable batteries for mobile phones, laptops, and electric cars, but fewer people will be aware that **lithium carbonate** (Li_2CO_3) is a drug used to treat **bipolar disorder**, a type of mental health condition. As an **antipsychotic** drug for bipolar disorder, lithium is very effective for some people, although how it works is not completely understood. Unlike other drugs in this book, lithium has not been patented by a pharmaceutical company. This is because lithium is a chemical element, and you cannot take out a patent on naturally-occurring products. Lithium can have severe side effects, including acute and chronic kidney damage. **Nephrogenic diabetes insipidus** is the most common of lithium's renal adverse effects.

A **monolith**, literally meaning "one stone," is a column or other structure made from a single large block of stone. There are monolithic human figures on Easter Island, and in England there are ancient stone monoliths at Stonehenge. **Monolithic** is often used to describe a society or company that is not diverse and is resistant to change.

*℮ People criticize Japan for being culturally and ethnically **monolithic**, but anyone who lives here will know that Japanese society is far from being homogenous.*

A word from archeology with a similar meaning to monolith is **megalith**, a very large stone used in ancient cultures. The prefix *mega~* means "large/great." Words and phrases with this prefix include **megaphone**, **mega rich**, **megapolis**, **megastore**, **megalomania**. The word **omega** (Ω) literally means "large "o." (While Ω is the final letter of Greek alphabet, **omicron**, the 15th letter of the Greek alphabet, means "little 'o'"; the Greek prefix *micro~* is used in many words including **microbe**, **microscope**, **microphone**, **microwave**, and **micromanage**). In maths, *mega~* is a prefix to represent 1 million (10^6). When you take a photo on your smartphone, how many **megabytes** (MB) is one photo?

While the atmosphere is the mixture of gases around the earth, the **lithosphere** is the rocky outer part of the Earth. Paleontologists, scientists who study fossils, can learn a lot about dinosaurs from their coprolites. A **coprolite** is fossilized animal poo. The suffix *~lite* is derived from *lithos* and *copro* means "animal feces." Rats are **coprophagic**, meaning they eat their own droppings, or the droppings of other rats (*phag* = "eat").

SD 2F: What is more painful than childbirth?

According to some women who have both given birth and experienced kidney stones, the pain from kidney stones is worse than the pain of childbirth. Pain is subjective and, unlike blood pressure or heart rate, cannot be directly observed by a person who is not experiencing it. For this reason, it would be difficult to objectively "prove" which is more painful. A more important question for this chapter is, Why are kidney stones so painful? A kidney stone that is in the kidney can cause intense pain, but pain from a kidney stone is often caused by the stone passing along the ureter to the bladder. Pain is also often caused by a kidney stone in the urinary tract blocking the flow of urine. This causes urine to back up into the kidney, leading to renal swelling. While the kidney itself does not have many pain receptors, the **renal capsule**, the connective tissue that surrounds each kidney, has many **stretch receptors**. When the capsule is stretched by the swollen kidney, messages are sent to the brain that is felt as pain. The pain caused by kidney stones is called **renal colic**. Rather than being a continuous, steady pain, renal colic pain is **intermittent**, meaning that it comes and goes in waves. Pain also results from muscle spasms of the ureter due to a blockage and from localized inflammation due to irritation from the kidney stone. The pain from a kidney stone often starts as a **flank pain** (i.e., pain in the upper abdomen or in the back and sides) and then **radiates** to the lower abdomen and **groin** (**radiating pain** is pain that starts one place and then spreads across a bigger area of the body).

Pain that arises from internal organs is known as **visceral pain**. The pain from kidney stones is **visceral pain**, as is the pain from a stomachache or from angina. The word "visceral" comes from "**viscera**," which are the internal organs of the body, especially those in the abdominal cavity. A key characteristic of visceral pain is that it is often **diffuse** (over a wide area) and is difficult to localize (i.e., the person with visceral pain will find it difficult to point to the location of the pain with a single finger). Another type of pain is **somatic pain**, from the Greek *soma*, meaning "body." This pain arises from bone, joints, muscles, skin, or connective tissue. Somatic pain is usually well localized and a person can often point to the location of the pain from, for example, a sprained ankle, muscle tear, or bone fracture.

One way that doctors diagnose **acute appendicitis** (inflammation of the appendix) is by how the location and nature of the pain changes. An early sign of appendicitis is pain around the area of the belly button (called **periumbilical pain**), or pain in the upper part of the abdomen (**epigastric pain**). This abdominal pain is visceral pain that is relatively diffuse. However, after around 24 hours, the pain sometimes shifts to the lower right side of the abdomen (**right lower-quadrant pain**), where the appendix is located. The pain on the right side of the abdomen is a well-localized, sharp pain that is easier for the patient to pinpoint. This sharp pain, which is somatic pain, is caused by the appendix swelling and irritating the peritoneum, the membrane lining the abdominal cavity. If you get severe abdominal pain, especially pain that shifts as described above, get medical attention. An infected appendix can rupture, often within 48 to 72 hours after the onset of symptoms. Infection from a **ruptured appendix** can spread to the peritoneum, causing **peritonitis**, a life-threatening condition.

10) *Ureters* **are the two tubes that transport urine from the kidney to the bladder.** The *urethra* carries urine from the bladder out of the body. One way to remember the difference between *ureter* and *urethra* is to count the number of *e's*: there are *two ureters* and two "*e's*," but only *one urethra* and only one "*e*." A **urinary tract infection** (UTI) is an infection in any part of the urinary system. As you know, the suffix *~itis* means "inflammation," which is the immune system's response to infection. So, **urethritis** is inflammation of the urethra, and **cystitis** is inflammation of the bladder, the muscular sac that stores urine. Cystitis is the most common form of UTI. Much less common, but the most serious UTI is **pyelonephritis**, which is a bacterial infection of one or both kidneys.

WFE: The WFE *ur* means "urine." **Uremia** literally means "urine in the blood". It is caused by substances, particularly urea, that are normally excreted in the urine accumulating in the blood. Many of the symptoms of kidney failure are due to uremia, including cognitive symptoms such as disorientation and confusion. **Nocturia** is excessive urination at night (*nocti* = "night"). It is often an early symptom of kidney failure and is due an impaired ability to concentrate urine. **Oliguria** is when a person only produces only a small amount of urine (less than 400 mL of urine a day). It can be sign that the kidneys are not working properly (*oligos* = "few"). In cystitis, "cyst" is from the Greek *kystis* meaning "sac." A **cystoscopy** is a procedure to look inside the bladder (*~scope* means "to look at").

The **gallbladder** is a small pear-shaped sac that sits under the liver. It is an **accessory organ** of the digestive system that stores bile, a fluid made by the liver that aids fat digestion. The medical term for inflammation of the gallbladder is **cholecystitis**. This word is made up of *chole*, the Greek for "bile," *cyst* (= "sac"), and the suffix *~itis* ("inflammation"). So, it literally means "inflammation of the sac that holds bile." One substance in bile is **bilirubin**, a reddish substance made from the breakdown of hemoglobin in old RBCs (*bili~* = "bile" + *rub* = "red" + *~in* = a suffix indicating chemical substances). Bacteria in the colon act on bilirubin and change it to a colorless pigment called **urobilinogen**. Some of this urobilinogen is absorbed into systemic circulation and is excreted in the urine. On exposure to air, urobilinogen is oxidized into a yellow pigment called **urobilin**. So, it is urobilin, also called **urochrome**, (*uro~* = "urine" + *chrome* = "color"), that makes urine yellow. In short, urine's yellow color (and the brown color of feces) results from the degradation of RBCs.

SD 2G: Why is cystitis more common in women?

Cystitis, inflammation of the urinary bladder is the most common type of UTI. It is usually caused when bacteria that live in the large intestine somehow enter the urethra, the tube that connects the bladder to the outside. Upon reaching the bladder, these bacteria grow quickly. Around 50 per cent of women will have cystitis at some time in their life. Men do get cystitis, but women are around ten times more likely to get it than men. The main reason that women are more prone to getting cystitis is related to anatomical differences. The urethra in women is shorter than in men. The female urethra is about 4 cm in length, while in men it is about 20 cm long. This means that in women bacteria have a much shorter distance to travel from the opening of the urethra to the bladder. In addition to having a shorter ureter, the urethra, anus, and vagina are very close together, facilitating the spread of bacteria from one opening to another. Most cases of cystitis are caused by *Escherichia coli* (E. coli), a type of bacteria that normally live in the colon. In the colon, E. coli are usually harmless, but if these bacteria enter the urinary tract, they can become pathogenic and cause infections.

Cystitis in men is more likely to be a symptom of an underlying problem such as kidney stones, BHP, or a narrowing of the urethra (**urethral stricture**). Many men get their first UTI in hospital. Most hospital-acquired UTIs are associated with a **urinary catheter**, a tube inserted through the urethra into the bladder, because it can introduce bacteria into a man's bladder. A urinary catheter is used after surgery and at other times when it is difficult for a person to urinate naturally. Symptoms of cystitis include a burning sensation when urinating (pain or discomfort when urinating is called **dysuria**), increased urge to urinate, and passing urine that is cloudy or smelly. Mild cystitis caused by a bacterial infection often clears up on its own, but it may require treatment with a course of antibiotics. If left untreated, there is a risk that infection from the bladder can move up the ureters to the kidney, causing a kidney infection.

SD 2H: What is one cause of urinary tract obstruction that is unique to men?

The urethra is much longer in males because it extends through the length of the penis. Talking of penises, I neglected to mention in the essay that in men the urethra is part of both the urinary system and of the **reproductive system**. While in women the urinary and reproductive systems are separate, in men the urethra is the channel used to carry both urine and sperm, contained in a fluid called semen. (Although the urethra is the common channel for both urine and semen, it is impossible for a man to ejaculate and urinate simultaneously.) **Urologists** not only deal with urinary problems in both men and women, but also problems of the male reproductive system, including **erectile dysfunction** and male **infertility**.

Another condition that urologists frequently treat is **BPH**, an abbreviation of **benign prostatic hyperplasia**. Simply put, BPH is an enlarged prostate. Most common in men over 50, BPH is thought to be caused by changes in male sex hormones associated with aging. About the size of a walnut, the **prostate gland** is located just below the bladder (pro~ = "in front" + stat = "stand", so, "standing in front [of the bladder]"). The main function of the prostate is to produce **seminal fluid**, the fluid that nourishes and transports sperm. In BPH, the "H" means "hyperplasia," an increase in the number of cells. Hyperplasia increases the size of the prostate gland, sometimes by five times the original size. This puts pressure on the bladder and urethra—the urethra runs through the center of the prostate—and blocks the flow of urine from the bladder. This leads to **urine retention** (i.e., urine remaining in the bladder rather than being excreted). The urine left in the bladder becomes **stagnant**, providing an environment for bacteria to **proliferate**, which is why BPH is a common cause of cystitis in men.

The "B" in BPH stands for "benign." If a growth or tumor is benign, it is not cancerous, meaning it does not invade nearby tissues or **metastasize** (spread) to other parts of the body. The prefix ben~ means "good" (e.g., benefit), while the prefix mal~ means "bad" (a **malignant tumor** is one that is cancerous). In BPH, there is an increase in the number of cells (**hyperplasia**), but microscopically the cells look normal. Cancer cells do not look normal under a microscope, and they behave differently from normal cells in various ways. Prostate cancer is the second leading cause of cancer death in men in the UK, and in Japan it is the leading cause of cancer death in males.

11) *Vet* **is an abbreviation for "veterinarian," a person qualified to give medical care to sick animals**. Vet is also an abbreviation for a "veteran," someone who served in the armed forces (this abbreviation is used more often in American English than British English). For example, an American who fought in the Vietnam War is called "Vietnam vet." A veteran also describes a person who has been in a particular job for a long time (e.g., *a veteran politician*).

WFE: The root of **veterinarian** and **veteran** is the Latin *vetus*, meaning "old/advanced in years." What is the connection between "old" and a "doctor of animals"? Well, the Latin word *veterinum* was used to describe animals, usually horses or cows, that pulled a cart or a plough. Young animals were not big enough to pull a heavy cart or plough; only older and more experienced animals could do this hard work. From *veterinum* came the word *veterinarius* to describe a person who provided health care to these older, hard-working animals. Over time the word's meaning broadened to mean a doctor for all animals. The word "veterinarian" (from the Latin *veterinarius*) entered English in the 16th century. There is also a verb "to vet," meaning "to carefully check or examine," which is derived from veterinarian. It originated with the action of carefully inspecting a horse before a race, and its meaning expanded to include carefully checking people, documents, and other things.

*& I am a British citizen, but if I wanted to become a naturalized Japanese citizen, the Legal Affairs Bureau would **vet** my application documents carefully.*

2-3 Dozen in Detail (D)　（12 の話題を詳しく）

1) Antidiabetic and antihypertensive pharmacotherapy: Diabetes and hypertension are major risk factors for CKD. There is a specific name for the kidney damage causes by diabetes: **diabetic nephropathy**, also known as **diabetic kidney disease**. High blood glucose (**hyperglycemia**), a characteristic of diabetes, damages the endothelium of blood vessels, promoting **atherosclerosis** (hardening of the arteries). In addition, glucose in the blood causes changes to the renal blood vessels, including thickening of capillaries in the kidney glomeruli. Such changes allow albumin to leak into the nephron tubule from where it is excreted. That is why people with diabetes are tested regularly for **proteinuria**. Excreting urine that is **foamy** could be a sign of proteinuria.

Hypertension is one of the causes of CKD, but CKD also **exacerbates** hypertension, partly because the extra fluid that accumulates because of renal dysfunction increases the blood volume. There are many **antihypertensive drugs** (medications for high blood pressure). **ACE inhibitors (angiotensin converting enzyme inhibitors)** and **ARBs (angiotensin receptor blockers)**, are **first-line treatments** for hypertension in people with CKD. Both these drugs act on the **renin-angiotensin-aldosterone system (RAAS)**. ACE inhibitors block angiotensin-converting enzyme (ACE), thus inhibiting the conversion of angiotensin I to angiotensin II. **Angiotensin II** is a peptide hormone that raises blood pressure in several ways, including by causing vasoconstriction. ARBs block receptors to which angiotensin II binds (specifically ARBs bind to AT1 receptors, which are highly concentrated on cells in the heart, blood vessels and kidneys). Preventing the formation of angiotensin II (ACE inhibitors), or blocking the action of angiotensin II (ARBs), helps to lower blood pressure.

Diuretics are another class of drugs used in CKD. Sodium (Na) is freely filtered in the glomerulus, but only a tiny fraction of the filtered sodium is excreted in the urine. This is because most (up to 99%) of sodium is reabsorbed from the nephron tubule into the peritubular capillaries, from where it is returned to the systemic circulation. Because water follows sodium passively by osmosis, the reabsorption of sodium is accompanied by water (this is called "**obligatory water reabsorption**," because water is "obliged" to follow the sodium). Most diuretics work by inhibiting the reabsorption of sodium. Water follows sodium, so if more sodium remains in the tubule, more water will also remain in the tubule, leading to **diuresis** (increased urination). Diuresis reduces the volume a blood in the circulatory system, lowering blood pressure and relieving edema. Different classes of diuretics exert their effects at different locations along the nephron. For example, **loop diuretics** inhibit sodium (and chloride) reabsorption in the loop of Henle (specifically, in the **thick ascending limb** of the loop of Henle). In addition to loop diuretics, other classes of diuretics include **thiazides** and **potassium-sparing diuretics**.

2) Blood urea nitrogen (BUN) and **creatinine:** Creatine phosphate is a storage form of energy in muscle tissue. When creatine phosphate is broken down, creatinine is produced. In other words, creatinine is a **byproduct** of energy metabolism in muscles. The creatinine produced by the muscles is freely filtered at the glomerulus, so almost all of it enters the nephron tubule. Moreover, almost none of it is reabsorbed back into the bloodstream. Because the kidneys are wholly responsible for getting rid of creatinine, if the GFR—the volume of blood that is filtered by the glomeruli per unit of time—declines, the amount of creatinine in the urine will also decline, and the level of creatinine in the blood will rise. For this reason, measuring blood creatinine levels can be a good indicator of renal function. Simply put, when the kidneys are not working well, more creatinine remains in the blood. However, the level of plasma creatinine alone does not give an accurate measure of GFR because creatinine is influenced by muscle mass; for example, a bodybuilder with healthy kidneys will have a higher blood creatinine than an elderly woman with **sarcopenia** (age-related muscle loss). For this reason, a person's age, sex, weight, and ethnicity are taken into account using certain mathematical calculations. The higher the plasma creatinine level, the lower the amount of creatinine filtered by the glomeruli and excreted in the urine. A blood test of creatinine only gives an estimate of the GFR, which is why it is called an **estimated GFR (eGFR)**.

　Another waste product in the blood is **urea**. Because it is the job of the kidneys to excrete urea, if there is kidney dysfunction, plasma urea will increase. Therefore, measuring plasma urea can give an indication of kidney failure. One kind of blood test called **BUN (blood urea nitrogen)** measures the nitrogen in the urea molecule (urea consists of carbon, nitrogen, and oxygen). A high BUN may indicate a decline in kidney function. I say "may" because a high BUN can be due to other reasons. It is the liver that produces urea. Excess amino acids are **catabolized**, or broken down, by the liver into energy and ammonia; the ammonia is then converted into urea, a compound that is less toxic than ammonia. Therefore, BUN is also a measure of liver function. An increased BUN could reflect increased production of urea in the liver for some reason (e.g., dehydration, or eating a high protein diet). Even bleeding in the stomach could also cause BUN to rise (blood is high in protein). Finally, a word about the pronunciation of BUN: pronounce each letter ("B.U.N"); don't say "bun", which is a small, round cake. "BUN" is an **initialism**, not an **acronym**.

SD 2I: Why do some people prefer to drink zero-purine beer?

Several makes of Japanese beer have "プリン体ゼロ" ["zero purines"] printed on the can. What are **purines**, and why would someone want to drink beer that contains no purines? Purines are one of two nitrogen-containing organic compounds (the other being pyrimidines) that are the building blocks DNA and RNA. There are five types of nitrogenous bases in **nucleic acids** (i.e., DNA and RNA), and two of these, **adenine** and **guanine**, are purines. Most of the purines in the body come from the breakdown of nucleic acids as old cells are degraded. Purines that originate from inside the body are called **endogenous purines**. Other purines, called **exogenous purines**, enter the body in the food and drink we ingest. Between 70% to 80% of the purines in the body are endogenous. Both endogenous and exogenous purines are mainly metabolized by the liver. In humans, the end-product of this purine metabolism is **uric acid**. About 60% of uric acid is excreted by the kidneys, and the rest is excreted in the feces. The metabolic pathway by which purines are metabolized is shown below ("XO" stands for **xanthine oxidase**, an enzyme that is essential in the production of uric acid. XO catalyzes the oxidation of hypoxanthine to xanthine, and of xanthine to uric acid):

$$\text{purines} \xrightarrow{} \text{hypoxanthine} \xrightarrow{XO} \text{xanthine} \xrightarrow{XO} \text{uric acid}$$

An elevated uric acid level in the blood is called **hyperuricemia**. In Japan, hyperuricemia is defined as a blood uric acid level of over 7mg/dl (milligrams per deciliter). Hyperuricemia is caused by an overproduction of uric acid, a decreased uric acid excretion, or a combination of both. The most obvious cause of overproduction is a purine-rich diet, but there are many rarer causes related to errors of purine metabolism and increased cell breakdown. Decreased uric acid excretion is sometimes associated with kidney disease. Many people with hyperuricemia will be asymptomatic, but it can lead to several diseases, including uric acid kidney stones and **gout**, a type of **inflammatory arthritis**.

Gout occurs when uric acid crystals **precipitate** out of the blood and are deposited in and around joints. These tiny, needle-like crystals trigger a response by the immune system, resulting in inflammation of the affected area. Joints become red, swollen, hot, and often **excruciatingly** painful. The Japanese name for gout, *tsufu* (痛風) is composed of characters for "pain" and "wind," expressing how only the pressure of wind on a joint inflamed by gout can cause pain.

Beer has long been associated as gout-causing because it is high in purines. This explains the popularity of beer that is free of purines. For people who have hyperuricemia, drinking such beer may help prevent them getting gout, and for people who have had a gout attack in the past, choosing a purine-free beer may help prevent another gout attack. The incidence and prevalence of gout is increasing in many countries, including Japan, where it is estimated that over 1 million people have gout and 10 million have hyperuricemia. It would, therefore, be useful to know a bit more about this condition:

- In the USA, gout affects about 4% of the adult population. Some studies show that gout is 10 times more common in men than in women—and the incidence in men increases over

30 years of age. It is thought that women are less **susceptible** to getting gout because **estrogen** promotes renal clearance of uric acid, and is thus protective against hyperuricemia. In **postmenopausal** women, the incidence of gout increases and the "gout gap" between the sexes begins to close.

- Gout can affect any joint, including the ankle, knees, elbows, and fingers, but it most often affects the big toe. The big toe is particularly **prone** to gout because it is cooler than other body areas (uric acid forms crystals more readily at lower temperatures—the solubility of solutes falls with lower temperatures).

- A gout attack will usually be most painful in the first 12-24 hours after onset. Without treatment, gout symptoms usually get better after one or two weeks. However, frequent attacks over several years can cause permanent damage to joints, leading to **deformity**. A complication of chronic gout is **tophi**, lumps under the skin due to accumulation of uric acid crystals. Tophi often develop at the end of fingers and on the outer ear.

- The prevalence of gout is higher in people with CKD than in people without kidney disease. In CKD, gout occurs as a result of under excretion of uric acid due to a decrease in glomerular filtration. This causes blood to become saturated with uric acid. Gout is not only a consequence of kidney disease, there is some evidence that hyperuricemia contributes to the onset and progression of CKD. Experiments on rat kidneys show hyperuricemia causes a decline in kidney function by promoting **glomerulosclerosis** (scarring and hardening of the glomeruli) and damaging renal blood vessels.

- Certain medications, for example diuretics and aspirin, can **precipitate** gout.

- For centuries, gout has been seen as a disease of overweight men who **overindulge** in luxury foods such as red meat and caviar and who drink too much alcohol. In the 19th century, gout was even considered a status symbol because of its associations with wealth. It was called the "disease of kings." However, this **stereotype** of gout is no longer accurate (and perhaps it never was). It is true that being overweight does increase the risk of gout, as does over-consumption of foods and drinks that are high in purines. Such foods include red meat, offal, seafood, sugar-sweetened soft drinks, and alcoholic beverages. Regarding alcohol, beer contains more purines than some other types of alcohol (e.g., wine) because of the brewer's yeast used in its fermentation. However, research in recent years suggests that **genetic factors** probably have a much greater influence on hyperuricemia than diet.

- It is likely that for people who are **genetically predisposed** to gout, eating a lot of high-purine foods could trigger or **aggravate** a gout attack. So, reducing the intake of these foods is likely to contribute to lowering blood uric acid levels. However, for many people with gout, diet, and other lifestyle changes (e.g., staying hydrated, losing excess weight) will not be sufficient to prevent gout attacks. Most people will also need to take a medication to lower uric acid levels. The most widely used medication to lower blood uric acid is called **allopurinol**, which is a **xanthine oxidase inhibitor**. Remember this from above:

$$\text{purines} \xrightarrow{\text{XO}} \text{hypoxanthine} \xrightarrow{\text{XO}} \text{xanthine} \rightarrow \text{uric acid}$$

Allopurinol inhibits **xanthine oxidase** (XO), the enzyme that converts hypoxanthine to xanthine and xanthine to uric acid. In this way, allopurinol reduces the amount of uric acid produced by the body. Allopurinol is used to prevent gout attacks (it is **prophylactic therapy**), but it cannot treat an attack that has already occurred. Allopurinol is a long-term treatment, and some people take it for life to manage uric acid levels. A common side effect of allopurinol is a surprising one: in the first few weeks of treatment, this drug sometimes actually causes a gout attack. This is an example of a **paradoxical reaction**, when a drug has the opposite reaction to what would be expected.

3) *Chronic heart failure* (CHF) is a progressive condition in which the heart is unable to pump enough blood to meet the body's needs. Each organ in the body is part of a system. For example, the brain is the main organ of the nervous system, the stomach is part of the digestive system, and the prostate gland is part of the male reproductive system. What about the heart and the kidneys? The heart is the key organ of the **circulatory system** (in fact, if you think about it, the heart is the only organ of the circulatory system), and the kidney is the center of the **urinary system**. The eleven organ systems of the body do not work in isolation, but are interconnected and dependent upon one another. This is especially true for the heart and kidney. My father had CHF, which is an important risk factor for both AKI and CKD. In CHF, the heart is no longer able to pump blood around the body efficiently. Low cardiac output leads to **renal ischemia**. In addition, fluid accumulation that occurs in CHF can cause **renal congestion** (the buildup of blood in the kidneys). Also, when the heart is not pumping strongly, blood pressure will fall, and this fall will be sensed by cells in the kidney, triggering the release of **renin** from **juxtaglomerular cells**. The release of renin activates the RAAS, resulting in systemic vasoconstriction and increased blood volume (due to increased sodium and water reabsorption in the kidney), both of which act to raise blood pressure. Thus, the heart will need to work harder, which over time will further weaker it. In this way, CHF can **exacerbate** CKD, and CKD can worsen CHF. The term **cardiorenal syndrome** describes the complex ways in which cardiac dysfunction can induce renal dysfunction, and vice versa.

4) Comparison of the composition of blood, filtrate, and urine: Table 2.4 shows the amounts of certain substances in the blood plasma, glomerular filtrate (filtrate is fluid that has passed through a filter, in this case the glomeruli), and urine. For now, don't worry about the meaning of "mEq/day" and other units of measurements; just look at the change in the amount of each substance. We see that almost all the water is reabsorbed, and that plasma protein and RBCs (red blood cells) do not pass through the glomerulus. Glucose, a substance needed by the body for energy, is readily filtered by the glomerulus, but all of it is reabsorbed. In a healthy person no glucose appears in the urine. You can also see that the electrolytes such as sodium (Na+), potassium (K+), and calcium (Ca+), are mostly reabsorbed. Very little bicarbonate (HCO3-) is excreted because the kidneys maintain the acid-base balance of the blood by reabsorbing HCO3-back into the blood.

Urea is a waste product of protein metabolism that is toxic if it is allowed to build up, so why does the kidney reabsorb some urea and not excrete all of it? The full explanation is beyond the scope of this book, but the reabsorption of urea is needed to produce concentrated urine (it is related to **osmotic gradients**). When the kidneys are damaged, the values shown in Table 2.4 will change. For example, RBCs, protein, and glucose, may appear in the urine.

Table 2.4

Comparison of Substances in Blood Plasma, Glomerular Filtrate, and Urine

（血しょう、原尿と尿に入っている成分の比較）

Substance (成分)	Blood Plasma (血しょう中)	Glomerular Filtrate (原尿中)	Urine (尿中)	Filtered Amount that is Reabsorbed (%) (再吸収した濾過量（糸球体で濾過された量の何%が血液に再吸収されたか）)
Water (L/day)	180	180	1.5	99.2
RBCs	Yes	No	No	
Protein (g/dl)	7	No	No	
Glucose (mmol/day)	800	800	0	100.0
Urea (g/day)	56	56	28	50.0
Na+ (mEq/day)	25,200	25,200	150	99.4
K+ (mEq/day)	720	720	100	86.1
HCO3- (mEq/day)	4320	4320	2	99.9
Ca+ (mEq/day)	540	540	10	98.2

Note. Modified from Koeppen, B.M, & Stanton, B. A. (2019). *Renal Physiology* (6th ed.). Elsevier.

5) CKD can be divided into 5 stages according to the degree of kidney damage, as shown in Table 2.5. Stage 1 indicates mild kidney damage and stage 5 is the most severe kidney damage. These stages are based on estimated **glomerular filtration rate** (eGFR), a measure of kidney function. The normal range for eGFR is 100-140 ml/min. An eGFR of 60 means that around 60% kidney function remains. As a person's kidney disease progresses (gets worse), eGFR declines. Symptoms of CKD often do not appear until stage 3b. Some people remain asymptomatic until stage 4 (severe loss of kidney function). CKD is often silent, despite significant kidney disease, because the kidney has much **redundancy**. Even if many nephrons have been damaged, the undamaged ones are able to take over and maintain normal renal function. However, redundancy has its limits. Once the kidneys are too damaged, not enough healthy nephrons will remain to take over and symptoms will emerge.

Table 2.5

Stages of Chronic Kidney Disease　（慢性腎臓病のステージ）

Stage	Degree of kidney function　（腎臓の働きの程度）	eGFR (ml/min)
1	Kidney damage present*, but normal function. Usually "silent" (asymptomatic)	≥90
2	Kidney damage. Mild loss of function.	60-89
3a	Mild to moderate function loss	45-59
3b	Moderate to severe function loss	30-44
4	Severe function loss	15-29
5	Kidney failure (End-stage renal disease)	< 15

*As indicated by high levels of protein in the urine (proteinuria).

6) CKD-MBD (chronic kidney disease-mineral and bone disorder) results from changes in the blood level of certain minerals and hormones. Electrolytes are minerals in the blood and other body fluids that carry a positive or negative electric charge. The main electrolytes in the body are sodium, calcium, potassium, chloride, phosphate, and magnesium. Let's look at two of these in relation to CKD. **Phosphate** (P) and **calcium** (Ca) are absorbed in the small intestine and stored in the bones. They have many important functions, including building strong bones and teeth. The bones store 99% and 80% of the body's whole store of calcium and phosphate, respectively. Blood calcium levels are regulated by **parathyroid hormone (PTH)** secreted from **parathyroid glands** located in the neck, near the **thyroid gland** (*para~* = "next to"). Low blood calcium levels stimulate the release of PTH, and the release of PTH leads to an increase in plasma calcium in the following ways:

- PTH promotes the breakdown of bone tissue and the release of calcium and phosphate from bone, a process called **bone resorption**.

- PTH decreases the reabsorption of phosphate in the nephron, thereby increasing the excretion of phosphate in the urine. Increased phosphate excretion leads to decreased blood phosphate and higher blood calcium levels.

- PTH acts on the kidneys causing them to release more **calcitriol** (active vitamin D) into the blood. Calcitriol acts on cells in the intestine, increasing the amount of calcium absorbed from the gut into the bloodstream.

People with CKD can suffer from bone problems. One reason this happens is because a decline in GFR means less phosphate is excreted, causing it to accumulate in the blood. A high blood phosphate level is known as **hyperphosphatemia**. Phosphate binds to calcium forming an insoluble salt, which reduces the amount of free calcium in the blood. This is why a rise in blood phosphate levels causes a decrease in blood calcium. Low calcium partly explains the **muscle cramps** and **spasms** experienced by some people with CKD (calcium is needed for the contraction of skeletal muscle).

As explained above, low blood calcium is detected by the parathyroid gland, which will secrete more PTH. Increased PTH secretion pulls more calcium from the bones so as to increase the calcium available in the bloodstream. Calcium is vital for the contraction of the heart and has other critical functions, so maintaining **homeostasis** of blood calcium is the priority for the body—even if this means sacrificing bone health. A loss of calcium from the bones can cause various **bone disorders**. Calcium and phosphate in the blood can also form deposits in the wall of blood vessels (**vascular calcification**), leading to **atherosclerosis**, and making people with CKD prone to cardiovascular complications such as stroke and heart attack. The risk of CKD-MBD can be reduced by a diet that is low in phosphate; with medications such as **phosphate binders**, which react with phosphate and reduce its absorption from the gastrointestinal tract; and with **vitamin D analogues** to supplement the vitamin D deficiency caused by CKD (vitamin D increases calcium absorption from the small intestine).

7) Disturbances of acid-base balance and electrolyte disorders: The abbreviation *pH* stands for "potential of hydrogen" (the "p" comes from the German *potenz*). For the body to function normally, blood pH needs to be maintained within a narrow range of 7.35 to 7.45. If the pH moves even slightly outside this range, it can have serious consequences. The problem for the body is that normal metabolic activities result in the continuous production of carbon dioxide (CO_2) and **hydrogen ions** (H+), both of which tend to reduce the pH (i.e., make the blood more acid). **Acid-base homeostasis** is a complex process involving the lungs, kidneys, and brain, as well as chemical buffers in the blood and red blood cells. By changing the speed and depth breathing, the lungs can make quick (within minutes or hours) adjustments to blood pH. The kidneys, however, make these adjustments more slowly (over days).

The kidneys adjust acid-base in two main ways. The first way is by secreting hydrogen ions from the blood into the nephron tubule, from where they are excreted in the urine. The second way is by the reabsorption of bicarbonate, which is alkaline, from the peritubular capillaries into the nephron tubule. Not only do nephrons reabsorb bicarbonate, certain nephron cells also produce it. Therefore, a decline in kidney function can lead to an increase in blood acidity, a condition called **metabolic acidosis**. Metabolic acidosis affects approximately 15%-19% of people with CKD. There are several consequences of metabolic acidosis, including a loss of minerals from bones (**bone demineralization**), a decline in insulin sensitivity (insulin resistance), and a worsening of CKD (it's a **vicious cycle**: a buildup of acid leads to a decline in kidney function, and as renal function declines, acid builds up).

8) *Drug excretion* is a process by which drugs are removed from the body. Pharmacy and medical students study **pharmacokinetics**, which, put simply, is what the body does to a drug. As expressed by the acronym **ADME**, the drug is **a**bsorbed by the body, it is then **d**istributed, metabolized, and excreted (or eliminated) by the body. The end of a drug's journey through the body is usually excretion, which is the process of removing a drug and its **metabolites** from the body. There are various **routes of excretion** for drugs (e.g., bile, breast milk, sweat, and tears), but the most important route is in the urine. There are several factors that affect the excretion of drugs in the urine by the kidney. For example, the size of the drug molecule is important: small drugs can readily pass through the glomerulus into the nephron tubule, but large-molecule drugs (e.g., heparin), and drugs that bind to albumin and other plasma proteins (**bound drugs**) are poorly filtered by the glomeruli (a drug bound to a protein has a large **molecular mass**, so it is unable to pass through cell membranes). Many drugs are **lipophilic** (lipid soluble), but are metabolized in the liver to make them more **hydrophilic** (water soluble). A drug metabolite that is more hydrophilic is more easily be excreted by the kidneys.

Some drugs, however, undergo minimal or no metabolization by the liver. For example, most penicillin is excreted in the urine unchanged. In the early 1940s when penicillin could only be made in small amounts, the drug was recycled from patients' urine and reused. In addition to drugs entering the nephron tubule by glomerular filtration, another way for drugs to enter is by **tubular secretion**. This is when drugs are transported from the **peritubular capillaries** into the proximal nephron tubule. Tubule secretion involves **active transport**, that is, the movement of dissolved drug molecules against a **concentration gradient**—from an area of low concentration to an area of high concentration—using energy. (In **simple diffusion**, particles move down a concentration gradient, from an area of higher concentration to an area of lower concentration, without requiring energy.) Tubular secretion involves two carrier systems in the cells of the proximal nephron. One of these carriers transports basic substances (e.g., dopamine, histamine), and the other carrier transports acidic substances (e.g., penicillin). Because penicillin readily enters the nephron by tubular secretion and is then excreted, it does not stay in the body for very long. In order to prolong the action of penicillin in the body, a medication called **probenecid** is sometimes used in combination with penicillin. Probenecid inhibits tubular secretion, thereby slowing the elimination of penicillin from the body.

Apart from the size of the drug molecule and whether the drug is bound to plasma proteins, other factors can affect renal drug excretion, including the amount of renal blood flow and the **pH of urine**. Changing the pH of the urine can be used to treat drug overdose. For example, if a man takes an aspirin overdose, he may be given **sodium bicarbonate**, which makes his urine more alkaline. In alkaline urine, an acid drug such as aspirin becomes **ionized**. When a substance is in its ionized form it is has a low solubility in lipids, but is more soluble in water. With a low lipid solubility, the ionized aspirin cannot readily diffuse across the plasma membranes of nephron cells, which contain a lot of lipids (around 50 % of the plasma membrane is composed of lipids). Therefore, more of the aspirin remains in the nephron tubule, from where it is excreted in the urine. This treatment, an example of **forced diuresis**, minimizes the aspirin that is reabsorbed from the nephron back into the bloodstream, resulting in a more rapid elimination of aspirin from the body.

   Kidney disease can affect the pharmacokinetics of drugs in various ways. For example, a decline in the GFR will reduce how much drug is excreted, so a drug will stay in the body for longer. Also, a decline in **albumin** in the blood, due to it being excreted in the urine, results in a greater amount of **free drug** in the bloodstream. It is only such free drug (i.e., drug not bound to albumin) that is able to diffuse through cell membranes and have an effect. Because impaired kidney function can have a big effect on pharmacokinetics, the drug dosage for people with kidney disease will often need to be adjusted, usually reduced. Finally, aging alone, without kidney disease, is accompanied by a decline in kidney function. This puts older people at greater risk of a drug accumulating in the body and causing adverse effects, which is one reason older people may require smaller doses of medicines.

9) Extracellular fluid: The body of an adult man is 60% water, while that of an adult woman is 55% water. However, this percentage varies depending on the proportion of muscle to fat: fat contains around 10% water, while muscle is approximately 75% water. Because they generally have less muscle, the elderly, women, and overweight people have lower total body water. Fluid in the body can be divided into fluid inside the cells and fluid outside of the cells.
   •   Fluid inside the cells is called **intracellular fluid (ICF)**. ICF makes up 66% of all the fluid in the body.
   •   Fluid outside the cells is called **extracellular fluid (ECF)**. The ECF comprises 33% of the total body fluid. ECF is divided into **plasma**, the fluid part of the blood, and **interstitial fluid (IF)**, the liquid that is found between the cells of the body. Plasma, which can also be considered **intravascular fluid** because it is inside blood vessels, makes up around 25% of ECF, while IF comprises 75% of the ECF.

   In the capillaries, water, ions, nutrient molecules, and waste molecules are exchanged through capillary pores between the plasma and IF. In order to ensure that cells function normally, the ECF must be at the correct pH and have the correct balance of electrolytes and water. By filtering the plasma and excreting waste products, excess water and electrolytes, the kidneys help to regulate the composition of the plasma. And because plasma is in exchange with the IF, the kidneys also regulate the IF.

   A common symptom of kidney failure is **edema**, which occurs when fluid accumulates in the IF. One factor that causes fluid to move from blood vessels into the IF is a decrease in the amount of protein in the blood, particularly **albumin**, the most abundant plasma protein. To see how a loss of albumin from the body, as can occur in kidney disease, can cause edema, it is important to understand that because the IF is derived from plasma, its solute content is very similar to plasma. The main difference between plasma and IF is that plasma contains more proteins than IF. Small molecules easily pass through the walls of capillaries, but protein molecules, which are much bigger, cannot pass through.

The presence of more protein in the plasma exerts a pressure, called **oncotic pressure**, that keeps fluid in the blood vessels. About 70% of the oncotic pressure is generated by albumin. Healthy kidneys retain (i.e., do not excrete) what is valuable to the body, including albumin. But when the capillaries in the glomeruli are damaged, they become more permeable, allowing albumin and other proteins to be filtered into the nephron tubules and then excreted in the urine. Protein in the urine is called **proteinuria** (or **albuminuria**). As protein is lost from the body, the plasma protein declines, leading to **hypoproteinemia** (or **hypoalbuminemia**), an abnormally low level of blood proteins. This hypoproteinemia will cause a fall in oncotic pressure (the pressure "pulling" fluid into the capillaries). With oncotic pressure reduced, **hydrostatic pressure** (i.e., the force of the blood pressure "pushing" fluid out of the capillaries), will become relatively stronger. As a result, fluid will leak out of the capillaries into the interstitial space, resulting in edema.

10) Hormones are intimately involved in renal function: Several hormones are involved in regulating kidney function. **Angiotensin II** and **aldosterone** are the two key hormones in the **renin-angiotensin-aldosterone system** (RAAS). A drop in blood pressure stimulates the release of angiotensin II, and this hormone induces **vasoconstriction**, which helps to maintain an adequate blood pressure. Aldosterone, a steroid hormone, promotes sodium reabsorption and, because water follows sodium, this results in increased water retention. Another important role of aldosterone is regulating potassium (aldosterone promotes K+ excretion). Aldosterone is released from the **adrenal cortex**, the outer part of the **adrenal gland**.

The adrenal gland is part of the **endocrine system**, but it is not only endocrine glands that release hormones. Several organs, whose main job is not hormone secretion, have a secondary endocrine function. Examples of such **secondary endocrine organs** are the stomach, kidney, and heart. The heart's main job is to pump blood around the body, but the atria also secrete **atrial natriuretic peptide** (ANP). This hormone inhibits sodium reabsorption by the kidneys and stimulates vasodilation. Its effect, therefore, is opposite to that of the RAAS.

Antidiuretic hormone (**ADH**) is another key hormone in kidney regulation. In the nephron tubule ADH promotes the reabsorption of water back into the blood by making the collecting duct of the nephron more **permeable**. ADH does this by triggering chemical reactions that lead to the activation of **aquaporins**, which are proteins in the plasma membrane of cells in the collecting duct. Aquaporins form tiny channels that carry water molecules across the plasma membrane. When fluid intake is inadequate and the body needs to conserve water, more ADH is produced, causing the activation of more aquaporins, and enabling more water to be reabsorbed. ADH is vital for concentrating the urine and thus protecting against dehydration. (The name "aquaporin" is composed of *aqua*, the Latin for "water," and *poros*, the Greek for "small hole"). There are also several other hormones that effect the kidney, including **parathyroid hormone** (PTH), and the female sex hormone **estrogen**, which is thought to have a role in repairing damaged kidney cells.

11) Prerenal, intrarenal, and postrenal: *Prerenal* causes of AKI are those that reduce blood flow to the kidneys. Factors that can reduce renal blood flow include a reduction in **cardiac output** due to heart failure, or a decrease in blood volume (**hypovolemia**) from blood loss or from severe dehydration. **Sepsis**, an extreme response by the body to bacteria or other pathogens, is also a major cause of AKI. Sepsis involves the release of cytokines to fight infection. These cytokines trigger **systemic vasodilation**, leading to a drastic fall in blood pressure and a decrease in blood flow to the organs, including the kidneys. Medications such as **NSAIDs** can also reduce renal blood flow. If renal blood flow is severely reduced, cells in the nephron can suffer **ischemic injury** (i.e., damage due to diminished or absent blood flow).

Intrarenal causes of AKI are within the kidney itself. Some drugs can directly damage the kidney, including certain antibiotics, chemotherapy drugs, and **contrast dyes** (solutions used to highlight certain structures in the body when having a CT or MRI scan). Direct kidney damage can also be caused by an infection of bacteria (e.g., salmonella), viruses (e.g., SARS-CoV-2), or nephrotoxins in plants and poisonous mushrooms. Regarding bacterial infection, certain strains of *Escherichia coli* (*E. coli*), such as E. coli O157, produce a toxin called **Shiga toxin**. This toxin can cause inflammation and damage to renal blood vessels. This damage can lead to the formation of blood clots that block glomeruli, interfering with the ability of the kidney to filter and eliminate waste products. This condition, called **hemolytic uremic syndrome** (HUS), can be life-threatening and requires prompt treatment in hospital.

Postrenal AKI, occurs when there is an obstruction in the urinary tract below the kidneys that blocks the flow of urine. Such an obstruction leads to increased pressure in the nephron tubules and a decline in GFR. Common causes of postrenal AKI are **kidney stones**, which can obstruct a ureter, or an **enlarged prostate** that squeezes on the urethra and impedes the flow of urine from the bladder. The most common cause of an enlarged prostate is **benign prostatic hyperplasia** (BPH). A complete obstruction of the urethra can lead to **anuria**, a cessation of urine output. Without treatment, such an obstruction can result in irreversible kidney damage. Some central nervous system (CNS) disorders (e.g., **multiple sclerosis**) that prevent the bladder from emptying can also cause postrenal AKI.

SD 2J: The effect of NSAIDs on renal blood flow

The first **non-steroidal anti-inflammatory drug (NSAID)** was aspirin, which was created in 1897 by Felix Hoffman of the Bayer company in Germany. Since then, more than 20 different

NSAIDs have been developed, including ibuprofen and naproxen. NSAIDs are widely used to relieve symptoms of various common conditions, including colds and flu, migraine, headaches, painful periods (**dysmenorrhea**), and injuries to ligaments, tendons, and muscles. Chronic pain conditions such as **rheumatoid arthritis** can also be treated with NSAIDs. The symptoms of these and other conditions can be relieved by NSAIDs because these medicines have **anti-inflammatory**, **analgesic** (i.e., pain relieving), and **antipyretic** (fever-reducing) effects. For almost 80 years, it was not known how aspirin worked, but in the 1970s a British scientist called John Vane (1927-2004) discovered aspirin's mechanism of action. For this discovery Vane and two other scientists received the 1982 Nobel Prize in Physiology or Medicine. Thanks to Vane's research we know that **prostaglandins**[*1], a group of lipid compounds, play a key role in the generation of the inflammatory response, part of the body's healing process. So, the **cardinal signs of inflammation** (i.e., heat, pain, redness, and swelling) that occur in, for example, a gout attack, result from the production of prostaglandins (as well as other chemical mediators in the body). Prostaglandins are also involved in causing **fever**, a common symptom of infection, and in controlling blood flow (prostaglandins cause **vasodilation**). Prostaglandins have a diverse range of other important roles, such as the control of blood clotting and smooth muscle contraction, and in women, the prostaglandin-induced contraction of the **uterus** is important in **menstruation** and in **inducing labor**.

Like hormones, prostaglandins are chemical messengers or mediators, but unlike hormones, which are carried throughout the body, prostaglandins are short-lived and stimulate a reaction in the tissue in which they are produced or in nearby tissues. For this reason, prostaglandins are sometimes referred to as **local hormones**. So, how are these local hormones produced? The precursor of prostaglandins is **arachidonic acid**, a fatty acid in the plasma membranes of cells. The conversion of arachidonic acid to prostaglandins is catalyzed by an enzyme called **cyclooxygenase (COX)**[*2]. Many medicines act by inhibiting enzymes, and NSAIDs also work in this way. By inhibiting COX, NSAIDs decrease prostaglandin synthesis, which in turn helps to relieve a person's headache, fever, or painful joints.

However, NSAIDs have various side effects, which is not surprising, considering the numerous important functions prostaglandins carry out in the body. The most well-known of the many side effects are **gastric irritation** and **gastric bleeding**, worsening of asthma symptoms, and problems with the kidney. One reason renal adverse effects can occur when taking NSAIDs is related to renal blood flow. Prostaglandins are potent vasodilators, and they cause vasodilation of the **afferent arterioles**, the small blood vessels that supply blood to the glomerulus. Vasodilation decreases resistance to blood flow in the afferent arteriole, thus increasing **renal perfusion**, and helping to maintain blood flow to the glomerulus. By inhibiting prostaglandins, NSAIDs reduce this vasodilation, and so decrease blood flow through the afferent arterioles[*3]. This can lead to a decline in how much blood is filtered by the glomeruli. In people with normal kidney function, a decline in renal blood flow due to taking an NSAID does not usually cause problems because healthy kidneys have a lot of extra capacity. But in people with pre-existing kidney disease, the inhibition of prostaglandin synthesis could lead to renal failure. NSAIDs can also cause serious renal problems in people whose kidneys are already under stress due to, for example, dehydration, or underlying conditions such as chronic heart failure or **liver cirrhosis** (scarring of the liver resulting in a decline in hepatic function).

*¹ In 1930 a substance was discovered in human semen. Ulf von Euler, a Swedish physiologist, concluded in 1935 that the new substance was a secretion of the prostate gland, so he named the substance "prostaglandin" (prostate + gland+~in, a suffix indicating a chemical substance). Subsequent research showed that prostaglandins are not found only in human semen, but are produced by almost all the body's cells.

*² There are three variants (**isoforms**) of COX (cyclooxygenase): **COX-1, COX-2**, and COX-3. Only COX-1 and COX-2 will be discussed here. Cyclooxygenase-1 is a **constitutive enzyme**, meaning that it is formed in a constant amount, regardless of the environment or metabolic state in the tissues. Put simply, COX-1 is continuously present in tissues, where it maintains normal body function. In the stomach, for example, COX-1 protects the gastric mucosa (stomach wall) by maintaining a healthy mucosal blood flow and by stimulating mucus and bicarbonate secretion. An **inducible enzyme** is an enzyme that is produced only under certain conditions; an example is COX-2, which is generally only produced in response to pro-inflammatory stimuli. Although it is COX-2 that is involved in the inflammatory response, aspirin inhibits both COX-1 and COX-2. It is the inhibition of COX-1 that causes many of the side effects associated with NSAIDs. Wouldn't it be ideal if a pharmaceutical company could develop an NSAID that inhibited COX-2 but left COX-1 relatively untouched? This, in fact, has been tried. In 1999, the first selective COX-2 inhibitor, called **celecoxib**, was introduced in the USA. Celecoxib and other COX-2 inhibitors do reduce, but do not eliminate, the risk of gastrointestinal bleeding compared to non-selective NSAIDs. However, because selectively inhibiting COX-2 is associated with increased cardiovascular risk, the use of these drugs is controversial.

*³ While NSAIDs inhibit the renal synthesis of prostaglandins, **loop diuretics** do the opposite. The primary use of loop diuretics is to increase elimination of sodium and water from the body, but they also **induce** the renal synthesis of prostaglandins, causing vasodilation, and so leading to increased renal blood flow.

12) *RAAS*, short for the *renin-angiotensin-aldosterone system*, plays a vital role in regulating sodium and water reabsorption by the kidneys, which in turn has a direct effect on the blood pressure of the whole body. The first stage of the RAAS is the release of renin from the kidneys (*ren* = "kidney"), a substance that is usually described as an enzyme, but is also considered to be a hormone. Renin is released from **juxtaglomerular cells** in the walls of the **afferent arterioles** (small arteries that deliver blood to the nephrons). The juxtaglomerular cells secrete renin when blood flow through the kidney falls, most often due to a drop in systemic blood pressure. Enzymes act on a **substrate**, and the substrate that renin acts on is a protein in the blood called **angiotensinogen**, produced by the liver. Renin acts on angiotensinogen, converting it into **angiotensin I**. Angiotensin I has no known function in the body, but it is a **precursor** of **angiotensin II**, a hormone with several important effects in the body. It is an enzyme called **ACE (angiotensin converting enzyme)**, produced mainly in the kidneys and the lungs, that converts angiotensin I into angiotensin II. (For those who are interested, angiotensin I is a **decapeptide**, a short peptide of 10 amino acids, and angiotensin

II is an **octapeptide**, composed of 8 amino acids. It is ACE that **cleaves** the two amino acids off angiotensin I).

Angiotensin II has important functions, for example it:

- acts on blood vessels to cause **vasoconstriction**.
- stimulates sodium reabsorption in the nephron tubule.
- causes the release of **aldosterone** from the adrenal cortex. Aldosterone is a steroid hormone that acts on the kidney to increase the amount of sodium reabsorbed from the nephron. (Remember that water follows sodium, so an increase in sodium reabsorption also causes more water to be reabsorbed into the blood.)
- stimulates the release of **antidiuretic hormone (ADH)** from the pituitary gland. ADH acts on collecting ducts in the nephrons, causing them to become more permeable to water, thereby increasing the reabsorption of water.
- stimulates **thirst centers** in the brain, motivating increased fluid intake.

Overall, the effect of angiotensin is to increase the volume of blood and to increase peripheral resistance, both of which lead to a rise in blood pressure. Considering that the RAAS is a key physiological system controlling blood pressure, it is not surprising that antihypertensive medications have been developed that target the RAAS. One such class of medications is **ACE inhibitors**.

Finally, it is useful to know that **alcohol** inhibits the secretion of ADH by the pituitary gland. ADH, as the name suggests, acts against **diuresis** (urination), leading to the conservation of water. Therefore, when there is less ADH acting on the collecting ducts, the amount of water reabsorbed by the nephron is reduced, resulting in more urine being excreted. The **diuretic effect** of alcohol explains why toilets in pubs are usually busy places. While alcohol reduces ADH levels in the body, sleep increases ADH. **Nocturnal** ADH secretion is higher than daytime ADH secretion. Increasing ADH levels in the body at night makes sense because we do not drink while sleeping; therefore, the body needs to minimize water loss from urination to conserve the body's fluid volume.

SD 2K: What condition can cause someone to pee over 30 liters of urine in a day?

Located at the base of the brain and about the size of a pea, the **pituitary gland** is a very important **endocrine gland**; in fact, the pituitary gland, together with the **hypothalamus**, which are connected to each other, are sometimes called the "master glands" because they control many of the body's other endocrine glands. One of the several hormones produced by the hypothalamus and released from the pituitary gland is **antidiuretic hormone** (ADH), also called **vasopressin** (so called because it is a **vasopressor**, a substance that constricts blood vessels and so raises blood pressure). The main function of ADH is the regulation of water in the body. Increased secretion of ADH results in more water being reabsorbed by the kidneys, while decreased ADH levels cause more water to be excreted by the kidneys. ADH acts mainly on the nephrons' collecting ducts, increasing their **permeability** to water, and allowing more water to be reabsorbed by osmosis from the collecting ducts and returned to the bloodstream.

Imagine that you are hiking through Death Valley in Southern California, the hottest place on earth. You are dripping with sweat and you are running short of bottled water. You are **dehydrated** (i.e., your body has lost more fluids than it has taken in) and very thirsty. **Baroreceptors** (in the walls of certain arteries and in the heart) and **osmoreceptors** (in the hypothalamus), two kinds of sensors in the body, detect a fall in blood volume and a rise in the level of plasma sodium. These changes stimulate the release of ADH from the pituitary gland. ADH is carried in the bloodstream to your kidneys, where it promotes water reabsorption. Water reabsorbed from the collecting ducts returns to the bloodstream, thereby increasing your blood volume, which helps to maintain your blood pressure, and diluting the concentration of sodium in your blood. When you stop to pee behind a rock, you produce only a small amount of urine, and you notice that the urine is dark yellow (this color indicates that the pee is highly concentrated). In Death Valley, your body needs to conserve water by reducing the amount of water lost in the urine, and this is what ADH helps to do. (Of course, while ADH slows down water loss, you can only completely restore fluid balance by increasing water intake).

Imagine how your life would change if your body did not produce any ADH. Without ADH, the collecting ducts would become impermeable to water, preventing water from being reabsorbed back into the blood. This would cause you to pass huge amounts of dilute urine. You would need to go to the toilet frequently, which could be embarrassing and very disruptive to your life. You would feel constantly thirsty (**polydipsia**), and, unless you drank fluids constantly to replace the water lost in urine, you would quickly become dangerously dehydrated. This is not a made-up disease; it is what happens to people with **diabetes insipidus** (DI), a disorder resulting from either a **deficiency** of ADH or from ADH not having an appropriate action. While most people urinate six to eight times in a 24-hour period, eliminating between 1L to 1.5L of urine, people with DI pass over 20 liters of urine per day, and need to visit the toilet up to 30 times a day. Diabetes insipidus can have neurogenic or nephrogenic causes. **Neurogenic DI** is when the brain doesn't produce enough ADH. This often results from damage to the pituitary gland or hypothalamus due to a head injury or surgery, or from brain inflammation due to **meningitis**. It can also be **idiopathic**, meaning that it occurs for no obvious reason. In **nephrogenic DI**, adequate amounts of ADH are produced, but the kidneys are partly or completely unresponsive to it. In children, nephrogenic DI is often due to an inherited disease that affects the nephron tubules, but in adults **acquired nephrogenic DI** is most often a side effect of drug treatment with **lithium**.

Diabetes insipidus is not related to **diabetes mellitus (DM)**[*1], which is a disorder of glucose metabolism. The word "diabetes" that both DI and DM share means "to go through." Diabetes refers to **polyuria**, or excessive urination, a symptom that is common to both conditions. However, while the urine of people with DI is tasteless ("insipid" means "without flavor"), the urine of people with DM tastes sweet ("mellitus" means "as sweet as honey") due to its high glucose content. Before urine and blood could be tested in biochemistry labs, doctors distinguished between the two conditions by tasting a patient's urine. Diabetes insipidus is a much less common condition than DM. In the USA, for example, the prevalence of DI is about 1 in 25, 000, compared to over 2800 in 25,000 for DM.

Diabetes insipidus is rarely fatal if a person drinks enough water to compensate for the water lost in the urine. But the danger of this condition is higher for people who may not recognize that they are thirsty or who ignore the thirst sensation (e.g., people with dementia or certain mental illnesses). A rare complication of brain cancer is **adipsia**, which is a complete lack of thirst despite being dehydrated. It would be highly unfortunate if a person with DI also developed adipsia because a lack of fluid intake can lead to **hypernatremia**. Hypernatremia, an abnormally high concentration of sodium in the blood—specifically, a plasma sodium level of over 160 mmol/L—occurs when water is lost from the body without losing an equal amount of sodium. Signs of hypernatremia include confusion, **lethargy**, irritability, and seizures. Without treatment, severe hypernatremia can lead to unconsciousness, coma, and death.

Japan is an earthquake prone country, which makes me wonder how long I could survive after an earthquake if I were trapped in my university office, unharmed and with adequate air, but without any water. If the earthquake occurred in October, when the temperature in Nagoya is quite mild, I could probably survive for around 3 days*2. But if I had DI, my body would be unable conserve water, and my survival time would likely be much shorter.

Neurogenic DI can be treated with a medication called **desmopressin**, a synthetic **analogue** of ADH (i.e., desmopressin has a similar chemical structure to natural ADH). However, this drug does not work for nephrogenic DI, which results from the kidneys being resistant to ADH, rather than from an ADH deficiency.

*1 Under normal circumstances, all the glucose filtered by the renal glomerulus is reabsorbed in the proximal convoluted tubule (PCT). This glucose reabsorption is a two-stage process that involves SGLT2, proteins that act as glucose pumps in the membrane of the cells lining the PCT, and GLUT2s, glucose transporters that ferry glucose from the cells into the blood. In people with chronic hyperglycemia, as occurs in uncontrolled DM, polyuria occurs because the amount of glucose that is filtered by the glomerulus overwhelms the glucose transport mechanisms in the PCT. Unable to be reabsorbed, the glucose remains in the **lumen** of the nephron tubule, where it exerts an osmotic pressure that keeps water within the lumen. This additional water is then excreted in the urine. This is an example of **osmotic diuresis**, or increased urination resulting from the impairment of water reabsorption due to solutes (e.g., glucose, urea) remaining in the glomerular filtrate.

*2If you do an outdoor-survival course, you will probably be told about the "rule of 3's":

You can survive for **3 minutes** without oxygen.

You can survive for **3 hours** without shelter in a harsh environment.

You can survive for **3 days** without water (if you have adequate shelter)

You can survive for **3 weeks** without food (if you have water and shelter)

The "rule of 3's" are not **hard and fast rules**, but a way to help people decide on priorities in a survival situation. For example, if you were lost on Mount Fuji in the middle of winter without any food or drink, your priority would be to find shelter. Without shelter, you would die of **hypothermia** before you died of thirst.

2-4 Well, what do you know?

（どのくらいわかるようになったか試してみよう）

Are the following statements true (T) or false (F)?

1. Creatinine is freely filtered by the glomerulus and is not reabsorbed.
2. By inhibiting the formation of angiotensin II, ACE inhibitors cause the smooth muscles of arterial walls to relax leading to vasodilation.
3. NSAIDs such as ibuprofen cause vasodilation of renal blood vessels.
4. A kidney stone that blocks a ureter can be a cause of AKI.
5. The plural form of "glomerulus" is "glomeruluses."

What is the meaning of the underlined WFE?

1. Each of the four **parathyroid** glands are only the size of a grain of rice, but they release a hormone that is very important in the regulation of calcium.
2. The renal system of birds has **evolved** to conserve water. Birds excrete droppings containing a lot of uric acid, a substance that requires very little water to be excreted.
3. In 1880, a German **anthropologist** went to Hokkaido to study the culture of the Ainu, the indigenous people of Hokkaido.
4. During the COVID-19 pandemic, people practiced physical-distancing because the risk of infection increases when people are in close **proximity** to each other.
5. The heart is enclosed in a fibrous sac called the **pericardium**, which protects the heart and has several other important functions.
6. The right kidney is lower than the left kidney because it needs to accommodate the liver, the body's largest internal organ, which sits **superior** to it.
7. All biological reactions within human cells depend on enzymes, so it should come as no surprise that many drugs work by inhibition of these vital **catalysts**.
8. **Acromegaly** is a disorder that occurs when the pituitary gland produces too much growth hormone, causing the excessive growth of bones and other body tissues.

Choose a word from below to replace the underlined word(s)

a) filtered b) hematuria c) excess d) reabsorbed e) metabolized
f) secreted g) renin h) rennet i) deficiency

1. The kidneys are responsible for converting calcidiol, a form of vitamin D produced in the liver, into calcitriol, the active form of vitamin D that can be used by the body.

Vitamin D increases absorption of calcium from the intestine; therefore, renal impairment can lead to calcium ☐.

2. Because creatinine is freely ☐ by the glomeruli and is not ☐ in the nephron tubule, we would expect blood creatinine to equal the amount of creatinine excreted in the urine. However, some creatinine is ☐ into the nephron tubule from the peritubular capillaries. This means that the amount of creatinine excreted in the urine is about 10% more than the amount in the blood.

3. There are two types of ☐, microscopic or gross. The former indicates blood in the urine that is only visible under a microscope; the latter is used for blood that is visible and turns the urine red, pink, or tea colored.

4. A mnemonic to help remember the functions of the kidney is "WET BREAD." **W** = Water balance regulation; **E** = Electrolyte balance; **T** = Toxin and waste excretion; **B** = Blood pressure control; **R** = ☐ synthesis; **E** = Erythropoietin synthesis; **A** = Acid-balance maintenance; **D** = Vitamin D activation

2-5 May Jo's Health-Podcast

（メイ・ジョーの健康ポッドキャスト）

Podcast presenter May Jo (MJ) and Dr Neil Smith (Dr) are talking about COVID-19-associated AKI.

MJ: On today's podcast is Dr Neil Smith, a nephrologist at Oak Hospital in Manchester. When the first wave of COVID-19 hit Britain in March 2020, he was on the pandemic-frontline working in intensive care. Most people associate COVID-19 with pneumonia, but COVID-19 can affect other organs besides the lungs. That's correct, isn't it, Dr Smith?

Dr: Yes, we know it can damage multiple organs, including the brain, heart, gastrointestinal tract, and the kidneys.

MJ: You're a kidney specialist, so I want to focus on COVID-19 and the kidneys. When did you start to notice that people hospitalized with this then new disease were having kidney problems?

Dr: Well, a week after Boris Johnson[1] announced the first nationwide lockdown.

MJ: That was on March 23, 2020.

Dr: Yes, a week after that we started to notice that several patients with COVID-19 had developed acute kidney injury, or AKI.

MJ: What exactly is AKI?

Dr: It's an abrupt decline in kidney function.

MJ: When you say "abrupt," how quick is the onset?

Dr: AKI can happen over a few days or even a few hours. Anyway, by February 2020, of the twenty COVID-19 patients in intensive care at Oak Hospital, eight required dialysis.

MJ: Was this only at your hospital?

Dr: No, COVID-19-associated AKI has been reported in hospitals in many countries, and AKI is now recognized as a common complication of severe COVID-19. Studies from the first year of the pandemic suggest that up to 30% of patients hospitalized with COVID-19 developed kidney injury.

MJ: What's the reason for this high incidence of AKI in COVID-19 patients?

Dr: Firstly, we should remember that many people hospitalized with COVID-19 will also have underlying conditions, such as hypertension and diabetes. These conditions leave people more at risk of developing kidney problems. But I have treated AKI in many COVID-19 patients who don't have any pre-existing conditions. In answer to your question, the mechanisms, or pathophysiology, of COVID-19-associated AKI is complicated and research is ongoing.

MJ: What are some of the possible causes that researchers are investigating?

Dr: Well, we know that SARS-CoV-2, the virus responsible for COVID-19, can infect kidney cells. There is a protein receptor called ACE2 located on the surface of many cells and tissues, and the virus uses ACE2 receptors as a doorway to enter cells. These receptors are highly expressed on kidney cells, which could explain why the kidneys are susceptible to being infected by SARS-CoV-2.

MJ: So, you're saying damage is caused by SARS-CoV-2 targeting kidney cells.

Dr: That's right, viral damage of kidney cells, particularly certain cells in the nephron tubule, is one likely cause. Another is hypoxia, a lack of oxygen reaching the body tissues.

MJ: And hypoxia can result from COVID-19 pneumonia, can't it?

Dr: Yes, it can. The kidney is very sensitive to insufficient oxygenation of renal tissue, and hypoxia can rapidly lead to a deterioration of kidney function.

MJ: Could you briefly talk about the cytokine storm?

Dr: Yes, of course. Well, cytokines are small proteins that control how immune cells communicate and interact. They are crucial in the normal immune response, but damage to the body results if there is too big a release of cytokines into the blood at one time.

MJ: And COVID-19 can trigger such a flood of cytokines?

Dr: Yes, infection by SARS-CoV-2 causes the immune system to react in way that is much too aggressive. Macrophages, T lymphocytes, and other immune cells release a tsunami of cytokines, triggering excessive inflammation. It is this systemic inflammatory response that damages healthy tissues and organs.

MJ: So, in the case of the cytokine storm, it's the immune system's overreaction to the virus, not the virus itself, that is responsible for the AKI.

Dr: Yes, exactly.

MJ: Thank you Dr Smith. I know that you also wanted to talk about COVID-19 and abnormalities in blood clotting and how blood clots can damage the kidneys, but I'm afraid we've run out of time today. Perhaps you could find some time next month to talk about this important topic.

Dr: I'd be happy to.

[1] Prime Minister of the UK from 24 July 2019 to 6 September 2022.

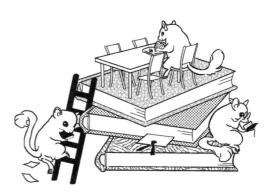

Chapter 3 Inflammatory bowel disease
（炎症性腸疾患）

Intestines

The one and only viscera piercing the body as the digestive conveyor

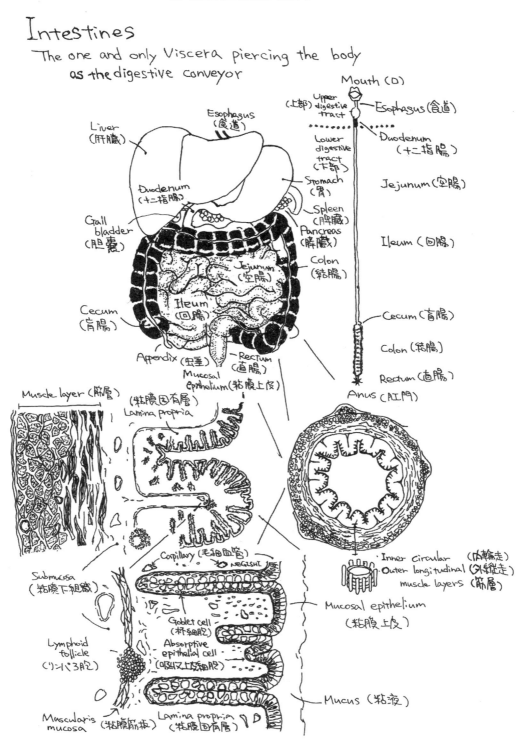

NAVvocab 60 （案内役の単語 60）

1. adverse reaction・有害反応（副作用）
2. aggravate・悪化させる
3. ameliorate・良くする
4. analgesic・鎮痛剤
5. anecdotal・逸話的な
6. biologics・生物学的製剤
7. biopsy・生体組織検査
8. bloating・膨脹
9. carcinogenesis・発癌
10. colectomy・結腸切除術
11. colonoscopy・大腸内視鏡
12. colorectal cancer・結腸直腸癌
13. commensal bacteria・共生細菌
14. constipation・便秘
15. curative・治癒的な
16. defecate・排便する
17. diarrhea・下痢
18. digestive system・消化器系
19. dysbiosis・腸内フローラの破綻
20. dysplasia・異形成
21. enema・注腸製剤
22. enteric nervous system・腸管神経系
23. epidemiological research・疫学的研究
24. etiology・病因学
25. exacerbation・増悪
26. extraintestinal・腸管外
27. fecal microbiota transplantation・糞便移植
28. fistula・瘻孔（ろうこう）
29. flare-up・急性増悪（再燃）
30. gastroenteritis・胃腸炎
31. gastroenterologist・消化器専門医
32. generic name・一般名
33. gut microbiota・腸内微生物叢
34. hematochezia・血便
35. high-grade dysplasia・高度異形成
36. immunosuppressive・免疫抑制剤
37. incidence・発生率
38. inflammatory bowel disease 炎症性腸疾患
39. integrity・完全性 (territorial integrity: 国の領土一体性)
40. interspersed with・〜がちりばめられている
41. malabsorption・吸収不良
42. metaplasia・化生
43. mucosa・粘膜
44. pancolitis・全大腸炎型
45. parenteral administration・非経口投与
46. pass blood・血便が出る
47. peptic ulcer・消化性潰瘍
48. positively correlated・正の相関
49. precancerous changes・前癌病変
50. prophylactic surgery・予防的手術
51. rectal administration・直腸投与
52. rectal bleeding・直腸出血
53. refractory・難溶性
54. second-degree relative・第二度近親者
55. stoma・ストーマ
56. symptomatic treatments・対症療法
57. systemic side effects・全身性副作用
58. tenesmus・しぶり
59. topical administration・局所投与
60. ulcerative colitis・潰瘍性大腸炎

3-1 Essay — Blood in the Toilet Bowl: IBD
（炎症性腸疾患：便器に血がつく）

[1]From 1996 to 1999, when I was in my early 30s, I lived in Takamatsu, the capital city of Kagawa Prefecture (the smallest of Japan's 47 prefectures). I was enjoying my work in the Kagawa Prefectural Government Office, but a few months after arriving, I noticed I was **passing blood** in my **stool**. Sometimes it was only a little bit of blood on the toilet paper, but often the water in the toilet would turn bright red (I later learned that the medical term for red blood in the stool is **hematochezia**). My **undergraduate degree** was in physical education, and I vaguely remembered learning that strenuous exercise could cause **rectal bleeding**. I was training hard at a karate *dojo* near my house in Takamatsu, so I **put** the blood **down to** the demanding exercise I was doing. One day, almost a year after the bleeding had started, my girlfriend at the time went into the toilet after me. She screamed because there was blood in the **toilet bowl** (perhaps I had not flushed the toilet properly!). It was then I realized I had been **fooling myself** by thinking that blood in the stools was nothing to worry about. Relying on half-remembered medical information, as I did, is not wise. As the proverb goes, **a little knowledge is a dangerous thing**.

[2]A few days later, I went to a hospital in Takamatsu to see a **gastroenterologist**, a doctor who specializes in conditions of the **digestive system**[D7]. The visit was **far from reassuring**. With a serious expression, the doctor, who spoke good English, said that rectal bleeding is a **red flag sign** for colon cancer, and that I would need to have my **large intestine** examined with an **endoscope** to check for anything "**sinister**." A **tide of anxiety** swept through me because I knew that "sinister" meant "cancer." The following week, I returned to hospital for a **colonoscopy**[E3]. To spot any abnormalities during the colonoscopy, the large intestine must be completely empty, so I had to **fast** from the evening before the procedure and take two kinds of **laxative**, a type of medicine that facilitates emptying of the bowels and is often used to treat **constipation**[D5].

[3]During the colonoscopy, **biopsies** (tissue samples) were taken from the innermost lining of the colon, called the **mucosa** (the **GI tract** is composed of **four layers**[D8]). The colonoscopy took around 30 minutes. Although uncomfortable and embarrassing, the experience was also fascinating because I could watch on a TV monitor as the endoscope traveled along the whole length of my large intestine. It was the first time I had seen deep inside my body, but I knew that something was wrong because my colon wall was bleeding and looked very inflamed.

[4]It was an anxious time waiting for the colonoscopy results; in fact, I was so sure I had

cancer that I wrote a **bucket list**. However, when I walked into the doctor's office a fortnight later, he reassured me that the **pathologist's** examination of the biopsies had not found cancer. But, he said, "You do have **ulcerative colitis**, a type of **inflammatory bowel disease**." It was the first time I had heard either of these terms (at that time **peptic ulcer** and **gastroenteritis**[E6] were probably the only conditions of the digestive system I knew).

[5]Inflammatory bowel disease (**IBD**) is an **umbrella term** for conditions characterized by chronic inflammation of the gastrointestinal (GI) tract with the formation of **ulcers**. This inflammation damages the gut wall (or, in medical language, it compromises the **integrity** of the gut's mucosal barrier), and adversely affects its function. The two most common types of IBD are ulcerative colitis (**UC**) and **Crohn's disease** (**CD**). While UC and CD are similar in many ways, they also have important differences. Some of these are summarized in Table 3.1.

Table 3.1

Differences Between Crohn's Disease and Ulcerative Colitis

（クローン病と潰瘍性大腸炎の違い）

	Crohn's Disease　（クローン病）	**Ulcerative Colitis**　（潰瘍性大腸炎）
What part of the GI tract is affected?	Any part	Confined to the large intestine
What is the depth of inflammation?	All layers of the bowel wall can be affected	Usually confined to the mucosa
What is the pattern of inflammation?	Patchy with healthy parts **interspersed**[E7] with inflamed areas	The inflammation is continuous
What about rectal bleeding and bloody diarrhea?	Not always a symptom	This is a classic symptom
Type of pain	Sharp pain is common	Abdominal cramping is common
Efficacy of 5-ASA drugs	Not considered very effective	Often effective; first-line medicines in UC
Is surgery curative?	No. Crohn's disease is likely to recur after surgery	Yes.

[6]A key difference between the two conditions is the extent of the GI tract affected. UC only affects the large intestine. In CD, on the other hand, the disease can occur anywhere in the GI tract, although it most commonly affects the **small intestine**. Also, in UC, inflammation is limited to the inner lining of the large intestine, but in CD the entire thickness of the gut wall may be affected. About one in three people with CD develop a **fistula**, which is when an ulcer **penetrates** through the bowel wall.

⁷The most common symptoms of UC are **bloody stools** and **<u>diarrhea</u>^{D6}**. The stools are often mixed with **mucus,** a substance secreted by the mucous membranes lining the cavities of the body (note the different spellings of the noun "mucus" and the adjective "mucous"). Even after going to the toilet, some people experience **tenesmus** (a feeling that one still needs to **defecate**, although the bowels are empty), caused by inflammation of the lining of the rectum. Other symptoms include **fatigue**, **nausea**, **loss of appetite**, and a dry mouth due to **dehydration**. Chronic bleeding from the inflamed colon can lead to **anemia**. Apart from the large intestine, UC can affect other parts of the body. **Arthritis**, inflammation of joints, is the most common **extraintestinal** manifestation of UC.

⁸Compared to people without the condition, those with IBD are **prone** to **depression** and **anxiety**. Such mental health disorders are no doubt caused partly by the pain and discomfort that people with IBD may experience, but the fact that there is **bidirectional** (two-way) communication between the gut and the brain (the so-called **gut-brain axis**) may also be a factor. The gut has evolved its own independent nervous system called the **enteric nervous system (ENS)**, which has so many nerves that it is known as the "**the second brain**." The ENS is known to influence mood and emotion, so it would not be surprising if the influence of inflammation on the ENS also contributed to mental health conditions. The intestines, especially the colon, is home to **gut microbiota**, a community of many types of bacteria and other microbes. A **dysbiosis** (imbalance) in the gut microbiota is thought to play an important role in the pathogenesis of IBD. In relation to mental health, it has been suggested this dysbiosis could also be involved in the development of depression in people with IBD.

⁹Symptoms of UC range from mild to severe depending on the extent and severity of the inflammation. A person with inflammation of only a small part of the colon will usually have less severe symptoms than someone with **pancolitis** (i.e., inflammation of the whole colon). Symptoms will also vary from person to person. For example, some people will suffer from uncomfortable **bloating**, while others will not. The condition is often accompanied by **bowel urgency,** a sudden and strong **urge** to defecate. Suddenly needing to go to the toilet can result in **<u>embarrassing accidents</u>^{E5}** that can harm self-esteem and **disrupt** normal life. I have never experienced pain as a symptom of UC, but for some people, this is the most **debilitating** symptom.

¹⁰People with IBD experience **flare-ups**, when symptoms become worse, and periods of **remission**, when the symptoms go away. Certain things can **exacerbate** symptoms; for example, spicy foods can trigger an **exacerbation** of symptoms in some people, as can a lack of sleep and psychological stress. Medications, such as **NSAIDs**, which includes commonly used **<u>analgesics</u>^{D2}**such as aspirin and ibuprofen, can **aggravate** symptoms, and should be used with caution. (For pain relief in people with IBD, the safest option is

paracetamol). A class of drugs called **proton pump inhibitors** (**PPIs**)[D11], which act to suppress gastric acid secretion, can also provoke flare ups in some people.

[11]**Smoking** is a risk factor for many conditions, but regarding UC it appears that smokers are actually *less* likely to develop the condition. There have also been **anecdotal**[D1] reports of UC symptoms improving when former smokers started smoking again. On the other hand, smoking seems to increase the risk for developing CD. The reasons for this so-called "**smoker's paradox**"[E10] are unclear.

[12]**Unintentional weight loss** is more common in people with CD compared to UC. This is because in CD the small intestine becomes inflamed. Around 90% of **digestion**[E4] and absorption takes place in the small intestine, so inflammation here can cause **malabsorption**[E8] of nutrients, leading to **malnutrition** and **vitamin K and vitamin D deficiency**[E11]. Some people with CD may require periods of **total parenteral nutrition** (TPN). Malnutrition is not usually a problem for people with UC, in which inflammation is limited to the large intestine, although it can occur during severe flare ups.

[13]The **pathogenesis,** or processes by which UC and CD develops, is still unclear. IBD is classed as an **autoimmune disease**[D4], in which the immune system mistakenly attacks healthy tissue. Research on the **intestinal immune system**[D9] in recent decades suggests that what causes the inflammation of IBD is the immune system "attacking" **commensal intestinal bacteria** (i.e., bacteria that normally live peacefully in the gut). This inappropriate inflammatory response to gut bacteria involves **leukocytes**[D10] migrating into the mucosa of the intestine.

[14]Although there has been considerable progress in IBD research, scientists are still unsure of its **etiology.** Most agree, however, that IBD is **multifactorial**, caused by a complex interaction of different factors. **Epidemiological research** has shown that a country's level of industrialization and urbanization is **positively correlated** with the prevalence of IBD. This suggests that **environmental factors** are important. Many environmental factors have been **implicated**, including the loss of **intestinal parasites** and the use of **antibiotics** during a child's first year of life.

[15]Crohn's disease is named after Dr Burrill Crohn. It was Dr Crohn who, in 1932, first reported on 14 patients with the disease at a hospital in New York. All these 14 patients were **Jewish**. At first Dr Crohn, who was himself Jewish, thought this was just a **coincidence**. However, studies carried out **subsequently** have confirmed that CD and UC are more **prevalent** in Jewish people, suggesting that this ethnic group could have an underlying **genetic predisposition** to IBD. That IBD has a strong genetic component of IBD is backed up by studies which have found over 10% of people diagnosed with IBD have a **family history** of the condition. In fact, after I was diagnosed in Japan, I found out that a **second-degree relative** of mine also has UC (a second-degree relative is an uncle,

aunt, nephew, niece, grandparent, grandchild or half-**sibling**; a **first-degree relative** is a mother, father, full-sibling, or child).

[16]Until the 1970s, UC was a rare disease in Japan. But from the 1970s its incidence began to rise. Fast forward to 2022, and the **prevalence** of UC in Japan had grown to over 220,000. Globally, the biggest increases in the **incidence** of UC are occurring in East Asia, particularly Japan and China, and the Middle East. The Japanese government now recognizes UC and CD as **intractable diseases**, and people with these conditions can apply to receive a subsidy to cover a part of their healthcare costs. (The root *tract* means "pull"—think of "tractor"; "intractable" literally means "unable to be pulled," but a more accurate definition is "not manageable").

[17]The fact there has been a rapid increase in the **prevalence** of IBD in just the last several decades cannot be explained by genetic changes in the population. There must be other factors at work. Many researchers think that a key reason is related to the westernization of the Japanese diet. In the same period that IBD has risen, the consumption of **meat** also rose. In 1960, the average Japanese consumed on average 3.5kg of meat a year (beef, pork, or chicken), but by 2016 this had risen to over 32kg. It is **speculated** that a westernized diet high in meat disrupts the gut microbiota, causing a dysregulated immune response in people with a **genetic susceptibility**. However, the fact that both meat consumption and the number of people developing IBD increased during the same period does not *prove* that meat was the **culprit** (remember that <u>**association does not prove causation**[D3]</u>).

[18]Compared to the general population, people with UC are at a higher **risk** of **colorectal cancer**. Chronic mucosal inflammation **predisposes** to the development of cancer and promotes **tumorigenesis** (i.e., the formation of a tumor). The mechanism by which chronic inflammation causes cancer is complex, but simply put inflammation causes cell damage, to which the body responds by constantly renewing cells. This makes the cells more **susceptible** to **mutations** that can become cancerous. I **dread** having a colonoscopy every five or so years, but I know that it can help in the **early detection** of cancer (tissue samples taken by biopsy are examined under a microscope by a pathologist to check for **precancerous changes** such as <u>**metaplasia**[E9]</u> and **dysplasia**).

[19]There is a wide range of pharmacological treatments for IBD. There are drugs that help relieve symptoms such as diarrhea, constipation, and pain. However, such **symptomatic treatments** will not reduce the underlying inflammation. When I was first diagnosed, I was put on **steroids** in order to get my symptoms under control. The doctor prescribed me a steroid **enema**, which allows the steroid to be administered directly into the rectum and colon. This is called **topical administration** (*topos~* is the Greek for "place")**.** Topical administration allows medicine to be delivered directly to the affected

area, and because less steroid is absorbed into the bloodstream, **systemic side effects** are usually reduced compared to **oral administration**. On the other hand, compared to oral administration, **rectal administration** with an enema is less convenient and **takes some getting used to**. When flare-ups are very severe, **parenteral administration** (e.g., **IV infusion**) of steroids may be necessary.

[20]While steroids can help greatly to **ameliorate** symptoms, they do not maintain remission. To **induce** and maintain remission, I was prescribed **Pentasa** tablets. Medicines, as you may know, have three names: a **chemical name** (describing the drug's atomic or molecular structure), a **generic name** (a shorter, easier to remember version of the drug's chemical name or structure), and a **brand name** (the name selected by the manufacturer). Pentasa—note that a drug's brand name is capitalized—contains the active ingredient **mesalamine** (generic name), which has the chemical name of 5-aminosalicylic acid (5-ASA). A Pentasa tablet is composed of tiny granules called **microgranules** that are covered by a semipermeable membrane. These microgranules are designed to release the mesalamine in a way that is dependent on the surrounding pH. The microgranules do not release the drug in the stomach, where the pH is low, but only when the tablet has entered the small and large intestine. Oral Pentasa is an example of a **delayed-release** medicine.

[21]Mesalamine has anti-inflammatory effects on intestinal **epithelial cells**, although the **mechanism of action** (MOA) is not fully understood. Because it is anti-inflammatory, long-term used of mesalamine has been shown to reduce the risk of developing colorectal cancer. (You may think it strange that a drug is such as mesalamine can be prescribed even though its MOA has not been completely elucidated. However, this is not really unusual. There are a number of drugs for which the MOA is not known or only partially known, including paracetamol and metformin. The MOA of aspirin, one of the most commonly used drugs in the world, was only discovered in 1971, over seven decades after aspirin first went on sale in 1897. Interestingly, a complete understanding of a drug's MOA is not required for it to be approved by the **FDA**, the government agency in the USA that authorizes new drugs).

[22]Mesalamine is usually **well tolerated**, but not all patients respond to it, and other drug types are sometimes needed. Increasingly being used to treat IBD is a class of drugs called **biologics**. A biologic is a drug with a large, complex molecular structure produced by processes that involve living cells. An example of a biologic used in IBD is **adalimumab** (**Humira**), an **anti-TNF-a** drug. Standing for **tumor necrosis factor alpha,** TNF-a is a signaling protein, produced by macrophages and other immune cells, that has a pivotal role in promoting inflammation. Adalimumab prevents TNF-alpha from binding to TNF receptors on cells, and inhibition of TNF-alpha by adalimumab reduces the inflammatory reaction. This improves the symptoms of IBD and also results in healing of the inflamed

intestine. Another anti-TNF-a drug that is commonly used in Japan is **infliximab** (**Remicade**). While adalimumab is administered by a subcutaneous injection that takes around 10 seconds, infliximab is given by an intravenous infusion that takes up to 4 hours. Another biologic, called **vedolizumab**, reduces inflammation by inhibiting the movement of lymphocytes, a type of white blood cell, across the lining of the gut.

[23]Because these biological drugs are **immunosuppressive** (i.e., they **suppress** the immune system), they can lower the ability to fight infections and leave people more **vulnerable** to **infection** and **susceptible** to certain cancers. Some people will need to stop these drugs because of **adverse reactions**[E2]. You may have noticed that the generic names adalimumab, infliximab, and vedolizumab end in "*~mab*", a suffix that stands for **monoclonal antibodies**. As well as the drugs described above, there are new IBD drugs **in the pipeline**. There is also research into less conventional treatments, in particular **fecal microbiota transplantation** and therapy with **parasitic worms** (**helminths**).

[24]Because UC and CD are chronic diseases, medications are often taken for life. **Without fail**, I take a daily dose of Pentasa tablets and I also use a **Pentasa enema** every night. I have had almost no symptoms for several years, so I am sometimes tempted to stop taking my medicine. But I know that it is thanks to the medication I take that I am in remission. Some people discontinue medication because they no longer have symptoms; however, stopping medication is a main cause of **relapse** (i.e., the return of symptoms after remission). Healthcare professionals can improve drug **adherence**[E1] by educating patients to appreciate that continuing medication is important for maintaining remission.

[25]While most people with UC will respond well to drugs, some will be **refractory** (i.e., not respond to treatment) or suffer **intolerable** drug side effects. For such people, surgery may be the only treatment to give freedom from the **debilitating** symptoms. A **colectomy** (surgery to remove part or all of the large intestine) may be required if cancer develops in the large intestine. Surgery may also be indicated if **high-grade dysplasia** is identified in a biopsy because cells with such precancerous changes are likely to become malignant (this is an example of **prophylactic surgery**, done to *prevent* cancer developing, rather than to treat cancer that is already present). People who have had a **total colectomy** (removal of the whole colon) will sometimes no longer be able to pass stools through the anus; instead, they eliminate waste through a **stoma** (an opening in the abdomen).

[26]A total colectomy is **curative** for UC. In other words, if I had my large intestine removed tomorrow, I would no longer have UC. But, as you can imagine, living without a colon brings its own problems. I would only choose to have such an operation as a **last resort**. For now, I am grateful that Pentasa, a relatively inexpensive medicine, is **keeping my UC at bay** without any obvious side effects.

3-2　Eleven Etymologies (E)　（11 の単語を詳しく）

1) Adherence: *Medication (drug) adherence* **is the extent to which a patient takes medication as instructed by a healthcare professional.** Not taking medications properly can result in poor treatment outcomes, hospital admission, and even death. It is important that healthcare professionals understand factors that **hinder** good adherence and how it can be improved. One barrier to achieving adherence is the cost of medications. Especially in the USA and other countries without a **universal healthcare system**, the high cost of drugs could, for example, lead to a person taking a medicine only once a day rather than twice as prescribed so as to make the medicine last longer. Other factors that can lower drug adherence include:

- *Low health literacy.* Not understanding basic health information is a barrier to adherence.
- *Insufficient patient education*: A healthcare provider not explaining about a condition properly or not giving clear instructions to a patient.
- *Mistrust*: A patient is less likely to follow instructions if they do not trust the doctor.
- *Unpleasant side effects* such as nausea or dizziness may be put a patient off taking a medication. Concern about side effects, or fear of becoming dependent or addicted to a prescribed drug, can lead to poor adherence.
- *Perceived lack of need or effect*: For example, hypertension usually does not have any symptoms, so a person prescribed an antihypertensive medication may not feel a real need to take it. In conditions that have periods of remission, adherence tends to decline in remission. Symptoms are a reminder of the need to take medication: as the proverb goes, **"out of sight out of mind."**
- *Complicated drug regimen*: Adherence is likely to decline if a drug has to be taken, for example, four times a day rather than once, or by injection rather than orally.
- *Forgetting*: People may forget to take a medication due to a busy lifestyle. Older people may forget due to **cognitive decline**.
- *Unpleasant or inconvenient*: A drug may taste bitter or be painful to administer.
- *Disease denial:* Not taking a medication may be a way to avoid accepting a diagnosis.

WFE: The root *here* in "adherence" means "stick," so **adhere** means "stick to" (*ad~* = "to").
*& Some seeds are dispersed by **adhering** to the feet of birds.*
*& Japan **adheres** to a policy of not possessing nuclear weapons, not producing them, and not allowing them to be brought into Japan.*

　Another word with this root is **coherent** (*co~* → *com~* = "together"). A **coherent argument** is one that "sticks together" (i.e., it is logical and consistent). This root is also found **inherent**, which means "being a natural or basic part of something."

*& That small island is considered by X country to be an **inherent** part of its territorial integrity. However, neighboring Y country also asserts that the island is an inherent part of its territory. Such territorial disputes need to be peacefully resolved or they can lead to war.*

The phrase "**territorial integrity**," in the above sentence, refers to the "oneness" or "wholeness" of a country's territory. If you keep up with international news in English, you will no doubt come across this phrase. In medical contexts, **integrity** means "completeness." In UC, inflammation and the formation of ulcers impairs **mucosal integrity** ("completeness or wholeness of the mucosa"), which adversely effects the barrier function of the intestinal wall. The root *teg* means "touch," and *in~* means "not," so integrity means "not touching/not whole." Integrity is an example of a word that is used in both medical English and everyday English. The more frequent, everyday use of the word means "honest and having strong moral principles."

*& Men and women who enter politics should have **integrity**, but the fact there are corruption scandals involving politicians suggests that some don't.*

Variations of *teg* are found in many words including **contact**, **contagious**, and **tangible**.

Finally, a variation of the root *here* (to stick) is *hes*, found in the words such as **adhesive** and **hesitate**.

*& When I have a small cut, I sometimes use a topical skin **adhesive**, a medical glue that closes a wound.*

*& I often tell my students this: "There's no such thing as a stupid question; questions show that you are thinking. Do not to **hesitate** to ask me any question at any time."*

2) Adverse reactions: The words **side effect** and **adverse reaction** are often used **interchangeably**, but they have different meanings. One key difference is that side effects can be desirable and therapeutic, but adverse reactions are never desired or therapeutic. Adverse reactions are considered more severe than side effects. Also, while side effects are expected and are often **dose dependent**, an adverse reaction is not expected and can occur at any dose. I saw at firsthand a desirable side effect. When my father was taking **finasteride**, a drug to treat **benign prostatic hyperplasia** (noncancerous enlargement of the prostate gland), it caused new hair to grow on his head. Where he had once been bald, hair was regrowing. **Adverse** is used in general English to mean "unfavorable" or "harmful."

*& I decided to get the train rather than drive because of the **adverse** driving conditions caused by the typhoon.*

WFE: The root *vers* (and variations *vert*, *vers*, *vors*) is from the Latin *vertere*, meaning "to turn." Adverse means "turn towards" (*ad~* = "towards"). Other words with this root include **convert** (*con~* → *com* = "together"), **extrovert** (lit. "turn outwards"), **introvert** (lit. "turn inwards"), **advert** ("turn [your attention] towards"), **universe** (lit. "turned into one"), and **divorce** (*di~* = "apart"; "turn away from each other").

3) *Colonoscopy* **is a procedure in which a flexible medical instrument is inserted through the anus into the colon in order to examine the colon for abnormalities and disease.** In Japan, to help patients relax and to reduce discomfort, a colonoscopy is usually done with the patient under light **sedation**; however, in the USA, colonoscopies are often carried out under full **anesthesia**. The length of a **colonoscope**, the instrument used in a colonoscopy, is 170 cm and its diameter is 1cm. A **sigmoidoscope** looks similar to a colonoscope, but it is shorter (70 cm) because it is designed only to examine the lower colon. Another name for colonoscopy is **lower GI endoscopy**. The lower GI (gastrointestinal) tract runs from the small intestine to the anus. (The **upper GI tract** includes the mouth, esophagus, stomach, and the duodenum.) An **endoscope** is the general name for an optical instrument that is used to look inside the body (*endo~* = "inside").

The small intestine is more difficult to examine than the colon. This is because the small intestine is around four times longer than the colon (around 6.5 meters, compared to 1.5 meters), and is much narrower (it is named "small" because of its smaller diameter, around 5cm, compared to the large intestine, which has a diameter of around 10cm). The large intestine is also straighter than the small intestine, which is highly **coiled** and has many bends. But it is possible to examine the small intestine using a **small bowel endoscopy**, in which the endoscope is moved through the small intestine with the help of a balloon.

With **capsule endoscopy** doctors can visualize the whole of the digestive system, including the small intestine, in a way that is easy and painless for the patient. Capsule endoscopy was approved by the FDA in 2000, and it has been covered by the Japanese health insurance since 2014. All the patient needs to do is swallow a capsule that is about the size of a large vitamin tablet. As the capsule travels along the GI tract, a camera in the capsule takes pictures. The pictures are transmitted to an external recording device. The capsule leaves the body when you do a poo. The capsule is **disposable**, so it does not have to be **retrieved** from the toilet. A disadvantage of capsule endoscopy is that **biopsies** cannot be taken,

WFE: In the word colonoscope, the root *scope* is from the Latin *specere*, meaning "to look at/observe." So, a colonoscope is an instrument to "look at the colon." Variations of the "*scope*" root are *spect* (e.g., **spectator**, **inspect**, **prospect**, and **suspect**; *sus~* = "under"; Lit "look under"), *spic* (e.g., **conspicuous**), and *spis* (e.g., **despise**; lit. "look down on"). *Scope* is found in **microscope**, **telescope**, and **horoscope** (*horo* = "hour"; Lit. "observe the hour [of a person's birth]"). "Scope" itself is also a word meaning "extent" or "opportunity/possibility to do something."

& Pharmacists in the USA can give vaccinations, take blood samples, and prescribe certain medications. In Japan, pharmacists are not permitted to do these things. There are calls in Japan to expand pharmacists' ***scope*** *of practice.*

& Do you understand the ***scope*** *of extinction being caused by humans? Humans are now*

*driving one million **species** to extinction.* (<u>speci</u>es → *spek* = "look"; animals that belong to the same species "look similar in form")

Biopsy literally means "view of the living" (*opsy* = "to see/view"). **Autopsy**, an examination of a dead body to find out the cause of death, literally means "view for oneself." A variation of *opsy* is the root *opt*, found words such as **optic** and **optician**.

SD 3A: Evidence-Based Medicine

For several years I have had almost no symptoms of UC. Doctors would say that I am in remission. My symptoms improved after a gastroenterologist, a Dr T, at Nagoya City University Hospital put me on a new course of treatment. Until then I had been taking Pentasa tablets daily and using a steroid enema when symptoms worsened. Dr T suggested that I should change to a combination of oral Pentasa and Pentasa enema. He explained that when Pentasa is taken orally, the medication reaches the proximal colon (the first and middle part of the colon), but not much drug is able to act on the wall of the distal colon (the last part of the colon) and rectum. However, adding a Pentasa enema would enable the medication to cover the wall of rectum and distal colon. Dr T drew a little diagram showing how combined oral and enema treatment "attacked" the colon with Pentasa from both ends, allowing the drug to cover the whole of the colon. I followed Dr T's recommendation, and after a few months of this therapy, rectal bleeding and other symptoms of UC had gone. Did Dr T recommend that I change my treatment just because he "had a feeling" that it could work? No, his decision was based on evidence from clinical research. Dr T showed me this 2005 article from a medical journal.

Combined oral and enema treatment with Pentasa (mesalazine) is superior to oral therapy alone in patients with extensive mild/moderate active ulcerative colitis: a randomised, double blind, placebo-controlled study. *Gut*, 54(7), 960–965.

Dr T had adopted Evidence-Based Medicine (EBM), an approach to medicine in which doctors and other health care professionals use the best current evidence from medical research to help them make decisions about the treatment of patients. I am very grateful that Dr T kept his eyes on the latest research. Talking of "eyes," the word "evidence" is from the Latin *videre*, meaning "to see" (so it is related in meaning to "scope," explained in E3). The prefix *e~* (from *ex~*), means "out," so, evidence literally means "seen easily from the outside" (i.e., "obvious/apparent"). The root *vid* and its variant *vis* are in many common words; for example: **video**, **provide** ("see before"), **divide** ("see apart"), **supervise** ("look around from above"), and **improvise** (*im~* = "not"+ *pre~* ="before"; lit. "unable to see in advance").

4) *Digestion* is the breaking down of food by the digestive system into a form that can be absorbed and used by the body.

WFE: Digest literally means "carry apart" (*di~* = "apart" + *gest* = "to carry"). The WFE *gest* is found in words such as **ingest** (lit.= "to carry into"); **congestion** (lit.= "carry/bring together"); and **indigestion** (*in~* = "not"). Indigestion is not a specific disease, but a term for various symptoms such as **epigastric pain,** or pain in the area of the upper abdomen (*epi~* =

"upon/above"), **acid reflux**, and feeling **bloated**. Indigestion can have various causes such as stress and anxiety, eating too fast, overeating, and eating foods that do not agree with you. Indigestion is not usually something to worry about, but persistent indigestion can be a symptom of an underlying illness. The medical term for indigestion is **dyspepsia** (*dys~* = "bad/difficult" + *peps*, from *peptos*, the Greek word for "digest"). **Pepsin**, an enzyme in gastric juice that digests proteins, is so called because it aids digestion.

A **digest** is a summary of something such as the news. Just as food is divided and separated in the stomach and intestine, so is the information in a digest. There are many news-digest sites on the internet. As a verb, digest also means "to think carefully and reflect on so as to understand better."

& *It is not good to leave test revision until the last minute. You need time to **digest** all the information that you have learnt so that you can really understand it deeply.*

& *Queen Elizabeth II died at the age of 96 on September 8, 2022. She had been on the throne for 70 years, and many British people needed time to **digest** the reality that she was no longer there.*

5) Embarrassing accidents: You have no doubt heard the word "accident" used in phrases such as "traffic accident" and "drop by accident." However, it can also be used as a **euphemism** for when a person urinates or **defecates** in a way that is not controlled or involuntary. A euphemism is a way to refer to something that is embarrassing, unpleasant or offensive in a softer, more pleasant way (*eu~* = "good" + *phem* = "to say"). For example, "She is big boned" is less offensive than "She is fat," and "I have to let you go" is a softer way to say "I have to fire you." A "**bucket list**" is a list of the things you want to do before dying. It comes from "**kick the bucket**," which is a euphemistic expression for "to die." Another euphemism for dying is "pass away" or just "pass."

& *John's grandfather passed last night.*

The medical term for when bowel movements cannot be controlled is **fecal incontinence**. Causes of fecal incontinence include muscle or nerve damage, neurological disease, and childbirth. In IBD, fecal incontinence is usually due to inflammation in the rectum and diarrhea (watery stools are more difficult to hold in the rectum than solid stools).

WFE: The root *cid* (e.g., **acc<u>id</u>ent**) and *cas* are from the Latin for "to fall" (*cadere*). These roots are found in many words such as **coincidence, case,** and **incidence**. In the sentence "*the incidence of IBD is increasing in Japan,*" "incidence" is the rate at which people develop a condition during a particular time period (e.g., in one year). However, it might help to think of incidence as meaning the number of new patients "falling on (= *in~*)" Japan in a year.

In the Essay, I wrote that the amount of meat eaten in Japan increased over the same period that the incidence of IBD rose. However, we cannot assume that there is a **causal association** between meat consumption and IBD. That meat consumption and IBD both increased together could just be a **coincidence** (lit. "fall together"; *com~*, meaning "together," is reduced to *co~* before vowels). During the same period that IBD cases increased, the percentage of students going to university in Japan increased from 10% in 1962 to around 55% in 2022, but nobody is suggesting that there is a causal relationship between university enrollment rates and the incidence of IBD. It is unlikely that increased meat consumption alone caused the increase in IBD, but an increase in meat consumption in many countries has also been accompanied by a rise in the consumption of highly processed foods (typically high in fat, sugar and salt), and a decrease in the amount of fiber being consumed (in the form of fresh fruit and vegetables). What a person eats alters the composition of the intestinal microbiota, and changes in the microbiota could well be a factor in the pathogenesis of IBD.

6) ***Gastroenteritis* is inflammation of the lining of the intestines caused by an infection by a pathogen.** Symptoms include **abdominal cramps**, **vomiting**, and **diarrhea**.
WFE: The word diarrhea contains the prefix *dia~* (= "through") and the suffix *~rrhea* (= "flow"); so, diarrhea literally means "to flow through." This suffix is found in other medical words such as **rhinorrhea**, more commonly known as a runny nose (*rhino* = "nose"), and **dysmenorrhea**, or painful menstrual periods (*meno* = "month"). **Verbal diarrhea** is not an illness, but an expression that means "speaking too much."

The suffix *~itis* in gastroenteritis means "inflammation," and the root *entero* is from the Greek *enteron*, meaning the "intestine." The **enteric nervous system** is the nervous system in the walls of the gastrointestinal tract. Some oral medications have an **enteric coating**, a chemical compound applied to a pill or tablet that protects against gastric acid, thereby preventing the active ingredient from being released until it enters the small intestine.

When talking about different routes by which medication can be administered, the word **parenteral** means "introduced into the body in a way that is not via the digestive system." An insulin injection is an example of **parenteral administration** because insulin is directly put into the bloodstream (rather than being absorbed into the bloodstream from the digestive tract after being swallowed). An inhaler delivers medication for asthma straight into the lungs, another example of parenteral administration. **Parenteral nutrition** is giving nutrition to a person intravenously. There are some cases where a person requires all nutrition to be given parenterally. This called **total parenteral nutrition** (TPN). The prefix in *para~* in parenteral means "beside" (a drug enters the body "besides" the GI tract, not via it).

7) *Interspersed* **means having something in several places among something else.**
℮ One of the features of CD is that the inflammation is patchy; that is, inflamed areas are ***interspersed*** *between healthy areas of the gut. In UC, the inflammation is usually continuous.*

*℮ Cells called the islets of Langerhans, which secrete insulin and glucagon, are **interspersed** within the exocrine tissue of the pancreas.*

*℮ The farmland was **interspersed** with small fragments of remaining forest.*

WFE: The prefix *inter~* means "between" and the root *sper* (and variations *spar*, *spor*) means to "spread out/scatter." Here are some examples of words with this root:

*℮ During the COVID-19 pandemic, health authorities encouraged people to open windows. This is because fresh air from the outside helps to quickly **disperse** viruses and prevent them lingering in the room. (dis~ = "apart")*

*℮ With a population density of 3 people per square kilometer, Australia is one of the most **sparsely** populated countries in the world.*

*℮ The world's largest community of people of Japanese descent is in Brazil. However, Brazil is only one part of the Japanese **diaspora**, or the spread of people of Japanese ancestry throughout the world. (dia~ = "across"; so, diaspora means "spread/scattered across")*

*℮ Some diseases of the lungs are caused by inhaling fungal **spores**.*

*℮ **Sperm** is produced in the **testicles**. A man's testicles make several million sperm each day.*

8) *Malabsorption* is a condition caused by the decreased ability to absorb nutrients from food. In IBD, an inflamed small intestine can impair the absorption of nutrients. For example, inflammation of the **ileum** (the lower part of the intestine), which is common in CD, often impedes the proper absorption of **vitamin B12**. Vitamin B12 is important for the synthesis of red blood cells, and a deficiency of this vitamin can lead to **pernicious anemia**. Malabsorption is one cause of **malnutrition** in IBD, especially CD. Malnutrition occurs when the diet does not contain the right amount or balance of nutrients. Signs of malnutrition in people with IBD include weight loss, slow healing of wounds, and fatigue.

WFE: The prefix *mal-* has a negative meaning of "abnormal/bad/wrong/evil." **Malaria** is from the Italian *mal aria*, which literally means "bad air." Until the middle of the 19th century (when the **miasma theory** was replaced by the **Germ theory** of diseases), it was thought that dirty air was the cause of the disease. In 1898, it was discovered that mosquitoes transmit the microscopic **protozoa** that cause malaria. The word **malaise** contains the WFE *~aise,* which is from "ease." Therefore, malaise means "not at ease," or having a general feeling of "discomfort" or "feeling unwell."

*℮ The initial symptoms of Ebola are non-specific and include flu-like symptoms such as fever, myalgia, and general **malaise**.*

The French word for "sick" is *malade*, and the English word **malady** can also mean a physical disease, although it is more often used figuratively to mean "a serious problem."

*℮ Opioid addiction is a serious social **malady** facing the USA.*

Malignant literally means "giving birth to badness" (*~gnant* comes from the WFE *gene*), but it can be defined as "tending to cause death or deterioration." A **malignant tumor** is another way to say "cancer." A word coined in the 1990s is **malware,** which is short for "malicious software."

The word **odor** means "a smell" (as in **deodorant**), and **malodorous** means "bad smell."

*& As the policeman opened the door, he was hit by **malodorous** wall of air. The old man had been lying dead in apartment for weeks. The policeman went home that night feeling **nauseous** and sad that such kodokushi (孤独死), or solitary deaths, are increasingly common in Japan.*

("Nauseous" is the adjective form of the noun "nausea." It is from the Latin for "seasickness." The root *neu* means "ship"; and an **astro<u>naut</u>** is a person who travels on a "star ship.")

Here are four more examples of words with the prefix *mal~*:

*& If taken during pregnancy, some drugs can cause fetal **malformations**.*

*& The doctor accidentally administered the patient an overdose of medicine, which led to the man's death. His family is now suing the doctor for medical **malpractice**.*

*& An electrical **malfunction** caused the fire that broke out in the elementary school.*

*& Yusuke was doing really well at high school, but he became addicted to video games and was unable to focus on his studies. His parents tried everything to get him to spend less time playing on his smartphone, but they couldn't. As expected, Yusuke got **dismal** results in his university entrance exams. (dis~ = "day"; lit. "evil day")*

9) *Metaplasia:* When I did weight training, I used to get thick **calluses** on the palms of my hands. These calluses were a result of skin cells increasing in number as a response to the friction caused by frequently lifting weights. This increase in the number of cells is called **hyperplasia** and is a normal **physiological** response. While hyperplasia is simply an increase in cell number, **metaplasia** is a process in which one cell type changes into a different type (or form) of cell. Metaplasia is often induced by some sort of abnormal stimulus, such as prolonged irritation or inflammation. In response to this abnormal stimulus, the cells in the exposed tissue change into a type of cell that is more **robust**, and thus more able to protect the tissue against that stimulus. In other words, metaplasia is an **adaptive response**. Although the metaplastic cells are better suited to withstand the abnormal stimulus, metaplasia may result in cells that have are at a greater risk of becoming cancerous.

An example of metaplasia is a condition called **Barrett's esophagus.** The lining (epithelium) of the esophagus is composed of **simple squamous cells**. These are flat cells that provide a smooth surface to help swallowed food pass easily into the stomach. However, in some people, gastric acid moves from the stomach and back into the esophagus. The squamous cells are easily damaged by this **acid reflux**, and they respond to the acid by changing into another type of cell called **simple columnar cells**. These simple columnar cells are the same as those lining the stomach, and they are more resistant to stomach acid. So, the change of esophageal cells into the same cells that are in the stomach is an adaptation to protect the esophagus (which is not normally exposed to a low pH) from gastric acid reflux. Unfortunately, the metaplastic replacement of squamous epithelium to columnar epithelium also increases the risk of **esophageal cancer**. In IBD, chronic inflammation is the abnormal stimulus that can induce metaplasia of intestinal cells.

Dysplasia is when cells change in a way that makes them abnormal. Dysplasia is not the same as cancer, but the abnormal changes in cells greatly increase the risk of developing cancer. In simple terms, metaplasia can be a **precursor** to dysplasia, and dysplasia can, in some cases, become cancer.

WFE: The root *plasia~* means "molding/formation." From this root we get the words **plasma** and **plastic**. The literal meaning of hyperplasia, dysplasia, and metaplasia are, respectively, "over formation," "abnormal formation," and "change in formation." Incidentally, doctors sometimes refer to changes in cells that suggest a **neoplasm** (lit. "new growth" = cancer) as "**sinister pathology**." The original Latin meaning of sinister is "left." It used to be thought that left-handed people were bad luck or even evil.

Let's now focus on *meta~*. This prefix has a wide range of meanings. It can indicate a change, as in **metaplasia** ("change in formation"), and **metamorphosis** ("change in shape or form"; *morph* = "form"), and **metabolism** (the chemical processes in the body). In the Essay, I wrote the expression "a tide of anxiety swept through me." This is an example of a **metaphor** (anxiety is compared to a tide). The prefix *meta~* means "over" and *phor* is "carry," so metaphor means "to carry the characteristics of one thing over to another thing." *Meta~* can also mean "beyond." In 2021, the American company Facebook changed its name to Meta. It was reported that this renaming was to signal that the company went *beyond* a single product and was working to "move *beyond*" what is possible today. An increasingly common use of meta is to indicate that something is referring to or describing the same thing. So, a meta-joke refers to another joke, and **metadata** provides information about other data. A **meta-analysis** uses statistical methods to analyze the data from multiple studies. By combining many smaller studies into one big meta-analysis, the total sample size is increased, which increases the accuracy of the results.

10) Paradox: A *paradox* is a situation that is difficult to understand because it contains two parts that seem to contradict, or be opposite, to each other.

*ℰ During 2020 people were talking about the "Japan **paradox**" in relation to COVID-19. Why were there relatively few people dying from the disease, despite Japan having loose restrictions compared to the UK and other countries? Various factors were suggested such as good general hygiene practices of the population, high acceptance of mask wearing, customs such as not shaking hands or hugging, and a lower prevalence of obesity.*

*& There is a **paradoxical** aspect to air conditioning because it can protect against heat stroke and other effects of climate change, but it also contributes to climate change.*

In relation to IBD, the "smoking paradox" refers to evidence that smoking tobacco appears protective against developing UC, but it is a risk factor for CD. The fact that smoking seems to protect against UC could also be considered a paradox, considering that smoking is a major risk factor for a number of cancers and is very harmful in other ways. It has been suggested that **nicotine**, the active ingredient in tobacco, offers some protection against UC. The way nicotine does this is not clear, but there is some evidence that it decreases the synthesis of pro-inflammatory **interleukins** (a type of cytokine) and increases the thickness of the protective mucus in the intestine wall.

It would, however, be crazy to start smoking because of the small chance that it may lower your risk of UC. The huge proven risks of smoking greatly outweigh the small possibility of a benefit. If I had become hooked on tobacco smoking in my early 20s—and it's easy to get hooked because nicotine is said be the third most addictive drug, after heroin and crack cocaine—it is possible that this could have protected me against UC. However, it is very much more likely that I would have developed a tobacco-induced disease. Having said this, it is important to conduct research into the mechanisms by which smoking appears to protect against UC because it may help to increase our understanding of IBD and lead to the development of new drugs.

A "**paradoxical drug reaction**" is when a drug has an effect that is the opposite to what would be expected. For example, the pharmacological effect of morphine is to relieve pain, but in some people, it paradoxically increases sensitivity to pain (this is called **opioid-induced hyperalgesia**). And a class of antidepressant drugs called **selective serotonin reuptake inhibitors** (SSRIs) are meant to treat depression, but they can actually worsen depression in some people, especially at the beginning of treatment.

WFE: The prefix *para~* has many meanings, including "beyond" (e.g., **paranormal**), and "besides" (e.g., the **parathyroids glands** are besides, or adjacent to, the thyroid gland). It can also mean "abnormal"; for example, **paralgesia** is an abnormal sensitivity to pain (*algia*) and **parosmia** is a distorted sense of smell (*osme* = "smell"; *~ia* = "condition"). In **paradox**, *para~* means "opposite to," and the root *doxa* means "opinion." A view or idea that is **orthodox** is one that is considered to be correct and is held by most people. A belief or idea that is different from what is generally accepted is called a **heterodoxy** (*hetero* = "different").

*& Nicolaus Copernicus (1473-1543) proposed that the Earth revolved around the sun. This was a **heterodoxy** at a time when the **orthodox view** was that the Earth was the center of the universe.*

Orthodox also means "traditional."

*& **Orthodox Jews** follow more traditional beliefs and adhere to stricter rules than non-orthodox Jews.*

11) Vitamin K and vitamin D deficiency: A *vitamin deficiency* occurs if there is a lack of a vitamin over an extended period of time. A vitamin deficiency can be primary or secondary. **Primary vitamin deficiency** is when not enough of a certain vitamin is consumed in the diet. For example, a student who eats nothing but cup noodles (and no fresh fruit or vegetables) for several months could develop primary vitamin C deficiency. **Secondary vitamin deficiency** is when the vitamin shortage is due to an underlying disease; for example, people with chronic liver disease can suffer from secondary vitamin D deficiency (the liver has an important role in vitamin D metabolism). People with IBD are prone to vitamin deficiencies for several reasons:

* Inflammation of the small intestine in CD interferes with the absorption of nutrients from the **lumen** of the intestine into **enterocytes** (cells of the intestinal lining). This poor absorption (**malabsorption**) can lead to nutritional deficiency.

* Gut bacteria are involved in the synthesis and absorption of several vitamins, so imbalances of the microbiota in IBD could contribute to deficiencies.

* Some medications for IBD can also affect vitamin levels; for example, a side effect of oral corticosteroids is vitamin D deficiency.

* Severe diarrhea causes the loss of fluids together with nutrients and electrolytes (e.g., sodium, and potassium), and rectal bleeding can lead to iron deficiency.

* The abdominal pain and nausea that is common in IBD can reduce appetite, making it more difficult for people to eat enough food to maintain good health.

* People with IBD sometimes require a **resection** (i.e., surgical removal of part of the intestine). Resection reduces the surface area of the intestine available for absorption.

WFE: The word "deficiency" contains the prefix *de~*. This prefix has several meanings. Here are just three:

* **To reverse or undo an action; examples:**

<u>de</u>activate *& Enzymes are **deactivated** by high temperatures.*

<u>de</u>clutter *& I had too much stuff in my room that I did not need. After watching a video on the "KonMari Method," I decided to **declutter** my room.*

<u>de</u>hydration *& Diarrhea can be especially dangerous in children because it can quickly cause dehydration. A loss of body fluid decreases the blood volume, and in severe cases can lead to life-threatening shock.*

<u>de</u>frost: *& If you freeze a turkey, you will need to **defrost** it before you put it in the oven.*

* **To take or move away** (e.g., <u>de</u>duct, <u>de</u>lete, <u>de</u>part, <u>de</u>bilitating, <u>de</u>ficiency)

  *& **AIDS** is an acronym for Acquired Immune **Deficiency** Syndrome.*

* **To go down or make less** (e.g., decrease; demote, **devalue**)

  *& A few months after the Russian invasion of Ukraine, the National Bank of Ukraine **devalued** the country's currency, the Hryvnia, by 25% against the U.S Dollar.*

The root *val* in "devalue" is from the Latin *valere*, meaning "strength/worth." This root is in words such as e**qui**valent, **val**id, **val**uable, and **pre**valence. The adjective **prevalent** means "common/widespread."

*& **Scurvy** is a debilitating disease caused by an absence of vitamin C in the diet for around 3 or more months. Vitamin C is vital for the formation of collagen, and a chronic lack of vitamin C causes the destruction of connective tissue and leads to symptoms such as lethargy, bleeding gums, wounds that do not heal, skin ulcers, and joint and muscle aches. During the 18th century, scurvy was so **prevalent** in British sailors that it killed more sailors than were killed fighting the enemy. From around 1800, sailors in the British navy started to be given a daily ration of lemon juice and the incidence of scurvy declined dramatically.*

The root *fic* in deficiency means "make/do." Variations of this root are *fict*, *fact,* and *fect*; for example: **suf**fi**cient**, **ef**fi**cient**, **pro**fit, **manu**fac**ture**, and **per**fect (*per~* = "through"; *fect* = "make"; lit. "to make completely").

Many people think that the fax machine is completely **obsolete** (outdated), but it is still quite widely used in Japan. For example, when I go to the hospital every few months, my prescription is sent from the hospital to my local pharmacy by fax machine. "Fax" is short for **fac**simile (lit. "to make similar").

SD 3B: Is vitamin C vital for all?

What do humans, other **primates**, fruit bats, and **guinea pigs** have in common? Answer: They are the only mammals that are unable to synthesize vitamin C. This means they must get vitamin C from their diet in order to prevent **scurvy**, which, as you read in E11, is a potentially fatal disease caused by vitamin C deficiency. Humans cannot make vitamin C because of a mutation in a certain a gene that is required in the complex pathway that biosynthesizes vitamin C. **Natural selection** favors traits that are advantageous to survival, but losing the ability to synthesize vitamin C does not appear to help survival. Why then has natural selection allowed this mutation to be passed on through the generations in humans (and some other mammals)? There are various interesting theories that you can check out on the internet (suggested **search query**: "why did human lose the ability to make vitamin C"). Rats, cats, and all other mammals have the ability to synthesize vitamin C in the liver, which is why you don't need to give orange juice to your pet dog or cat! However, a dog or cat with liver disease can suffer from vitamin C deficiency.

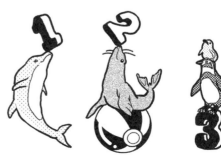

3-3 Dozen in Detail (D) （12 の話題を詳しく）

1) *Anecdotal:* In everyday English, an **anecdote** is a short story that is often amusing. **Anecdotal evidence** is evidence from personal experience. For example, since I started to regularly eat *natto* (fermented soy beans) around five years ago my UC symptoms have improved. I told my gastroenterologist about this and he was interested, but based just on the experience of a single patient, he could not start recommending a "*natto diet*" to people with IBD. To find out if *natto* really did improve IBD symptoms, a well-run **randomized controlled trial (RCT)** would be necessary. Anecdotal evidence provides only weak evidence compared to an RCT, which has a much greater strength of evidence. Anecdotes are not always reliable, but this does not mean that anecdotal evidence is of no value. For example, being told a similar anecdote by several patients could encourage a doctor to start asking questions, and this could eventually lead to a **quantitative study**.

SD 3C: "The Dose Makes the Poison"

The word **anecdote** literally means "something unpublished." The *dote* part of the word is from the Greek root *do*, meaning to give. This root is in two words that appear elsewhere in this book. The first is **antidote**, which literally means "give against." An antidote is a medicine that is given to counteract a poison. Okinawa, Japan's southernmost prefecture, is home to a venomous snake called a *habu* (pit viper). If you are bitten by a *habu*, it is important to get to hospital quickly so that you can be given an antidote. The other word is **dose**. This is the amount of a drug that is prescribed to be taken. In the 15th century, a Swiss doctor called Paracelsus wrote the following: "All things are poison and nothing is without poison; only the dose makes a thing not a poison." This is a very important concept in pharmacology and toxicology. This means that any chemical can be toxic if too much of it is ingested or absorbed into the body. Oxygen and water can be toxic, and, if given in overdose, an antidote itself can become a poison.

2) *Analgesics* are drugs that can relieve pain. Many of you are probably familiar with **NSAIDs** such as **aspirin** and **ibuprofen**. NSAIDs stands for nonsteroidal anti-inflammatory drugs. They are so called because they reduce inflammation as **corticosteroids** do, but they are not related to corticosteroids. Another popular analgesic is **acetaminophen** (called **paracetamol** in the UK), but because it has little or no anti-inflammatory action, it is not usually classed as an NSAID.

Opioid analgesics such as **morphine** provide stronger pain medication and are effective for relieving cancer pain and for chest pain from **myocardial infarction** (commonly called heart attack). However, the use of opioids to treat chronic pain can lead to serious addiction problems. In the USA, misuse of opioids has killed many people in the last few decades. In 2018, out of the 70,000 people who died from drug overdoses in the USA, 68% of these deaths were caused by an opioid (to find out more, search for "**US opioid epidemic**"). Another drug with analgesic properties is **cannabis**, which has been shown to be effective in treating some types of chronic pain. (Medical use of cannabis is currently not permitted in Japan, although this may change in the future.)

If you have had a tooth pulled out by a dentist, the dentist probably injected something into your gums to stop you feeling pain. What is injected at the dentist is not an analgesic but a **local anesthetic**. The difference between the two is that an anesthetic not only blocks pain but also causes a loss of **sensation.** An NSAID will not have this effect on sensation. In fact, the word **anesthesia** is from the Greek "without sensation." A patient under **general anesthesia** loses **consciousness** as well as all sensation.

SD 3D: The pain of homesickness

The word **analgesic** is made up from the prefix *an~* ("without"), *algesia* ("pain") and the suffix *~ic* used to from adjectives. The word **nostalgia** (ノスタルジー) also contains the root for pain. The WFE *nostos* means "homecoming." Nostalgia was **coined** in the 17th century and originally meant a painful longing for one's native country. We would now call this "homesickness."

SD 3E What's the point of chronic pain?

If you sprain your ankle, it will hurt and you will not be able to walk without a lot of pain. This pain is your body saying, "Your ligaments are damaged, take a rest to let the ligaments heal." The pain after this kind of injury is **acute pain**. It serves a valuable role and usually lasts a short time. Acute pain goes away once the body has healed or when the cause of the damage has gone. On the other hand, **chronic pain** continues even after the body has healed itself or the cause of the pain is no longer there. Importantly, chronic pain serves no useful purpose. Chronic pain is often defined as pain lasting more than 3 months. Because long-term use of analgesics can lead to drug dependence and other problems, there is now more emphasis on **non-pharmacological pain therapy** (interventions such as yoga, physical therapy, and **acupuncture** that do not involve medications).

Pain is a common symptom of IBD, with up to 70% of IBD patients reporting abdominal pain. People with IBD can experience both acute and chronic pain. The most common cause of acute pain is active inflammation in the intestines. Chronic abdominal pain can result from the scar tissue causing **strictures** (narrowing) of the gut lumen. Other causes of chronic pain are **visceral hypersensitivity** (increased sensitivity of the nerves in the gut causing a lower **pain threshold**), and pain from **extraintestinal complications** such as inflamed joints. Partly because of the **gut-brain axis** (the nerve connections between the gut and the brain), people with IBD are more likely to experience psychological stress, anxiety, and depression, all of which can heighten the perception of pain.

3) *Association does not prove causation* **means that an association (correlation) between two events does not necessarily mean that one event has caused the other**. Many studies have now determined beyond a doubt that there is a **causal relationship** between smoking tobacco and lung cancer (which is not surprising considering that tobacco is highly toxic and contains at least 60 chemicals that are known to be **carcinogenic**). However, before scientific evidence proving the dangers of tobacco became overwhelming, tobacco companies blamed the increase in lung cancer from the 1940s not on the increase in smoking, but on other factors that had increased in the same period of time. These factors included dust from newly tarred roads and industrial air pollution. For many years, tobacco companies fought to protect their profits by arguing that the association between smoking and lung cancer did not prove causation.

4) *Autoimmune disease* **occurs when the body's immune system mistakenly attacks healthy body tissue**. The immune system is able to distinguish between **self** (the body's own cells) and **non-self** (such as invading pathogens and cancer cells). How the immune system does this is complex, but it involves **antigens** on the surface of cells (an antigen is a substance, often a protein, that triggers the immune system to produce antibodies). These antigens act as labels. The immune system "checks out" these labels and decides whether or not to attack. Cells with **self-antigens** do not initiate an immune response and are left alone, but **non-self-antigens** on the surface of a bacterium, for example, do initiate one. As part of this immune response, invading bacteria are attacked and destroyed.

The ability of the immune system to recognize self-antigens as not being a threat and leaving them alone, while directing an immune response against non self-antigens is called **self-tolerance**. An autoimmune disease occurs when an immune response is directed against self-antigens. In other words, self-tolerance breaks down and the immune system (specifically, B and T lymphocytes) "sees" the body's own antigens as a threat and attacks them. There are over 100 autoimmune diseases, including **type 1 diabetes**, **rheumatoid arthritis**, and **multiple sclerosis**. The immune response is vital to protect the body, but the damage caused in autoimmune diseases shows that the immune system can be **a double-edged sword**.

SD 3F: What's your blood type?

Self-antigens are very important in **blood transfusions**. Antigens are on the surface of all cells, including red blood cells (RBCs). A person should only receive a blood transfusion from donor blood with the same type of antigen. If the antigens on the donated RBCs have a surface antigen that are recognized as non-self, the immune system will produce antibodies against these foreign antigens and trigger what is called an **incompatibility reaction**. My blood type is B. If I was mistakenly given a transfusion of blood type A, the anti-A antibodies in my blood would attack and destroy the new RBCs (this destruction of blood cells is called

hemolysis). Such acute **hemolytic transfusion reactions** can be fatal, but they are rare because blood of both donor and recipient is carefully checked.

In organ donations too, the blood type of the donor must be compatible with the recipient. Transplants between people with incompatible blood types is one cause of **organ rejection**. In 2022, researchers successfully altered the blood type of donor kidneys (to find out about how the researchers did this, and the implications of this breakthrough for organ transplantation, do an Internet search: "Cambridge university + alter blood type + kidney").

5) *Constipation* is when bowel movements become less frequent and passing stools becomes more difficult ("pass a stool" and "bowel movement" are euphemisms for "defecate"). Of course, the frequency of bowel movements varies a lot from person to person, so what is considered "less frequent" will depend on the person. But fewer than three bowel movements a week would typically be diagnosed as constipation. Constipation often occurs when what we have **ingested** moves too slowly through the digestive tract. The colon functions to absorb water from waste, so the more time the waste stays in colon, the more time there is for water to be absorbed. Spending too much time inside the colon causes the stool to become dry, hard, and difficult to push out. A person with constipation may experience associated symptoms such as **abdominal cramps** and **bloating**.

An increase in **colonic transit time** (i.e., the time it takes for waste to move through the colon) is often due to a decline in **gastrointestinal motility** (i.e., movements of the GI tract that mix and transport the food/waste within it). One key type of gut motility is **peristalsis**, which propels the food/waste along the GI tract. If peristalsis slows, absorption of water from stools increases. There are various causes of constipation, including:

- **A low fiber diet**: Dietary fiber is composed of **cellulose**, the complex carbohydrate in the cell walls of plants, which humans are unable to digest. Dietary fiber increases the size of the stool, thereby promoting peristalsis and speeding up the transit of food through the GI tract. Foods that are high in dietary fiber include fruit, vegetables, and legumes. Eating more fiber helps prevent constipation.
- **Irregular eating habits**: Eating meals at regular times can help prevent constipation.
- **Dehydration**: Drinking enough water keeps stools from drying out.
- **Lack of exercise**: Exercise, particularly aerobic exercise such as jogging, helps prevent constipation by speeding up transit time.
- **Ignoring the urge to defecate**: When stool moves into the rectum it stretches the wall of the rectum and triggers a **defecation reflex** (an urge to pass a stool). Ignoring or resisting the urge to pass a stool can cause the stool to accumulate in the rectum. A mass of dry, hard stool can become stuck in the rectum (**fecal impaction**). Also, ignoring the urge to defecate many times can result in the reflex becoming weaker or being lost altogether, resulting in long-term constipation.

- **Medicines**: Some drugs cause constipation as a side effect. Opioids such as morphine are well known for causing constipation. **Opioid-induced constipation** happens mainly because opioids bind to receptors in the GI tract resulting in reduced peristalsis.
- **Complete or partial obstruction**. For example, a **stricture** (narrowing) in a section of the intestine can occur in CD. A malignant tumor (i.e., cancer) in the colon can also obstruct or narrow the bowel, leading to slow or absent gut motility.

Medications to treat constipation are called **laxatives**. There are four main types: (1)**bulk forming**: contains fiber that soaks up water, making stools softer and bulkier. A larger stool stimulates peristalsis; (2)**stimulant**: irritates the lining of the intestine, which stimulates peristalsis; (3)**stool softeners**: soften stools and lubricates them so that they can be passed more easily; (4)**osmotic**: draws water into the stool by **osmosis** from surrounding tissues, making the stools softer. The type of laxative used will depend on the cause of the constipation. For example, a stimulant laxative is indicated for use in opioid-induced constipation, but should not be used if an intestinal obstruction is suspected. Laxatives should only be used if lifestyle changes have had no effect. Personally, I almost never get constipation because I eat a lot of fruit and vegetables, make sure I get enough sleep, and exercise regularly. If I do feel a bit blocked up, I eat a bowel of **prunes** with yogurt. Prunes, which are dried plums, have a laxative effect. Prunes will relax your bowels! (The root *lax* in laxative means "loose"; this root is also in the word "re**lax**").

6) *Diarrhea* **is the passage of loose or watery stools three or more times a day, or more frequently than is usual for that person**. Many people think diarrhea is just an inconvenient symptom of a cold or the manifestation of nervousness before an exam, but diarrhea and the severe dehydration it can cause is actually the second leading cause of death among children under the age of five in developing countries. Diarrhea is often a symptom of a GI tract infection. Viral and bacterial infections are the most common causes in high-income countries, but parasites are frequently responsible for diarrhea in parts of the world with poor **sanitation**. There are four main types of diarrhea.
- **Osmotic diarrhea**: Osmosis is the movement of water from a less concentrated solution to a more concentrated solution through a semi-permeable membrane. An increase in the concentration of solutes in the intestinal lumen will cause water to be drawn into the GI tract from the blood. Diarrhea will result if too much water collects in the intestinal lumen. One cause of osmotic diarrhea that I have experienced is eating too many prunes. Prunes contain **sorbitol**, a sugar alcohol that is difficult for the body to absorb. Sorbitol remains in the lumen, making the contents of the lumen **hypertonic** (i.e., having a greater osmotic pressure) compared to the surrounding tissue. A more serious, but much rarer

cause of osmotic diarrhea is damage to the pancreas. The exocrine cells of the pancreas produce enzymes that digest proteins, carbohydrates, and fats. If the production of these digestive enzymes is reduced or ceases, food cannot be completely digested or absorbed. As unabsorbed food passes along the GI tract, it draws water into the lumen by osmosis. Insufficient production of pancreatic enzymes often results from damage to the pancreas.

- **Secretory diarrhea**: This occurs when secretion of water into the lumen by intestinal epithelial cells exceeds the amount of water these cells absorb. **Cholera**, a bacterial infection, causes secretory diarrhea that is so severe it can kill within hours.

- **Exudative diarrhea**: Inflammation of the intestinal mucosa, for example in IBD, will result in fluid leaking out from the tissues (this fluid is called **exudate**). Consisting of mucus, blood and plasma protein, this exudate increases the fluid content of the stool, and also causes more water to move into the lumen by osmosis. Moreover, damage to the intestinal wall by inflammation makes it less able to absorb water, which adds to the amount of water that collects in the lumen.

- **Abnormal GI motility**: When the contents move too quickly through the GI tract, there is insufficient time for normal water reabsorption to take place. This increases the water content of the stool. **Hypermotility** (peristalsis that is too rapid) is associated with **irritable bowel syndrome,** or **IBS** for short (be careful not to confuse IBS with IBD).

Antidiarrheal medicines reduce diarrhea by slowing down peristalsis, resulting in food taking longer to move along the GI tract, and so allowing more water to be absorbed by the colon. One of the effects of **opioid drugs** is constipation. This occurs because activation of endogenous opioid receptors, called **μ-receptors** (pronounced "mu"), inhibits peristalsis. This bothersome side effect of opioids has actually been utilized therapeutically. **Loperamide** is a μ-receptor agonist (i.e., it stimulates these receptors) that is commonly used to treat diarrhea. Unlike other opioids, loperamide does not cross the blood-brain barrier, so it has minimal effects on the **central nervous system** (addiction to morphine and other opioids occurs due to their effects on the brain). It is important to remember that antidiarrheal medicines do not treat the underlying cause of the diarrhea. Also, in GI tract infections, diarrhea plays a crucial role in clearing the pathogens from the intestine. So, in certain cases, use of antidiarrheals could prolong an infection and actually be dangerous.

7) Digestive system: The function of the digestive system is to break down nutrients into parts that are small enough to be absorbed into the bloodstream and then used by body cells for energy, growth, and repair. The digestive system is made up of the **gastrointestinal tract (GI tract)**, as well as the **accessory organs of digestion** (i.e., salivary glands, pancreas, liver, and gallbladder). Accessory organs are not part of the GI tract, but they have essential roles in digestion. Around one hour ago I ate a delicious smoked salmon sandwich for lunch. What happened to that sandwich once I put it into my mouth, and what will happen to it over the following hours and days?

In my mouth, the sandwich was broken down using my teeth (this physical breakdown of food is called **mechanical digestion**). The **saliva** produced by the **salivary glands** in the mouth contains **mucus**, which acts as to **lubricate** and **bind** food so it can be easily swallowed. Saliva also contains **amylase**, an enzyme that breaks down starch into smaller carbohydrate molecules, so the chemical digestion of the bread actually began in my mouth. I then swallowed the **bolus**, the soft mass of the chewed food, moving it into the **esophagus**, a tube that carries the bolus of food to the stomach. The bolus was pushed towards the stomach by **peristalsis**, a series of wave-like contractions of the smooth muscle in the wall of digestive tract. These contractions start in the esophagus and occur throughout the GI tract. As well as moving food through the GI tract, peristalsis helps the digestion and absorption of food. Between the esophagus and the stomach is the **lower esophageal sphincter** (LOS), composed of a ring of muscle. Contraction of this muscle closes the opening to the stomach, thereby preventing the **reflux** of the stomach contents. The rest of the sandwich's journey through the GI tract, from stomach to anus, is summarized in Table 3.2.

SD 3G: Why nature often calls after eating

There are toilets in front of my university office. I have noticed that the time these toilets are busiest is between 12:30 to 13:00. Why the rush at this time? Could it be that the food students eat for lunch passes through the digestive system in around 30 minutes? Knowledge of the process of digestion would tell you that this is not a likely explanation (it usually takes over 24 hours for food to move through the digestive system). One reason that the toilets have most visitors soon after lunch is the **gastrocolic reflex**. When we eat something, food goes down the esophagus and enters the stomach, causing the stomach to stretch. This stretch of the stomach stimulates peristalsis in the colon, and this pushes the content of the colon towards the rectum. As the rectum fills, the urge to defecate is stimulated. Between eating and getting the urge takes around 30 minutes, so a person who eats lunch at 12:30, may make a visit to the toilet at around 13:00. The intensity of the gastrocolic reflex varies between people, and some people feel little or no urge to have a bowel movement soon after eating. On the other hand, certain conditions, including **IBS** (irritable bowel syndrome), IBD, as well as anxiety can increase the strength of the gastrocolic reflex. The purpose of this reflex is to make room for newly consumed food by moving already digested food out of the body.

Table: 3.2

The Digestive System from the Stomach to the Anus　（胃から肛門までの消化器系）

Organ（器官）	Main function（おもな機能）	Comments（コメント）
Stomach　（胃）	Muscles in the stomach wall churn the bolus (**mechanical digestion**), mixing it with gastric juices that break down the nutrients (**chemical digestion**). The bolus becomes **chyme** (a partially digested liquid). The **pyloric sphincter** controls movement of food out of the stomach.	Included in gastric juice are: **hydrochloric acid** (breaks down food and destroys harmful microorganisms); **pepsin** (enzyme that breaks down protein), and **lipase** (breaks down lipids). **Transit time** is 4-6 hours.
Small intestine (小腸)	Comprises the **duodenum**, **jejunum**, and **ileum**. Location of most digestion and absorption of nutrients. Cells in the wall of the small intestine secrete digestive enzymes. Intestine wall is lined with **villi** that increase the surface area for absorption of nutrients.	Absorption of nutrients is through a fine network of **capillaries** and **lacteals** in each villus. Lacteals are lymphatic vessels that absorb lipids into the lymphatic system.
Duodenum (十二指腸)	Most chemical digestion takes place here. Chyme is mixed with bile from the gallbladder and enzymes from the pancreas. **Pancreatic juice** contains enzymes that break down macromolecules (proteins, fats, and carbohydrates) into smaller building blocks (amino acids, fatty acids, and simple sugars). **Bicarbonate** secreted into the duodenum from the pancreas neutralizes stomach acid.	Enzymes in pancreatic juice include: **trypsin** (protein digestion), **amylase** (carbohydrate digestion), and **lipase** (lipid digestion). **Bile**, produced by the liver and stored in the gall bladder, **emulsifies** lipids, aiding chemical digestion of lipids by lipase.
Jejunum (空腸)	Most absorption takes place here.	Middle portion of small intestine.
Ileum　（回腸）	Absorbs remaining products of digestion. Key location for absorption of vitamin B12.	Connects the small intestine to the large intestine. Often affected in CD.
Large intestine (大腸)	Most nutrients and up to 90% of the water has already been absorbed by the small intestine. Primary role is absorption of water and salt from the intestinal contents. Feces are formed. Home to most of the **microbiome**. Bacteria break down carbohydrates and synthesize several vitamins (e.g., vit B, vit K). The vitamins are absorbed into the blood.	1.5 meters long. Has no villi. Plays almost no role in digestion (unlike epithelial cells in the small intestine, those in the large intestine do not produce digestive enzymes). Divided into the: **proximal colon:** cecum, ascending colon, transverse colon. **distal colon:** descending colon, sigmoid colon, rectum.
Cecum　（盲腸）	Receives material from the ileum. Most of remaining water and ions are absorbed.	Attached to the cecum is the **appendix** (also called **vermiform** process). It could be a **vestigial organ**, but some evidence that it stores beneficial bacteria.
Ascending colon →Transverse colon: Absorption continues.　（上行結腸　→　横行結腸）		
Descending colon (下行結腸)	Stores feces. When full, stool pass into the rectum.	
Sigmoid colon (S 状結腸)	Pushes the feces into the rectum.	Derives its name from the fact that it is curved in the form of an "S".
Rectum　（直腸）	Expands to hold stool. When feces enter, it causes an urge to defecate.	Around 15 cm long. Straight, tube-like structure. Inflammation in UC usually starts here.
Anus　（肛門）	Opening through which feces leave the body.	Composition of feces: 75% water, 25% solid matter. Of solid matter, 30% is dead bacteria.

8) Four layers: The GI tract is composed of four layers:

I. The **mucosa** is the innermost layer that lines the GI tract. The surface of the mucosa is made up of the **epithelial cells**, a layer of cells that separates the underlying cells from the contents of the lumen. The **lumen**, or open space of the GI tract, is part of the outside environment. The type of epithelial cell varies according to the location in the GI tract; for example, **stratified squamous tissue**, which provides protection against abrasion, lines the mouth and anus, while the stomach and intestines are lined with **simple columnar epithelial cells**, which are adapted for secretion and absorption. The cells of the epithelium divide rapidly. It takes only three to five days for the intestinal epithelium to completely renew itself, making it one of the most rapidly dividing areas in the body. This very high rate of cell renewal is vital because the epithelium needs to withstand the constant wear and tear of the processes of digestion and absorption. Epithelial cells must also renew quickly to maintain a normal gut barrier function. The epithelium is supported by an underlying layer of connective tissue called the **lamina propria**, which contains blood vessels, nerves, and glands. Underneath the lamina propria is a thin layer of smooth muscle called the **muscularis mucosa**.

Located in the mucosa are the cells that secrete mucus, digestive enzymes, and hormones. **Mucus** is secreted by modified epithelial cells called **goblet cells**. The mucus that is secreted onto the surface of the GI tract has various functions: it lubricates and binds food so that it can easily move over membranes; in the stomach, the mucus layer protects the mucosa from the acidic environment; and in the colon, mucus forms a barrier against direct contact between epithelial cells and bacteria, thereby reducing the risk of infection. One component of mucus is **mucins**, which are **glycoproteins** (a protein structure with a dense sugar-coating) that give mucus its slippery characteristic and are effective at binding together to form gels. Mucins enable mucus to create a strong barrier.

II. The **submucosa layer** is under the muscularis mucosa. It consists of fat, connective tissue, blood vessels, lymphatic vessels, and nerves.

III. The **muscularis propria** is comprised of two layers of smooth muscle that are responsible for peristalsis, the wave-like muscle contractions that move food through the digestive tract.

IV. The outer layer of the GI tract is the **serosa**. It is composed of connective tissue. The main function of the serosa is to protect the underlying tissue and to attach the intestinal organs to the posterior abdominal wall. The esophagus lacks a serosa, which is one reason esophageal cancer spreads more quickly to other organs compared to tumors in other areas of the GI tract.

The GI tract has its own local nervous system, called the **enteric nervous system**, that helps control activities of the digestive system. The GI tract is also controlled extrinsically (i.e., from the outside) by nerves from the CNS. In addition to intrinsic and extrinsic neural control, the GI tract is regulated by hormones released from the wall of the GI tract itself. One example of the many gastrointestinal hormones is **secretin**. Produced by cells in the duodenum, secretin stimulates secretion of pancreatic fluid, which is vital for digestion, and of bicarbonate. This bicarbonate neutralizes **chyme** (partially digested food that leaves the stomach). You can see that digestion is controlled by a combination of nervous innervation and hormones.

9) *Intestinal immune system*: This is a "hot" area of medical research because there is increasing evidence that many diseases, such as IBD, diabetes, allergies, obesity, and some cancers, are influenced, or even caused by an imbalance in the **gut microbiota** (i.e., the community of bacteria and other microbes that inhabit the intestine, especially the colon), and/or a **mistaken immune response to intestinal microbes**. The immune system in the gut is fundamentally different from the immune system in other parts of the body. For example, if bacteria infect a cut on the skin, the body's immune system will respond with an aggressive inflammatory response. However, the tissue of the gut wall is surrounded by trillions of microbes, so if the intestinal immune system reacted with an inflammatory response each time gut bacteria entered the gut wall, the intestine would be constantly inflamed. There is so much that is not known about the intestinal immune system, but a lot has been found out in the last few decades. Here is a little of what is known:

- About 100 trillion bacteria, of at least 500 different types, live inside the intestines (the total weight of these bacteria in an adult is around 2 kilograms!). The bacteria and other microbes that inhabit the gut (known as the **gut microbiota**) have such an important influence on human physiology that some researchers consider the microbiota to be another organ. Most of the gut bacteria are **commensal bacteria** that have a mutually beneficial relationship with the host.

- Commensal bacteria have various important functions. For example, they produce enzymes capable of breaking down certain types of fiber that cannot be digested by human cells. One metabolite produced by bacteria in the colon through the fermentation of dietary fiber is **short-chain fatty acids**. These metabolites maintain gut health in various ways; for example, they are a source of energy for intestinal epithelial cells in the colon, they increase mucus production, and improve the integrity of the gut barrier.

- Some commensal bacteria produce vitamins that we need to stay healthy. In addition, commensal bacteria protect against pathogens because they produce antibacterial compounds that kill or inhibit invading pathogens. Also, commensal bacteria are so well adapted to living in the gut that they inhibit the growth of pathogens by **out-competing** them for nutrients.

- Although the commensal bacteria are beneficial in many ways, they need to be kept within the gut. If they were able to freely pass through the gut wall and enter the bloodstream, they could trigger life-threatening systemic infections. Bacteria are inhibited from entering the tissues of the gut wall by a single layer of cells called the **epithelium**. In the epithelium, **goblet cells** secrete **mucus** that forms an extra barrier over the epithelium. The gel-like mucus layer traps bacteria; moreover, the mucus is rich in antibacterial proteins, which inhibit or kill bacteria.

- The intestinal epithelium with its mucosal layer forms an effective barrier, but it is not a perfect one. There are so many bacteria, and the surface area of the intestine is so big, that some commensal bacteria are bound to get through this barrier and enter the **lamina propria**, the tissue that surrounds the intestine. In fact, such an invasion of gut bacteria is happening all the time. If the immune system in the gut reacted to this invasion with an aggressive inflammatory response, the gut would be constantly inflamed. For this reason, the "**default** response" of the intestinal immune system is a gentle, non-inflammatory one.

- One reason the intestinal immune system is **tolerant** to commensal bacteria that **breach** the mucus and epithelium barrier is that the lamina propria is home to a large number of **regulatory T cells** (also called **Tregs**), a type of leukocyte. Tregs "calm down" the immune system by releasing **anti-inflammatory cytokines**.

- Another reason for the tolerance of the intestinal immune system is the presence of non-inflammatory macrophages. When a cut in the skin is infected with bacteria, macrophages are recruited. These macrophages not only "eat" the invading bacteria by **phagocytosis**, but they also secrete cytokines that attract neutrophils from the blood to help fight the battle. This results in inflammation at the site of bacteria invasion. However, in the lamina propria of the gut wall, the anti-inflammatory cytokines secreted by Tregs inhibit the macrophages from releasing cytokines. This means the macrophages in the gut wall remain efficient hunters that engulf bacteria entering the gut tissue, but they do not trigger widespread inflammation.

- IBD is thought to result from the normally tolerant intestinal immune system attacking commensal bacteria, triggering an inflammatory response in the gut. Knowledge of the microbiome and the intestinal immune system could help to develop new IBD treatments.

SD 3H: A possible treatment for IBD (1): Poo transplants

Various studies have shown that in the gut of people with IBD, the diversity of bacteria is reduced. In particular, there is a marked decline in bacteria with anti-inflammatory properties and an increase in more inflammatory bacteria. One way to fix this **dysbiosis**, or imbalance in the microbiota, could be by transferring the stool from a healthy donor into the colon of a person with IBD. Such a procedure is called **fecal microbiota transplantation (FMT)**. Stool from a healthy person is transferred to a patient (recipient) in an enema or through a colonoscopy. FMT is an effective treatment for recurrent infection by a bacteria called **Clostridioides difficile (C. difficile)**. C. difficile infection can cause severe diarrhea, inflammation, and other debilitating symptoms. In some cases, it can be fatal. One of the main causes of C. difficile infection is the use of antibiotics, which can suppress the commensal bacteria in the gut, allowing the pathogenic C. difficile to overrun the intestine. FMT reintroduces the commensal bacteria, reestablishing a healthy microbiota. While FMT has been established as an effective therapy for C. difficile infection, the results of studies on the efficacy of FMT for IBD are not so clear. FMT temporarily improves symptoms in some IBD patients, but it has no effect in others. More research is required to determine whether FMT can become a regular treatment for IBD.

SD 3I: A possible treatment for IBD (2): Parasitic worms

If you think that FMT sounds a bit disgusting, how about swallowing **helminths*** (parasitic worms)? Helminth therapy, in which people are intentionally infected with parasitic worms, has been used as an experimental treatment for IBD. For millions of years, humans evolved together with parasitic helminths. For most of human evolution, it is likely that humans had parasitic worms living in their guts. In order to protect themselves against being destroyed by the human immune system, these worms evolved ways to suppress the host's immune system. How they do this is complex, but one way is by inducing an increase in the number of **regulatory T cells** that suppress the inflammatory response. These worms help maintain an anti-inflammatory environment in the host's body.

Epidemiologists have noticed for a long time that asthma, hay fever, and autoimmune diseases, are much more prevalent in rich western countries compared to less developed countries where chronic helminth infection is **endemic**. In pre-war Japan, around 70% of Japanese people were infected with parasitic worms. After World War II, there was a campaign to eradicate these worms. A combination of mass treatment with **anthelmintics** (medicines that kill parasitic worms), improvements in **sanitation**, and more hygienic living conditions has greatly reduced intestinal infections with **hook worms** and other parasitic worms. In Japan, the USA, and other developed countries such infections are now rare. However, the decline in such infections has coincided with a rapid increase in autoimmune diseases and allergies. It has been proposed that an increase in these diseases is because we are no longer exposed to chronic infections by helminths.

Losing helminths and other "old friends" (i.e., microbes and parasites with which our ancestors co-evolved for millions of years) may have left our immune systems more susceptible to becoming overactive, causing IBD and other conditions. For details of this fascinating topic, check out **"old friends hypothesis"** on the internet.

* Some types of parasitic worms cause fatal diseases, and even hookworms, which are said to live "harmlessly" in the gut, can cause anemia, malnutrition, fatigue, and other unpleasant symptoms.

10) *Leukocytes*, commonly known as white blood cells, are a key part of the immune system that play a vital role in protecting the body from infection and disease. The five different types of leukocytes have different functions. As you can see from the list below, neutrophils are the most abundant type (the number in parentheses is the percentage of the total amount of leukocytes).

• **Neutrophils** (60 – 70%): Destroy pathogens and cancer cells by engulfing them in a process called **phagocytosis** (*phago~* = "swallow").

•**Lymphocytes** 20 – 30%): Produce antibodies.

•**Monocytes** (1 – 6%): The largest of all leukocytes. They migrate from the bloodstream to tissues and then develop into phagocytic macrophages and **dendritic cells**. Dendritic cells are **antigen-presenting cells**. These cells engulf invading pathogens and present the antigen material from the invaders to T lymphocytes. The T lymphocytes remember the presented antigens, enabling them to attack and destroy pathogens with the same antigen the next time they enter the body.

•**Eosinophils** (1 – 3%): Important role in the regulation of allergic reactions.

•**Basophils** (< 1%): Release histamine and other chemicals that medicate inflammation.

A useful mnemonic to help remember the different kind of leukocytes is "**N**ever **L**et **M**onkeys **E**at **B**ananas." Neutrophils are so called because they can be stained by neutral dyes (*~phil* = "prefer/affinity to"), while lymphocytes get their name because they are the main cell type in **lymph** (the fluid in the **lymphatic system**). If you are curious about the naming of the other three leukocytes, a quick internet search will give you the etymology.

Unlike mature red blood cells (**erythrocytes**), which do not have a nucleus, leukocytes are **nucleated** (i.e., they have a nucleus). Most leukocytes are produced in the bone marrow, but the **lymph nodes**, **spleen**, and **thymus gland** are the sites of production for lymphocytes. Some white blood cells flow through the blood, but most are found outside of the blood vessels within the tissues. Leukocytes pass from blood vessels into the tissues by moving through spaces between the cells that make up the wall of blood vessels (this migration of blood cells through the wall of blood vessels is called **diapedesis**). Leukocytes are attracted to move towards the site of an infection by inflammatory chemicals. On reaching the site, they release more substances to attract other leukocytes.

The movement of leukocytes to inflamed tissues has an essential role in fighting infection and in promoting wound healing. However, in autoimmune diseases, leukocytes moving into tissues contributes to inappropriate inflammation that causes tissue damage and dysfunction. In IBD, leukocytes promote inflammation and there is a treatment for UC that involves removing certain leukocytes from the blood. This treatment, which was developed in Japan, is called **leukocyte apheresis** (*apheresis* is from a Latin word meaning "to take away").

You may have heard of **cytokines**, a large group of small proteins that enable different cells of the immune to interact and communicate with each other. Cytokines have **immunomodulatory** functions (i.e., they affect and adjust the immune system). Within the large group of cytokines, there are various "families" of different cytokines such as **tumor necrosis factors**, **interferons**, and **interleukins**. You may have spotted that the word "interleukin" contains *leuk*. This is because these molecules were discovered in leukocytes and were found to act on other leukocytes (so, they act "between leukocytes"; hence, the prefix "*inter~*"). Since the discovery in 1977 of IL-1 (interleukin 1), the first interleukin, at least 15 other interleukins have been found. It is also now known that interleukins are produced by many other cells apart from leukocytes and that they have many other roles other than modulating immune responses.

I hope that this brief section on <u>leukocytes</u> was <u>lucid</u> ("clear and easy to understand") and <u>illum</u>inating (both *luc* and *lum* are related to the root *leuk*, meaning "white/light/bright").

11) *Proton pump inhibitors* **(PPIs) are a class of medication that work by reducing acid secretion in the stomach.** What makes the stomach environment acidic is **hydrochloric acid** (HCl) that is secreted into the lumen of the stomach by **parietal cells** (specialized cells in the gastric epithelium). Gastric acid has various important functions, including:

- A low pH (1.5 to 2) is necessary to change the **pepsinogen** (the inactive **precursor** of pepsin) into **pepsin**, a powerful enzyme that breaks down protein.
- An acid environment in the stomach **denatures** proteins (i.e., it makes them lose their structure), so that they can be more easily broken down by pepsin.
- A low pH kills or inhibits the growth of microorganisms that are ingested with food, helping to prevent infection.

Although gastric acid has important functions, excessive secretion of gastric acid is a key factor contributing to the development of **peptic ulcer**, which is an ulcer (open sore) in the mucosa of the stomach. Another contributing factor is **erosion** of the mucosa by the enzyme pepsin. Some of the signs of peptic ulcer are **indigestion** (the medical term for which is **dyspepsia**), heartburn (**pyrosis**), pain in the upper middle area of the abdomen (known as **epigastric pain**), **belching**, nausea, and, if the ulcer bleeds, blood in the vomit (**hematemesis**). If peptic ulcers formed only due to exposure to gastric acid and pepsin, you would expect everybody to have ulcers. However, peptic ulcers do not develop under normal conditions because there is a balance between factors that protect the wall of the stomach and factors that attack it. The most important **protective factor** is the mucus that forms a barrier on the surface of the stomach. The mucus is secreted by cells in the epithelium, which also releases **bicarbonate** (HCO3), meaning that the mucus is rich in bicarbonate (and HCO3 helps to **buffer** the acid). Another important protective factor is a healthy blood flow. Good blood flow to the mucosa maintains mucosal health by delivering oxygen and nutrients, and by removing acid and any toxins.

On the other hand, a decline in mucus production and/or an increase in acid secretion leaves the mucosa vulnerable to ulcers. There are numerous ulcer-producing factors, including smoking, alcohol, and chronic stress. But the two most important causes of ulcers are infection with **Helicobacter pylori** (***H. pylori***) and long-term use of NSAIDs (Non-Steroidal Anti-Inflammatory Drugs).

H. pylori is a spiral-shaped bacterium that is adapted to inhabit the mucus and epithelial layer in the stomach. *H. pylori* can happily survive without oxygen (i.e., it is an **anaerobic** bacteria), and it is able to neutralize the acid in the stomach by producing large amounts of an enzyme called **urease**. Urease breaks down urea (which is normally in the stomach) to carbon dioxide and **ammonia**. The ammonia acts to neutralize gastric acid, allowing the bacteria to survive. The bacteria cause damage to the gastric mucosa in several ways. One way is the toxic effect of ammonia on the epithelial cells. Also, *H. pylori* secretes enzymes (e.g., protease and lipase) that harm the mucosa. The damage done to the gastric mucosa leaves people infected with *H. pylori* more likely to develop peptic ulcers. In fact, studies in developed countries have shown that over 85% of people diagnosed with gastric ulcers are infected with *H. pylori*. The 2005 Nobel Prize in Physiology or Medicine was awarded to two Australian doctors for their discovery of *H. pylori* and its role in causing gastritis and peptic ulcers. The story of how these doctors, Robin Warren and Barry Marshall, made their discovery is very famous because it involves **self-experimentation**. If you are curious, check on the internet.

NSAIDs are widely used drugs with **analgesic** (pain killing), **antipyretic** (fever reducing), and anti-inflammatory effects. Unfortunately, a potentially serious side effect of NSAIDs is damage to the gastric mucosa and ulcer formation. The main reason that NSAIDs can damage the stomach wall is that they work by inhibiting **prostaglandins**. Prostaglandins are chemical messengers ("local hormones") that promote inflammation, pain, and fever. Inhibiting prostaglandins can, therefore, help to reduce joint inflammation, relieve the pain of a headache, or reduce fever from an infection. But prostaglandins also play an important role in protecting and healing the mucosa of the GI tract. They do this by stimulating the secretion of mucus and bicarbonate and increasing blood flow to the mucosa. Inhibition of prostaglandins with NSAIDs will reduce these protective and healing mechanisms (i.e., NSAID use will tend to increase acid secretion, decrease mucus and bicarbonate production, and decrease blood flow). In addition to damage caused by prostaglandin inhibition, NSAIDs can also cause topical injury to the mucosa (i.e., the irritant or toxic effect of direct contact with the mucosa).

The risk of gastrointestinal bleeding, peptic ulcers and other GI side effects is not the same for all NSAIDs, with a lower risk associated with ibuprofen compared to aspirin and naproxen. There is also a **dose-response relationship**, meaning that the higher the dose of the NSAID administered, the greater the likelihood of GI side effects. Higher doses are also associated with an increase in intensity and duration of symptoms. Although the risk of GI symptoms with NSAIDs is **dose-dependent**, they can still occur even at low doses. Particularly in people with IBD, even one or two doses of certain NSAIDs (e.g., naproxen) cause relapse of previously **quiescent** disease.

If left untreated, a peptic ulcer can completely erode through the stomach wall, allowing the contents of the stomach to leak into the abdominal cavity. This complication, called a **perforated ulcer**, is a medical emergency. To prevent this and other complications of a stomach ulcer, and to relieve unpleasant symptoms, people with a peptic ulcer are usually prescribed a **PPI (proton pump inhibitor)** such as lansoprazole or omeprazole (the generic names of PPI drugs end with the suffix ~*prazole*). PPIs reduce acid secretion in the stomach by inhibiting the **proton pump**. A proton pump is a protein enzyme in the cell membrane of parietal cells that push hydrogen ions (protons) from the parietal cells into the lumen of the stomach. This enzyme is called **H+/K+ ATPase** (hydrogen potassium ATPase), and it is the final step of acid production in the stomach. PPIs block this acid production by blocking proton pumps, thereby inhibiting them from secreting hydrogen ions into the stomach (basic chemistry: high concentrations of hydrogen ions cause a low pH). Although PPIs are quickly metabolized by the liver, one dose will reduce acid secretion for days. This is because they **irreversibly** block proton pumps, meaning that the only way acid production can start again is by the body regenerating new proton pumps. By reducing acid secretion, PPIs give the stomach lining time to heal. In peptic ulcers caused by *H. pylori,* treatment is by a combination of antibiotics to kill the bacteria and a PPI.

PPIs are one of the most widely prescribed class of medications in the world. In addition, they are now available OTC (over the counter) in many countries. Apart from peptic ulcers, PPIs are indicated for the treatment of **gastroesophageal reflux disease (GERD)**, **esophagitis** (inflammation of the esophagus), **Barrett's esophagus**, and other conditions. PPIs generally have few side effects and are usually **well tolerated**. However, there are concerns about the consequences of long-term use. Because PPIs are used by so many people, studies on serious adverse effects associated with PPIs are often reported in the media. For example, it has been reported that PPIs could:

- increase the risk of bacterial infections in the GI tract, including an increased risk of *Clostridium difficile* infections. Mechanism: Decreasing gut acidity due to PPIs allows the overgrowth of certain bacteria in the GI tract.
- increase in the risk of IBD. Mechanism: Long-term gastric acid suppression decreases the diversity of bacteria in the intestine or alters the microbiota in some other way. This could negatively affect the intestinal immune system.
- increase the risk of bone fractures. Mechanism: **Hypochlorhydria** (a low level of hydrochloric acid in the stomach) interferes with calcium absorption from the GI tract.
- cause iron deficiency. Mechanism: Gastric acid converts iron from the diet into a form that can be absorbed.

In addition, studies have reported an association between PPIs and increased risk of kidney disease, pneumonia, myocardial infarction, dementia, and other conditions. People reading the above may be put off using PPIs, but it is important to note that an association between, for example, PPI use and dementia does not mean that PPIs have been *proven* to cause dementia. Also, short-term use of PPIs is unlikely to have serious long-term consequences. PPIs are effective drugs and, if used as instructed, the benefits are likely to outweigh any risks there may be. Thanks partly to PPI treatment, serious complication from peptic ulcers are nowadays rare. Nevertheless, we should be aware that artificially suppressing gastric acid secretion could have **unintended consequences**.

SD 3J: Unintended Consequences of NSAIDs

When my father returned from a month-long trip to India in the late 1970s, he showed me a photo he had taken of some vultures feeding on a **carcass** (dead body) of a cow. I wondered how these **scavengers** were able to eat dead animals without getting sick. I found out from an encyclopedia that these birds could eat the decaying flesh of animals infected with pathogenic bacteria (e.g., bacteria that cause **botulism**, **anthrax**, cholera, and salmonella) partly because of their extremely acidic stomachs. In humans, the lumen of the stomach is around pH 1.5 (the pH near the gastric mucosa is nearer pH 7.0 because gastric acid is neutralized by bicarbonate secreted continuously by epithelial cells). In the vulture's stomach, however, the pH is close to 0 (battery acid is pH 0.8). This near-zero pH environment destroys most bacteria and parasites before they can reach the intestine. Vultures have many other adaptations to their scavenging lifestyle; for example, a vulture's head has no feathers (a naked head helps prevent blood and bacteria from sticking to it when the bird feeds). When my father went to India in the late 1970s there were about 40 million vultures in the country. Now there are few than 20,000. The main reason that a once common bird has almost become extinct is an NSAID called **diclofenac**. In the 1980s, farmers began to give diclofenac to cows. When these cows died, they were left by the road for vultures to eat. To humans and other mammals NSAIDs are relatively safe, but for vultures even small doses of an NSAID is extremely toxic. After ingesting contaminated dead cows, many vultures died from kidney damage. The widespread administration of a cheap NSAID to cows had the **unintended consequence** of killing most of India's vultures.

Another unintended consequence was an increase in the risk of diseases spreading to humans because, without vultures, millions of animal carcasses were left decaying in fields. Also, other scavengers such as rats and **feral dogs** were left with more **carrion** to eat, causing their populations to explode. A rise in the number of feral dogs resulted in more people suffering dog bites and subsequently dying from **rabies**.

12) Red flag sign: The red flag is a sign of danger. If you see a red flag at a beach it means it's dangerous to swim. A red flag sign or symptom in medicine is a sign or symptom that could indicate a serious condition. Here is an example. Supposing you go out for lunch to an Indian restaurant with an older colleague and you notice he is not eating. You ask him, "Don't you like Indian food?" He replies, "I love Indian food, but these last few months I've found it difficult to swallow food. Food just seems to stick in my throat. I'm a bit worried, but I've been too busy to go to the doctor." Trouble swallowing (called **dysphagia**), especially a feeling of food getting stuck in the throat or chest, is a red flag for **esophageal cancer** (it could be caused by a tumor partially obsructing the esophagus). If you or someone you know has this symptom, it is important not to **procrastinate,** but to see a doctor.

I ignored rectal bleeding for almost a year, which was stupid of me because it is a red flag for cancer of the colon and rectum (**colorectal cancer**). The color of the blood from the rectum can indicate where the bleeding is coming from. If the blood is bright red it probably originates from lower in the colon or in the rectum. Dark red blood usually indicates bleeding from higher in the large intestine or from the small intestine. The dark color is caused by digestive enzymes acting on the hemoglobin. A stool that is black (like the color of tar) can indicate bleeding in the stomach and is red flag for **stomach cancer** or a stomach ulcer. A black stool is called **melena** (*melano* = "black", as in **melanin**, the skin pigment that determines the color of the skin, hair, and eyes). Rectal bleeding that is not visible to the naked eye is called **fecal occult blood**. The **fecal occult blood test** is a screening test for colon cancer that is often part of annual healthchecks in Japan. There are other red flags that could indicate colon cancer, including **narrow stools** (possibly caused by narrowing or obstruction of the colon by a tumor), **persistent** abdominal pain, and **unintentional** weight loss.

Vomiting blood, or **hematemesis**, is something that, fortunately, I have never experienced, but it must be very shocking (the root *hemato* means "blood" and *emesis* is "to vomit"). Hematemesis is a red flag for peptic ulcer and stomach cancer. On the subject of being sick, an **emetic** is a drug that induces vomiting. Such drugs are sometimes used as an emergency treatment for poisoning. **Antiemetics** are drugs that prevent or reduce nausea and vomiting. They have various uses, including as treatments for **motion sickness**, **morning sickness**, and to prevent nausea and vomiting caused by chemotherapy.

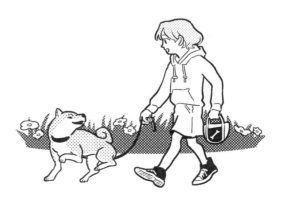

3-4 Well, what do you know?

（どのくらいわかるようになったか試してみよう）

Are the following statements true (T) or false (F)?
1. An enema is the administration of a medication into the rectum.
2. An ultrasound examination is an example of an invasive examination.
3. UC is characterized by inflammation in both the large intestine and small intestine.
4. IBD can manifest in places outside the GI tract, including the joints and eyes.
5. The rapid increase in the incidence of IBD over only a few decades suggests that genetic factors alone are involved in the pathogenesis of IBD.

What is the meaning of the underlined WFE?
1. I heard about a child who suffered a **perforated** stomach because he **ingested** a button battery from a toy.
2. In a few countries, people caught having **extramarital** sex can be punished with death.
3. I do not have **sufficient** space to include all the topics that I would have liked to.
4. Japan went through a long period of economic **malaise** after the end of the bubble economy in 1992.
5. Most courses in academic writing will teach you how to write **coherently** (i.e., in a way that ideas are logically connected).
6. **Melanin** is a pigment that determines our skin and hair color.
7. In 1817, a young German pharmacist called Friedrich Sertürner isolated morphine from opium. This was the first time an active ingredient had been isolated from a plant. Morphine and other many other opioids are now widely used to provide **analgesia**.

Choose a word from below to replace the underlined word(s)
    a) vasodilation   **b)** leukocytes   **c)** colonoscopy   **d)** malware   **e)** duodenum

1. I had a <u>medical procedure to examine the rectum and lower bowel</u> for abnormalities and disease.
2. In the name "Helicobacter pylori," *helico* refers to the helix, or twisted shape of this bacteria (the word "helicopter" is also derived from this root). The *pylori* part of the name refers to the pylorus, which is the part of the stomach that connects with the

first part of the small intestine. It was in the pylorus that that *H. pylori* was first discovered.

3. Shortly after opening the Email attachment, his computer became infected with a software program that is intended to damage or disable a computer.

4/5. Inflammation is the body's response to harmful stimuli such as infection by pathogens, physical injury, heat, and toxins. Inflammation is vital for removing harmful stimuli and for initiating the healing process. An area of inflammation will often be hot to the touch, painful, red, and have swelling. The redness and swelling are due to the action of histamine, which causes dilatation of blood vessels and increases the permeability of capillaries so that white blood cells can be transported to infected areas.

3-5 May Jo's Health-Podcast

（メイ・ジョーの健康ポッドキャスト）

Podcast presenter May Jo (MJ) and Dr Eugene Yamada (Dr) are talking about IBD.

MJ: Today, we're talking to Dr Eugene Yamada, a gastroenterologist from Nagoya in Japan who's currently a clinical researcher at Parkhill Hospital in London. Dr Yamada's area of research is inflammatory bowel disease, or IBD for short, and he recently published a paper on IBD in pregnancy. Welcome to the show.

Dr: Hello Jo. It's great to be here.

MJ: Thank you. Some listeners may not be familiar with IBD. What is it?

Dr: Well, as the name suggests, inflammatory bowel disease refers to conditions that involve chronic inflammation of the digestive tract. The two main IBD conditions are ulcerative colitis and Crohn's disease. Both are autoimmune conditions, but there are important differences between the two.

MJ: What kind of differences?

Dr: Well, in the case of Crohn's disease, there can be inflammation anywhere in the digestive tract, from the mouth to the anus. Many people with Crohn's disease have inflammation in both the small intestine and large intestine. But in ulcerative colitis, inflammation is limited to the large intestine. Another important difference is that Crohn's disease affects the whole thickness of the gut wall, but in ulcerative colitis only the lining of the gut wall is affected.

MJ: You mentioned that ulcerative colitis and Crohn's disease are autoimmune diseases. I understand that women are typically more likely to suffer from autoimmune diseases.

Is this also the case with IBD?

Dr: Some epidemiological studies have found that women are more likely to get Crohn's disease than men, but more men develop ulcerative colitis than women. However, other studies have found no gender differences in the incidence of ulcerative colitis.

MJ: Staying on the topic of sex differences, it is well known that in rheumatoid arthritis, another autoimmune disease, symptoms often improve during pregnancy. Is this also the case for IBD?

Dr: The studies on the effect of pregnancy on IBD show conflicting results, but some of my female patients have told me that their IBD symptoms improved during pregnancy. Of course, this is just anecdotal data.

MJ: Could this improvement be related to hormones?

Dr: It could be, but it may also be because the fetus is essentially a foreign body.

MJ: A foreign body?

Dr: Yes. The fetus has half the father's DNA, so you would expect the woman's immune system to attack it. But in pregnancy, the immune system is somehow dampened down so that it does not attack the baby growing in the womb.

MJ: And this suppression of the immune system to prevent rejection of the fetus could also be beneficial for IBD and other autoimmune diseases.

Dr: Yes. That could be the mechanism.

MJ: Well, thank you for taking time to talk on the show today.

Dr: It was a pleasure.

Chapter 4　**Stroke**

（脳卒中）

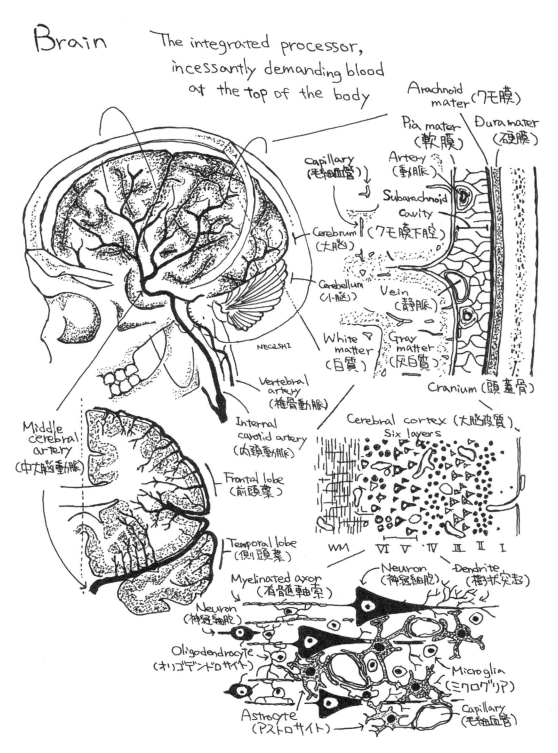

NAVvocab 60 （案内役の単語 60）

1. amphetamine・覚醒剤
2. aneurysm・動脈瘤
3. anticoagulant・抗凝固薬
4. antiseizure medication・
   抗けいれん薬, 抗発作薬
5. aphasia・失語症
6. arachnoid mater・クモ膜
7. astrocytes・アストロサイト(星状膠細胞)
8. atheromatous plaque・動脈硬化プラーク
9. bedridden・寝たきりの
10. bifurcate・分岐する
11. cardiogenic cerebral embolism・
    原性脳塞栓
12. carotid artery stenosis・頸動脈狭窄
13. cavernous angioma・海綿状血管腫
14. cerebral edema・脳浮腫
15. cerebral infarction・脳梗塞
16. cerebrospinal fluid・脳脊髄液
17. cerebrovascular disease・脳血管障害
18. contralateral control・対側制御
19. craniotomy・開頭手術
20. deep vein thrombosis・深部静脈血栓症
21. diplopia・複視
22. embolus・塞栓
23. extravasation・血管外漏出
24. glial cell・グリア細胞
25. hemostasis・止血
26. hematoma・血腫
27. hemiparesis・片側不全麻痺
28. hemodynamic shear stress・
    血流力学のずり応力
29. hemorrhagic stroke・脳出血
30. hypercoagulable state・凝固能亢進状態

31. infarct・梗塞
32. intracerebral hemorrhage・脳内出血
33. intracranial arterial stenosis・
    頭蓋内動脈の狭窄性病変
34. intracranial pressure・頭蓋内圧
35. ischemic stroke・虚血性脳卒中
36. lacunar stroke・ラクナ梗塞
37. meninges・髄膜
38. migraine・片頭痛
39. myocardial infarction・心筋梗塞
40. neurosurgery ward・脳神経外科病棟
41. neurosurgeon・神経外科医
42. neurotoxic・神経毒性
43. nonmodifiable risk factor・
    変更不可能な危険因子
44. numbness・しびれ
45. occlusion・閉塞
46. paralysis・麻痺
47. parenchyma・〔臓器の〕実質
48. pathogenesis・発症機序
49. posterior circulation stroke・
    後方循環脳卒中
50. primary motor cortex・一次運動野
51. prophylactic surgery・予防的手術
52. sickle cell disease・鎌状赤血球症
53. sleep apnea・睡眠時無呼吸
54. subarachnoid hemorrhage・クモ膜下出血
55. systemic hypoperfusion stroke・
    全身の低かん流による脳卒中
56. thrombogenic・血栓形成性の
57. thrombolytic drug・血栓溶解薬
58. TIA・一過性脳虚血発作
59. vascular dementia・脳血管性認知症
60. vascular malformation・血管奇形

4-1 Essay—Stroke: Disruption in the Brain's Blood Supply

（脳卒中：脳の血流が妨げられる）

¹I spent almost a month on the **neurosurgery ward** of Fujita Health University Hospital (FHUH), a hospital in Aichi Prefecture, Japan. I have a poor memory for dates, but I do remember that I was hospitalized in the summer of 2006 because my wife was pregnant with our first child at the time. I was in FHUH for an operation to remove a **cavernous angioma**, a type of intracranial **vascular malformation** (in simple English: a cluster of abnormal blood vessels in my brain). The cavernous angioma had **ruptured**[E7] and was leaking blood into my brain. This bleeding (or **hemorrhage**) was causing partial **paralysis** on the left side of my face and **numbness** in my left hand. (The bleeding was in the **primary motor cortex** in the brain's right **hemisphere**, but because of a phenomenon called **contralateral control,** it was the opposite side of my body—the left side—that was affected.) Worse of all, because of the bleeding, I was also having frequent **seizures**.

²The head of the medical team who was to perform the operation was a highly respected **neurosurgeon** called doctor Hirotoshi Sano(佐野公俊). Dr Sano had appeared on Japanese TV many times because of his amazing surgery skills—it was said he had "God Hands" (神の手)—and he even has his own Wikipedia entry! (Does it sound like I'm **bragging** about having my brain cut into by such a famous man?) Before the operation, Dr Sano used an MRI scan of my brain to point out the location of the cavernous angioma and the **hematoma**, a mass of clotted blood caused by the bleeding from the cavernous angioma. He told me he was confident that my symptoms would improve if the cavernous angioma was **resected** (cut out). Dr Sano doctor was right: the operation was a success. The paralysis on one side of my face **resolved**, and I suffered no **aftereffects**. However, the seizures did not completely disappear, and I still take **antiseizure medication**. Also, I was left with a big scar on my scalp from the **craniotomy**[E2], an operation to open the skull (but as long as I don't go completely bald, nobody will notice it).

³While hospitalized in FHUH, I saw patients who were not so fortunate as me. Some left hospital unable to walk or speak, and no doubt some did not leave hospital alive. Many of these people had suffered a **stroke**. During my time on the neurology ward, I stayed in three different multi-bed rooms. In the first room, my bed was opposite a man who was in a **coma**. The man was in his 30s, and every day his wife visited his bedside, sometimes accompanied by two young children. The children would say, "Papa, *okite*" ["Daddy, wake up"], and his wife would place headphones on her husband. I assumed she was playing music that she hoped would make him wake from his coma. When I asked a

nurse about the man, she said he had suffered a massive bleed in the brain one morning on his way to work.

⁴In the second room to which I was moved, the man in the bed next to mine was a Mr. Tanaka. He had just turned 67, and had been a *sarariman* (a white-collar company employee) until he retired two years previously. Mr. Tanaka told me that a week earlier he had been making his morning coffee, when suddenly his right arm went weak and he dropped the kettle. His wife suspected that he was having a stroke and phoned for an ambulance. In Mr. Tanaka's case, his stroke was caused by a blockage of a blood vessel in the brain. The stroke had left Mr. Tanaka with weakness of one side of the body (called **hemiparesis**E4), but he had already started **rehabilitation**D1 to improve his mobility. It was nice to chat to Mr. Tanaka during the day, but his snoring at night drove me crazy, and I was glad when I was moved for a third time.

⁵In the third room, my bed was next to a patient called Mr. Suzuki, who was in hospital not to treat a stroke, but to prevent one. He told me that a large **aneurysm**, a weak spot in an artery in the brain that balloons and fills with blood, had been discovered during an annual ***ningendokku***E8, a comprehensive annual medical check. Aneurysms typically form where arteries **bifurcate** (branch) because at such points the artery walls tend to be thinner and weaker and exposed to high **hemodynamic stresses** (i.e., stresses from blood flow). To prevent the aneurysm from rupturing, Mr. Suzuki had decided to undergo **clipping surgery**, which involves placing a small metal clip across the base of the aneurysm to stop blood flowing into it. If an aneurysm ruptures, it can bleed into the space between the brain and the thin membranes covering the brain, causing a **subarachnoid hemorrhage (SAH)**. This type of stroke has a high risk of mortality and disability in survivors.

⁶These three fellow patients illustrate three important points about strokes. Firstly, there are different stroke types, and secondly, a stroke can happen suddenly. In fact, the word "stroke" is short for "stroke of God's hand": the onset of symptoms such as **paralysis** was so sudden that, before modern medicine, strokes were considered the work of God. Imagine walking down the street feeling fine when you are suddenly punched hard in the face by a complete stranger. That is how a stroke often strikes—without warning. It is why a stroke is sometimes called a **"brain attack"** or **"cerebrovascular accident."** Thirdly, stroke is a condition that involves blood vessels, which is why strokes are included in the general categories of **cardiovascular disease** (conditions affecting the heart and blood vessels) or **cerebrovascular disease** (*cerebro* refers to the brain and *vascular* refers to the vessels that carry blood around the body).

⁷Let's look in detail at stroke types. Mr. Tanaka, mentioned above, had suffered an **ischemic stroke** (also called a **cerebral infarction**). It is the most common type, accounting for about 85% of all strokes. An ischemic stroke occurs when an artery

supplying blood to the brain is **occluded** (blocked), stopping blood flow to brain cells **downstream** from the **occlusion**.

[8]The man in the coma had suffered the other main type of stroke called a **hemorrhagic stroke**[E5]. Hemorrhagic strokes account for only about 15% of all strokes, but the fatality rate for them is higher—around 40% of stroke deaths are due to hemorrhagic stroke. Hemorrhagic strokes usually occur when a blood vessel in the brain ruptures and blood spills into surrounding brain tissue. This bleeding can be damaging for several reasons. Firstly, the hemorrhage reduces the blood supply that can be delivered to brain tissue. Secondly, blood that has escaped from blood vessel exerts damaging pressure on the surrounding brain cells. Thirdly, inflammation and swelling of the brain can result from a hemorrhagic stroke. This swelling, caused by fluid trapped in the brain, is known as **cerebral edema.** Untreated, the buildup of pressure in the skull can be fatal. Fourthly, as escaped red blood cells break down, hemoglobin is released into the surrounding brain tissue. And this **extracellular** free hemoglobin (i.e., hemoglobin not contained in red blood cells) is **neurotoxic** (i.e., it causes injury to nerve cells).

[9]Both ischemic and hemorrhagic strokes disrupt cerebral blood supply and cause **ischemia**, an inadequate supply of blood to a part of the body. Without an adequate blood supply, brain cells will soon start to die because it is blood that brings oxygen and glucose to the cells and then removes carbon dioxide produced during cellular respiration. Compared to other cells in the body, **neurons** are much less able to store glucose, so they require a continuous supply of it from the blood. Without glucose, neurons soon begin to die. (Another cell found in the brain called **astrocytes**, a type of **glial cell**, can store some glucose in the form of **glycogen**, making them more resistant to an insufficient supply of blood than neurons.)

[10]We have seen that strokes are broadly divided into those caused by blockage and those caused by bleeding. But within these two broad categories, there are several **subtypes** of stroke. Firstly, let's look at ischemic stroke. A main cause of this type of stroke is a process called **atherosclerosis**, in which fatty deposits—composed mainly of cholesterol, calcium, and white blood cells—build up in the **endothelium** (inner lining) of arteries. These deposits are known as **atheromatous plaques**, or **atheroma**. Healthy arteries are strong, yet flexible and elastic, and their endothelium is as smooth as glass, allowing blood to flow smoothly. But atherosclerosis causes arteries to harden—the *scler* of atherosclerosis means "hardening"—and to lose their elasticity. Also, over time, this buildup causes narrowing of arteries, reducing blood flow. One of the major causes of ischemic stroke is **intracranial arterial stenosis**, which is when a major artery in the brain becomes severely narrowed by atherosclerosis. Such narrowing due to atherosclerosis can also develop in one of the **cervical arteries**[E1], particularly the **carotid artery**.

Carotid artery stenosis, a narrowing of one or both of the carotid arteries in the neck, can lead to a stroke. It is not only large blood vessels in the brain that can get blocked by atherosclerosis. A **lacunar stroke**[D9] results from occlusion of small blood vessels in the brain. This type of stroke causes **infarcts** (areas of brain tissue that have died due to being starved of blood). Recurrent lacunar strokes can lead to **vascular dementia**, a common type of dementia caused by reduced blood flow to the brain.

[11]The organ systems of the body are all interconnected, and another type of stroke can happen if the heart fails to pump enough blood to **perfuse** (supply) the brain. This type of ischemic stroke due to low blood flow is called **systemic hypoperfusion stroke**[E10]. It can also occur because of blood loss from the body, the result of, for example, a stab or gunshot wound. A dramatic fall in blood pressure (**hypotension**) that can happen in **anaphylactic shock** is another possible cause of systemic hypoperfusion stroke.

[12]Above I have described how atherosclerosis, which develops inside blood vessels, can cause the **lumen** of those blood vessels to become narrowed or completely occluded. But, actually, the main cause of blood-vessel occlusion is **blood clots**. A blood clot is blood that has been converted from a liquid to a semi-solid state. Blood clotting, also known as **coagulation**, is a vital process because without coagulation, **hemostasis** (stopping of blood loss from a damaged blood vessel) could not occur. If we cut a finger, for example, it is coagulation that quickly stops bleeding from the injured blood vessels and allows repair to occur. However, if a blood clot forms within a blood vessel, it can lead to strokes and other life-threatening conditions such as **myocardial infarction** and **deep vein thrombosis**[D5] (**DVT**). A blood clot that forms inside the vascular system is called a **thrombus**[D3].

[13]A thrombus is often caused when an atheroma breaks off or ruptures. The rupturing of the cap of an atheroma exposes the atheroma's **core** to the blood. Because this core is highly **thrombogenic** (i.e., it promotes the formation of a thrombus), rupturing of an atheroma triggers blood clotting and the formation of a thrombus at the site of the ruptured plaque. Some plaques, called **unstable plaques**[D12], have certain characteristics that makes them at higher risk of rupturing. A blood clot can lead to two main stroke types: **thrombotic strokes** and **embolic strokes.** A thrombotic stroke is caused by a clot forming in one of the brain's arteries. Generally, the larger the artery that is blocked, the larger the area of the brain deprived of blood, and the greater the disability that results. In a thrombotic stroke, the clot blocking an artery remains **in situ**, that is, it stays attached to its place of origin. In contrast, an embolic stroke is caused by a clot that breaks free from its place of origin and is carried by the bloodstream to the brain. If this "floating clot," called an **embolus**, gets lodged in a cerebral blood vessel, an embolic stroke can occur.

[14]The most frequent cause of an embolic stroke is the formation of a clot in the left **atrium** (upper chamber) of the heart. This clot is then pumped out of the heart, and is carried in the bloodstream until it gets lodged in a cerebral blood vessel. An embolic stroke caused by a clot originating in the heart is called a **cardiogenic cerebral embolism**[D4] (or **cardioembolic stroke**). This stroke type accounts for around 20% of all ischemic strokes. A key risk factor for a cardioembolic stroke is **atrial fibrillation**, a type of **arrhythmia** (abnormal heart rhythm). In atrial fibrillation, the left and right atria **quiver** rapidly instead of beating regularly and effectively. This **unsynchronized** quivering causes blood to pool in the atria, and clots readily form in such **stagnant** blood.

[15]Hemorrhagic strokes are, as was mentioned earlier, less frequent than ischemic strokes, but they are associated with a higher mortality rate and with more severe disability in people who survive the stroke. There are two types of hemorrhagic stroke. The first type, **intracerebral hemorrhage,** is the most common. It occurs when an artery in the brain ruptures, flooding the surrounding tissue with blood. As in ischemic stroke, atherosclerosis is a key cause of intracerebral hemorrhage because arteries hardened and stiffened by atherosclerosis are more susceptible to rupturing when under high blood pressure.

[16]The other type of hemorrhagic strokes is a **subarachnoid hemorrhage**[E9] (**SAH**), which involves bleeding in the space that surrounds the brain. Specifically, blood collects in the **subarachnoid space**, the space between the **pia mater** and the **arachnoid mater**. The pia mater and arachnoid mater are two of the three layers of membranes, called **meninges**, that surround and protect the **CNS** (i.e., the brain and spinal cord). The subarachnoid space is usually filled only with **cerebrospinal fluid** (**CSF**), a colorless fluid that cushions the CNS and provides it with nutrients. Bleeding into the subarachnoid space not only damages brain cells near the site of the bleed, but it also results in a rapid increase in **intracranial pressure**. Such an increase can result in serious damage to brain tissue. This kind of stroke is sometimes the result of a traumatic brain injury, but the most common cause is an **aneurysm** that leaks or ruptures. Mr. Suzuki, whom I met in hospital, underwent **prophylactic surgery**[E6] to clip an aneurysm and so prevent it from bleeding. A SAH caused by a ruptured aneurysm is fatal in between 20% to 50% of cases.

[17]Many people get **headaches** or **migraine**, and they are not usually a sign of an **underlying illness** (such headaches are called **primary headaches**). However, certain headaches, termed **secondary headaches**, are caused by an underlying medical problem. A severe headache of sudden onset (a so-called "**thunderclap**" headache) may be the first symptom of a ruptured aneurysm.

[18]For both ischemic and hemorrhagic strokes there are a number of modifiable and nonmodifiable risk factors. **Nonmodifiable risk factors** (i.e., those that cannot be

changed) include age (the majority of strokes occur in people who are 65 or older); sex (the incidence is higher in men); and **ethnicity** (in the USA, people of African descent have a higher prevalence of stroke than any other ethnic group). **Modifiable risk factors** are those that can, in theory, be changed by taking certain measures; for example, smoking greatly increases the risk of stroke, but this risk factor can be reduced by quitting smoking (of course, this is **easier said than done** considering the fact that nicotine is highly addictive). The following modifiable risk factors are thought to account for the majority strokes: **hypertension, tobacco smoking, diabetes, dyslipidemia, obesity, unhealthy diet**, and a **sedentary lifestyle**. Of these, hypertension is considered the single most important stroke risk factor. Awareness of the modifiable risk factors can help people to make lifestyle changes that reduce stroke risk.

[19]The mechanisms by which the above risk factors contribute to the **pathogenesis** of stroke are complex and much is still unknown. Moreover, the risk factors are often interrelated; for example, obesity leads to **chronic inflammation**, which plays a central role in the initiation and progression of atherosclerosis. In addition, obesity increases the risk of developing **type 2 diabetes**[D6] and **sleep apnea**, both of which are risk factors for stroke. Table 4.1 summarizes the main stroke risk factors. (As you read the table, consider how these risk factors could be modified; for example, being physically inactive can be modified by incorporating **incidental exercise** into your daily routine. This is unplanned exercise, such as climbing the stairs instead of taking the escalator, or doing squats while watching TV.)

[20]In addition to the ones in Table 4.1, there are various other modifiable risk factors for stroke. Drug use, for example, can be a significant risk. Heavy use of alcohol, a legal drug, can greatly increase the risk of hemorrhagic stroke. **Illicit drugs** that can cause stroke include **cocaine** (a drug derived from the coca leaf) and **amphetamines**. Poor sleep is also linked to a higher stroke risk, as is **psychosocial stress**. (Many politicians seem to die of stroke, perhaps partly because of the stress of the job: the Allied war leaders, Roosevelt, Stalin, and Churchill all died from stroke in 1945, 1953, and 1965 respectively.)

[21]Certain underlying conditions can also increase the risk of stroke, including **diabetes** and arrythmia. **Hematologic disorders**[D8], particularly **sickle cell disease** (SCD), is another risk factor. In SCD, red blood cells become stiff and misshapen, and therefore prone to getting stuck in blood vessels. It has been estimated that without **prophylactic treatment**, 25% of people with SCD suffer an ischemic stroke by the age of 45. COVID-19, the viral disease that emerged in 2019 in China and became a pandemic, is not only a respiratory disease, and one of its complications is ischemic stroke. One reason for this complication is that, in **susceptible** people, COVID-19 induces a **hypercoagulable state** (i.e., one that increases the tendency of clots to form).

Table 4.1

Some Modifiable Risk Factors for Stroke （脳卒中の修正可能な危険因子）

Risk Factor (危険因子)	Mechanisms （メカニズム）
Hypertension (高血圧(高血圧 症))	• Higher blood pressure exerts more force against the wall of blood vessels[*1]. This force weakens blood vessels, making them more **prone** to rupturing. • Mechanical injury to endothelial cells promotes atherosclerosis. • Hypertension can cause plaques to detach from atheroma and block a cerebral artery.
Smoking (喫煙)	• Toxic chemicals in tobacco smoke damage the endothelium of blood vessel walls, leading to atherosclerosis. • Reduces levels of HDL cholesterol ("good" cholesterol that helps prevent atherosclerosis by removing cholesterol from blood vessel walls and transporting it to the liver). • Raises levels of LDL cholesterol ("bad" cholesterol that is **atherogenic**[*2]). • Chemicals in tobacco smoke make platelets more likely to aggregate, increasing the risk of clots forming. • Nicotine raises blood pressure.
Unhealthy diet （不健康な食生活)	• Increases risk of hypertension, dyslipidemia, obesity, type 2 diabetes.
Diabetes mellitus (糖尿病)	Chronic hyperglycemia promotes atherosclerosis by causing systemic inflammation and damaging changes to blood vessels.
Dyslipidemia (脂質異常症)	An unhealthy imbalance of lipids in the blood promotes atherosclerosis.
Obesity (肥満)	Obesity, particularly **visceral obesity** (fat around the internal organs), causes systemic inflammation that contributes to atherosclerosis. Contributes to type 2 diabetes, hypertension, atrial fibrillation, and sleep apnea.
Physical inactivity (運動不足)	A **sedentary lifestyle** promotes oxidative stress, which triggers vascular dysfunction and drives atherosclerosis. Increases the risk of dyslipidemia, hypertension, and insulin resistance. **Regular exercise helps**: Maintain a healthy weight and blood pressure; control blood glucose levels; lower blood cholesterol; promote vasodilation by increasing the production of **nitric oxide.**

[*1]The frictional force acting on the inner walls of an artery as a result of blood flow is called **hemodynamic shear stress**.

[*2]*Atherogenic* means "driving the development of atherosclerosis." After entering the artery wall, LDL cholesterol particles attract **macrophages** (a type of immune cell). These macrophages ingest the LDL particles to form fat-laden cells called **foam cells.** These cells secrete substances that promote atheroma growth. Moreover, the death of foam cells causes inflammation, further driving atherosclerosis.

[22]Symptoms of a stroke vary according to which part of the brain is affected. For example, problems with balance, dizziness, **vertigo**, and **diplopia** (seeing double) tend to occur with blockage of a blood vessel in the back part of the brain (this is called a **posterior circulation stroke**), while headache and **aphasia** (loss or impairment of the

ability to use or understand language) is more common with a blockage in a blood vessel in the front of the brain (**anterior circulation stroke**). The size of the blood vessel affected will also determine the type and severity of symptoms. Almost 90% of all ischemic strokes occur due to a blockage of the **middle cerebral artery** (a key artery supplying blood to the cerebrum). If the main stem of the middle cerebral artery is occluded, a large area of the brain will be deprived of blood, resulting in a large area of **necrosis** (tissue death). The consequence of this is likely to be severe disability or death. On the other hand, if a blockage occurs in a smaller branch of this artery, the stroke will probably not be as damaging because less brain tissue is affected.

[23]Although ischemic and hemorrhagic stroke share many symptoms, certain symptoms are more common in one type of stroke compared to another. For example, hemorrhagic strokes are more often accompanied by severe headaches and **seizures** than are ischemic stroke (seizures occur in up to 28% of hemorrhagic strokes, and a seizure in someone with no previous history of them is a **red flag sign** of a brain hemorrhage).

[24]The symptoms of a stroke usually occur rapidly, over minutes or hours. A useful **mnemonic** to help remember and spot three typical symptoms of a stroke is **FAST**[D7]. The "F" of FAST stands for "Face"; Is one side of the face **drooping**? Ask the person to smile. The "A" stands for "Arm weakness"; Is the person unable to raise one arm completely? Ask the person to lift their arms. The "S" is for "Speech"; Is the person's speech **slurred** or strange? Ask the person to repeat a simple phrase. The last letter of this acronym is not a symptom, but an instruction on how to respond if you think that you or someone else is having a stroke: "T" is "Time," meaning that if you see any one of the above signs you should call an ambulance right away.

[25]Sometimes the symptoms of a stroke may disappear after a few minutes. Because the symptoms **resolve**, people may ignore them, but such temporary symptoms could be a "warning stroke" or **TIA** (**transient ischemic attack**). This type of stroke occurs when a blood vessel is blocked, usually by a blood clot, causing stroke symptoms; however, the blood vessel quickly becomes unblocked, allowing blood flow to resume. Unlike a full-blown ischemic stroke, a TIA does not cause permanent brain injury. A TIA should be treated as a medical emergency because the risk of having a full stroke after a TIA is about 5% within the following 48 hours and 8% at one week. The risk of a major stroke after a TIA can be greatly reduced by taking an **antiplatelet medication,** such as aspirin. Antiplatelet therapy needs to be started as soon as possible after diagnosis, ideally within 12 hours of the onset of TIA symptoms. In the weeks following a TIA, aspirin therapy can reduce the risk of a major stroke by up to 90%.

[26]People who have had one ischemic stroke often take medication for **secondary prevention**[D10]. As well as **statins**, which are drugs to lower blood cholesterol, and

antihypertensives, secondary-prevention usually includes an antiplatelet agent and/or an oral **anticoagulant** such as **warfarin** or a **DOAC**. However, it is important to note that while drugs that prevent blood clotting reduce the risk of another ischemic stroke, they also increase the risk of bleeding in the brain. Simply put, antiplatelet and anticoagulant therapies are risk factors for hemorrhagic stroke.

[27]The "T" in FAST reminds people not to **brush off** symptoms, but to act without delay. Getting a suspected stroke patient to hospital rapidly is important because certain stroke treatments are effective only if started within a few hours. For every minute following an ischemic stroke, around two million neurons die, so the quicker the blockage in a blood vessel is removed and blood flow restored, the more of the brain that can be saved. One way to restore blood flow is by administering a **thrombolytic drug**[E11] that dissolves the clot. The most frequently used thrombolytic drug (or "**clot buster**," as this kind of treatment is commonly known) is **tissue plasminogen activator**[D11] (**tPA**), known by the generic name of **alteplase**.

[28]Since tPA was approved by the FDA in 1995 for the treatment of ischemic stroke, it has allowed many people, who otherwise would have died or been severely disabled, to leave hospital and recover with less severe post-stroke disability, or even no aftereffects at all. However, tPA is only effective if used within a **time window** of around 4 hours, and it is not without side effects. A serious, potentially fatal, complication of tPA is bleeding in the brain. Not all stroke patients are **eligible** for clot busting drugs, so as soon as a patient arrives at hospital, doctors will check whether the patient has any **exclusion criterion**. Here are three of the many reasons a stroke patient could be excluded from tPA treatment: the person's CT scan shows an intracranial hemorrhage; the person has suffered severe head trauma within the last 3 months; and the person has taken an anticoagulant within the last 48 hours. A blood clot can also be removed mechanically with a procedure called **stent retriever thrombectomy**. Once a clot has been removed by pharmacological or mechanical means, the patient is usually prescribed **antiplatelet and/or anticoagulant drugs**[D2] to reduce the risk of another blood clot developing.

[29]Emergency treatment of hemorrhagic stroke involves the administration of drugs to lower intracranial pressure and prevent **vasospasm**, a strong contraction of vascular smooth muscle. The pathogenesis of cerebral vasospasm is not fully understood, but one hypothesis is that it is caused by irritation of blood vessels by substances released from hemoglobin as the hemorrhage **degrades**. Vasospasm narrows the inside diameter of an artery, resulting in reduced blood flow to that part of the brain. This can induce a **secondary ischemic stroke** (which is not great news for someone recovering from a hemorrhagic stroke). After a hemorrhagic stroke, surgery may be needed to decrease pressure on the brain and to remove the mass of blood (**hematoma**) that forms from

extravasation of blood into brain parenchyma[E3]. The pressure exerted on surrounding brain tissue by a hematoma can cause life-threatening secondary brain injury (the effect due to a bleed, tumor, or other mass is known as **mass effect**).

[30]From 1951 to 1980 stroke was the leading cause of death in Japan. For various reasons, including advances in acute stroke treatment, stroke has dropped to the fourth leading cause. However, it is now the top cause of long-term disability. More people become **bedridden** due to stroke than from dementia. Maintaining a healthy body weight, taking regular exercise, and **refraining** from smoking and overconsumption of alcohol are a few things that can be done to lower the risk of a stroke. And acting FAST if stroke does strike can save lives and reduce the severity of complications. Knowing about strokes can contribute to increasing our **lifespan,** and, more importantly, extending our **healthspan**, the period of life when we are in good health and free from major disability.

4-2 Eleven Etymologies (E) （11 の単語を詳しく）

1) *Cervical arteries***:** The human brain is so metabolically active that it receives around 20% of the body's blood supply, despite the fact it is only about 2% of the total body weight. There are two pairs of arteries on each side of your neck that carry oxygenated blood to the brain. On each side of the neck there is a **carotid artery**, which supplies the front of the brain, and also a **vertebral artery**, which carries blood to the back of the brain. (When you check a pulse in a person's neck, you are feeling for the **carotid pulse**.)　Collectively these arteries are known as **cervical arteries**. A **carotid dissection**, a tear of the inner layer of the wall of one of the carotid arteries, is a cause of ischemic stroke, especially in people under the age of 50.

WFE: The word *cervical* is from a Latin word that means "neck." This Latin word is also used to refer to the **cervix**, a part of the female reproductive system. The cervix is the neck-like passage at the base of the **uterus** that opens into the vagina. According to WHO, **cervical cancer** is the fourth most common cancer in women. In Japan, this cancer is increasing in younger women in their 20s and 30s. However, in other higher income countries, particularly Australia, cervical cancer is decreasing due to many girls being vaccinated against the **human papillomavirus** (HPV), the main cause of cervical cancer.

2) *Craniotomy* **is the surgical removal of part of the skull to expose the brain.**
WFE: *Cranio* refers to the "skull," and the suffix *~tomy* means to "cut." This suffix is in the names of many operations (another example is **tracheotomy**, which is an incision, or cut, made into the trachea in order to allow a person to breathe). The medical term for skull is

cranium, and an **intercranial hemorrhage** is bleeding between the brain and the skull or within the brain tissue. The word **migraine** (a type of a severe headache) is from the Greek *hemicrania*, which means "half the skull" (the pain of migraine is usually greater on one side of the head than the other). The WFE *tomy* is part of the following words: **anatomy** (*ana~* = "up"; so "cut up"); **atom** (*a~* = "not" +, so "cannot be cut"; it was believed that the atom was the smallest particle and that it could not be split); and **entomology** (*en~* = "in"; so, "cut into"). Entomology is the study of insects, which are animals with segmented body parts. One possible aftereffect of a stroke is **dysphagia** (difficulty swallowing), with *phag* meaning "to swallow." If you combine *entomo* + *phag* you get **entomophagy**, the technical term for eating insects, which is much more environmentally friendly than consuming beef or other meat.

The word **insect** is the Latin translation of the Greek word *entomon*. The Latin root *sek* means "cut," so insect means "cut into" (the body of adult insects is cut or divided into three body sections: head, thorax, and abdomen). In the term carotid dissection (see E1), **dissection** literally means "cut apart" (*dis~* = "apart").

3) *Extravasation of blood into brain parenchyma*: In simple English, this sentence means "escape of blood from blood vessels into surrounding brain tissue." **Parenchyma** refers to the tissue that actually performs the functions of the organ. Connective tissue, blood vessels, and other parts that do not perform the specific functions of that organ are not parenchyma.
WFE: The word **extravasation** can be understood if you know that *extra~* means "outside" and *vas* means "vessel." So, *extravasation* means "outside a [blood] vessel." Another word in the Essay with *vas* is **vasospasm**. The word *spasm* is from the Latin *spasmus*, a sudden involuntary contraction of a muscle, blood vessel, or a hollow organ such as the gut.

4) *Hemiparesis* is weakness on one side of the body that often affects the arms, hands, legs, and face. If a stroke damages the left side of the brain, the hemiparesis will be on the body's right side and vice versa. This happens because the left side of the brain mainly controls the right side of the body, and the right side of the brain mainly controls the left side of the body. So, when you scratch your nose with your left hand, it is the right side of the brain controlling this movement. This is termed **contralateral control** of the brain (*contra* = "opposite").
WFE: In hemiparesis, the prefix *hemi~* means "half." Another word with this WFE is **hemisphere**, which means "half of a sphere." The brain is divided into two halves, the left hemisphere and right hemisphere. The two halves of the brain are not exactly the same because certain functions are located mainly in one half of the brain compared to another. For example, the right hemisphere controls the ability to recognize things we see, hear or touch. This is why a stroke on the right side of the brain (**right-sided stroke**) is more likely to cause **anomia** (*a~* = "no" + *nom* = "name"), or the inability to recall the names of everyday objects.

This localizing of a certain function on one side of the brain in preference to the other side is called **lateralization of brain function**. The word **lateral** means "side." **Multilateral** literally means "many sides," but it is usually used to mean "between three or more countries" (e.g., *multilateral discussions on trade*). Some people are good at **lateral thinking**, meaning they are able to solve a problem by approaching the problem from the side; in other words, thinking about it in a new or creative way.

SD 4A: The structure of possibly the most complex thing in the universe

The brain is the most complex organ in our body, perhaps the most complex thing in the whole universe. It is the seat of intelligence and thought, controls all the body's functions, interprets information from the environment, and has many other functions. The brain is who we are. It is said that the brain has the same **consistency** as tofu, and this tofu-like brain floats in **cerebrospinal fluid** (CSF)—the tofu sold in a supermarket is also bathed in a fluid (water). This floating brain is protected by the **skull** (which can be compared to the strong plastic packet packaging in which tofu is packed). The brain can be divided into three parts: the forebrain, the midbrain, and the hindbrain.

- The **hindbrain** connects the brain to the spinal cord. It includes the **brain stem**, and the **cerebellum**. The hindbrain's main role is controlling the body's vital functions such as breathing and heart rate.
- The **midbrain** plays a crucial role in visual and auditory (hearing) reflexes.
- The **forebrain** consists of **cerebrum** and the structures beneath it. This the largest part of the brain. The cerebrum is split into two **hemispheres** by a deep groove (fissure), but the two cerebral hemispheres communicate with each other via a tract of fibers called the **corpus callosum** that is between the hemispheres.

While the surface of packaged tofu is smooth, the other layer of the brain, the **cerebral cortex**, is highly folded. These folds greatly increase the surface area of the brain. And while tofu is usually an attractive white color, the cortex is gray (not a very appetizing color). It is gray because neurons in this area lack **myelin**, a lipid-rich material that covers certain nerves and insulates them. Deep within the brain are very important structures such as the **hypothalamus**, which maintains homeostasis in the body by influencing the **autonomic nervous system** and producing and secreting many hormones, and the **hippocampus**, a structure that is principally involved in storing long-term memory. On a soccer team, each player (e.g., defender, striker, goalkeeper) has special skills and specific roles, but they all work together to win the match. In the same way, different parts of the brain also have special properties, but they coordinate their activities and work together.

The severity of a stroke depends greatly on its location. For example, a stroke in the brainstem, the location of the body's "life-support" functions, can quickly **impair** breathing and heart functions. Some functions of the brain, including **handedness** and speech production, are controlled more by one side of the brain than the other (**hemispheric lateralization**). For example, language is dealt with more by the left hemisphere, so left-sided strokes tend to cause **aphasia** and other language problems.

5) *Hemorrhagic stroke* **is bleeding into the brain caused by the rupture of a blood vessel.**
WFE: The WFE *hem* means "blood" and the suffix *~rhage* means "heavy flow." Hemorrhage usually means severe or abnormal bleeding. (If I pricked my finger on a rose thorn, I wouldn't say "my finger is hemorrhaging," but "my finger is bleeding.") Be careful of the spelling: there are two r's in hemo**rr**hage. Another word with a double "r" is **diarrhea**. The WFE *~rhea* means to "flow," so its meaning is related to *~rhage*.

Other words with the WFE *hemo* are **hemostasi**s, meaning "to stop bleeding" (*stasis* means "stop") and **hematoma**, which is a mass of clotted blood, caused by blood leaking outside of a broken blood vessel. A hematoma can form in almost any organ, tissue, or body space. For example, a **subcutaneous hematoma** appears just under the skin (*sub~* = "under"; *cutis* = "skin"). A **subdural hematoma** is when blood pools between the brain and the skull; specifically, blood leaks into the space under the **dura mater**, the outermost membrane of the meninges. A subdural hematoma is usually caused by a head injury that causes a tear in an intracranial blood vessel. It can lead to a dangerous increase in pressure inside the skull. Because babies have weak neck muscles and large heads in proportion to the rest of their body, they are vulnerable to a subdural hematoma if they are violently shaken. Raising children can be very stressful, but never forcefully shake a baby. Doing so may cause a baby to suffer **shaken baby syndrome**, resulting in serious brain damage.

In hematoma, the WFE *~oma* means "swelling/tumor." **Melanoma** is cancer that develops in the melanocytes, the cells that produce the pigment **melanin**. In **atheroma**, *~oma* does not indicate cancer, but an abnormal growth caused by a buildup of materials on artery walls. The Greek word *athere* means "porridge," so atheroma is a "tumor that contains a porridge-like substance." Porridge, by the way, is a breakfast dish made from oatmeal heated in water or milk. It is a traditional dish of Scotland, but oatmeal is now widely available in Japan. Porridge is tasty and healthy (e.g., it helps to lower blood cholesterol levels), and as you eat it, you can imagine the porridge-like deposits that have probably already accumulated in the walls of your arteries (atheromas start forming early in life, often in the teenage years).

SD 4B: Did the ancient Romans have hypertension?

I get a monthly salary from my employer, one of the largest universities in the Chubu (central) area of Japan. The salary I receive is in Japanese yen, but in the time of the Roman Empire, the Roman soldiers were sometimes paid each month with salt instead of money. This payment in salt was called a *salarium*, with *sal* being the Latin word for "salt." By the 19th century, the word "salary" had entered English with the modern meaning. The Japanese word *sarariman*, meaning a "male salaried worker," was already being used in Japan by the 1920s. Salt is plentiful now, and no one I know would want their salary paid in salt instead of money, but in Roman times salt was a valuable commodity. Salt was so valuable mainly because it was used for preserving food, especially fish. Like the Japanese, the ancient Romans loved fresh fish, but they also ate a lot of salted or **fermented** fish. Also, they consumed several types of salty fish sauce, the most popular of which was called *garum*. Another dish popular with the ancient Romans was vegetables, such as lettuce, dipped in salt. This dish was called *herba salata*, and is the origin of the word "salad." Two other food-related words derived from the Latin *sal* are "sausage" and "sauce."

Hypertension was not recognized as a medical problem until the invention of the **sphygmomanometer**, a device to measure **blood pressure (BP)**, by an Italian doctor in 1896, so we cannot know for sure if people in ancient Rome had hypertension. However, because of all the salty food the ancient Romans seem to have eaten, it is likely that some of them would have been diagnosed with it by our modern-day criteria. Whether or not people who lived over 1500 years ago (the Roman Empire fell in 476) had hypertension could be an interesting research topic for medical historians, but it is not so important for the readers of this book. What is more important are answers to some basic questions about BP.

Q1. What is BP? It is the force **exerted** against the walls of the arteries by blood pumped out of the heart. Blood pressure is highest when the ventricles of the heart contract. This is called **systemic pressure**. The lowest BP is between contractions—when the heart relaxes and fills with blood—and is called **diastolic pressure**. BP depends on **cardiac output (CO)** and **peripheral resistance (PR)**, which can be expressed with this formula: $BP = CO \times PR$.

Cardiac output is the volume of blood pumped out of the heart (measured in liters per minute). Cardiac output in turn depends on **stroke volume (SV)**, the volume of blood pumped out of the heart in one beat, and the **heart rate** (HR), the number of heartbeats per unit of time, usually per minute. Factors that increase SV include **adrenaline**, a hormone that causes the heart to contract more strongly and so pump more blood out. Another factor is **venous return**, the return of blood by the veins from the body's **periphery** to the right atrium of the heart. Venous return depends partly on **blood volume** (i.e., the total amount of fluid circulating within the various blood vessels and within the chambers of the heart). An increase in blood volume leads to an increase in venous return to the heart. More blood flowing into the heart causes greater stretching of the **cardiomyocytes** (heart muscle fibers), and this extra stretching makes the heart contract more strongly and pump more blood out (do a search for **"Frank-Starling law"** to find out more about the relationship between venous return and **cardiac contractility**, the strength of contraction of the heart muscle cells).

Peripheral Resistance is the resistance of the arterial blood vessels to blood flow. As the arteries constrict, the resistance increases, and as they dilate, resistance decreases. One factor that increases PR is activation of blood vessels by the sympathetic nervous system. Such activation causes **vasoconstriction** (narrowing of blood vessels due to contraction of smooth muscle in the wall of blood vessels). **Compliance** also has a big effect on PR. Compliance is the ability of a space, such as a **lumen** of a blood vessel, to expand in order to hold an increased content (e.g., more blood). Because they have thick muscular walls, arteries tend to have a lower compliance compared to veins, which have thin walls that are less muscular. The compliance of arteries is reduced by stiffening due to atherosclerosis. So, vasoconstriction and lower vascular compliance increase PR.

Another factor affecting PR is **blood viscosity**, a measure of a fluid's resistance to flow (water has low viscosity, whereas the viscosity of maple syrup is higher). The more viscous blood is the harder the heart has to work to pump blood around the body. This creates more pressure within blood vessels. Viscosity is increased by factors such as **dehydration**, high blood sugar concentration (**hyperglycemia**), and an increase in **hematocrit** (the proportion of red blood cells in the blood; an increase in hematocrit occurs after several days of living at high altitude).

The regulation of BP is a complex process, involving **baroreceptors** that monitor arterial blood pressure, and cardiovascular, neural, renal, and endocrine systems working together to maintain a state of homeostasis. Table 4.2 lists some of the main mechanisms that help to regulate blood pressure.

Q2. What is hypertension? Blood pressure **fluctuates** throughout the day; it is never constant. Our blood pressure varies depending on factors such as **posture**, physical activity, emotional stress, how hydrated we are, and medications we have taken. When we get up after a night's sleep, blood pressure falls slightly (this is because when we stand, gravity causes blood to pool in the legs, which lowers the venous return). Because BP can be affected by many factors, hypertension is not diagnosed after a single high reading on a blood-pressure monitor, but after several separate measurements. So, hypertension is a condition in which the pressure of blood in the arteries is **persistently elevated**.

In the USA, blood pressure is defined 130/80 mm Hg or higher (read this as "130 *over* 80 millimeters of mercury"; the higher number is the **systolic BP** measurement, and the lower one is the **diastolic** BP). The Japanese Society of Hypertension defines hypertension as 140/90 mm Hg or higher when measured in a clinical setting, and 135/85 mm Hg when measured on a blood pressure monitor at home. Although hypertension can lead to stroke and other serious complications, it does not usually cause obvious symptoms. The **asymptomatic** nature of hypertension is why it is sometimes called a "**silent killer.**" It should be noted that severe hypertension can cause headaches, nosebleeds, and other symptoms in some people.

Q3. Why does salt raise BP? Salt (NaCl) is a chemical compound made up of sodium (40%) and chloride (60%). The word "sodium" was coined in 1807 by Humphry Davy, an English chemist. Sodium was so called because it was isolated from caustic soda (sodium hydroxide). The symbol Na is from the Latin *natrium*, meaning "soda." The Japanese word *natoriumu* (ナトリウム) has its roots in Greek and Latin, but was adopted from the German word *Natrium*.

We need salt because it performs various vital functions in the body. For example, sodium is required to conduct nerve impulses, contract and relax muscles, and to maintain fluid balance in the body. But the amount of salt that most people need for these vital functions is less than 500 mg a day. The WHO recommends a daily salt intake of less than 5 grams (which is about 2g sodium—it is sodium rather than chloride that is the major cause of hypertension). In Japan, however, the average consumption of salt is more than twice this at 11 g/day. A lot of the salt people consume is in the form of "**hidden salt**" in processed foods (e.g., breakfast cereals contain a lot of salt).

Our kidneys are usually efficient at regulating the levels of water and sodium in the blood. But for some people, eating too much salt over a long period can lead to the kidneys no longer being able to sufficiently process it. The body is sensitive to levels of sodium in the blood that are too high (or low), and it works to lower blood sodium levels by retaining water. This **retention** of water leads to an increase of fluid in the blood vessels, expanding the BV and increasing the venous return, CO, and BP. It is important to note that there are individual differences in salt sensitivity. For some people high salt consumption is associated with a significant rise in BP, while other people do not seem to be greatly affected.

One strong piece of evidence that high salt consumption is an important cause of hypertension is from research on the **Yanomami Indians**, indigenous people in the Venezuelan jungle. These people still lead a **hunter-gatherer** life. All the salt they consume is contained in the food they eat; for example, if they kill a monkey, they eat the bone marrow and **offal** (internal organs) of the animal, which naturally contain salt. But the amount of salt they consume each day is much less than half a gram. The average systolic BP of Yanomami people is 96mmHg, and the average diastolic BP is 60 mmHg. Moreover, their BP does not generally rise with age (in societies with a western lifestyle, increasing age is a key factor for hypertension). In short, for Yanomami Indians living a traditional hunter-gather life, hypertension does not seem to exist and stroke and other vascular diseases are almost unknown. This protection is not genetic because when Yanomami people migrate to urban areas and adopt a western lifestyle, they develop hypertension, type 2 diabetes, and early cardiovascular disease.

Finally for this section, I'd like to ask you question about a hypothetical situation: **If you had no choice, would you rather drink, within one hour, a liter of urine or a liter of soy sauce?** When I ask this question to first-year pharmacy students, most choose the soy sauce—or *shoyu* (醤油), as this **condiment** is called in Japan. This choice of *shoyu*, I tell my students, is a potentially fatal one. Here's why. Firstly, the urine from a person who is hydrated and healthy is sterile and 95% water, so in the short-term it is perfectly safe to drink. On the other hand, soy sauce contains between 15 to 18% salt (sea water is about 3.5% salt). A liter of soy sauce contains around 170 grams of salt. This amount of salt ingested in a short-period of time would cause **hypernatremia**, an abnormally high concentration of sodium in the blood and in the **intercellular fluid**, the fluid that surrounds the cells. (All the fluid outside of cells—in the blood and the intercellular fluid—is called **extracellular fluid**). Water will move according to the principle of **osmosis**, which means it will move across a **semi-permeable membrane** from an area of low solute concentration (i.e., **hypotonic solution**) to an area of high solute concentration (i.e., **hypertonic solution**). So, after drinking a bottle of soy sauce, water will move from the intracellular fluid (i.e., from inside body cells), across the plasma membrane, and move into the extracellular fluid. This movement will occur until the fluids within the cells and outside the cells have the same salt concentration (i.e., are **isotonic**).

Hypernatremia can cause problems to the heart, kidneys, and other body organs, but the rapid loss of water from cells is particularly damaging to brain cells. As brain cells lose water they shrink. This brain shrinkage induced by hypernatremia causes blood vessels in the brain to rupture, leading to cerebral bleeding and **cerebral edema** (swelling of the brain). Neurological symptoms of hypernatremia include confusion, seizures, and coma. There have been cases of people dying or being left with permanent brain damage after overdosing on soy sauce. A drop or two of soy sauce on sashimi is delicious, but in large amounts it becomes a poison. All things, including oxygen and water, can be toxic in excess. As Paracelsus, a Swiss doctor, wrote over 500 years ago: "The dose makes the poison."

Table 4.2

The Body's Main Mechanisms of Blood Pressure Control （血圧調節のおもな機構）

	Sensors of BP （血圧受容器（血圧の体内センサー））	CNS and PNS （中枢神経系と末梢神経系）	Kidneys　（腎臓）	Other Hormones （他のホルモン）
Overall function （総合的機能）	**Baroreceptors:** sensory neurons located in the carotid artery, aorta, and other places. They sense BP and pass information to the **cardiovascular center**.	**Cardiovascular center** in the **medulla** of brain stem controls CO and adjusts the diameter of blood vessels.[*1]	**Renin** (hormone released by cells in the kidneys) is part of the **RAAS (renin-angiotensin-aldosterone system)**.	**Adrenaline and noradrenaline**[*2] ↑HR+↑CC→↑BP. Causes vasoconstriction. **Antidiuretic hormone** causes kidneys to retain H_2O →↑BV→↑CO→↑BP.
Cardiac Effect （心臓の役割）	Rapid regulation of BP by: a) Stimulating heart via **sympathetic nerves** →↑HR+↑CC→↑CO→↑BP. b) Inhibiting heart via **parasympathetic nerves** →↓HR+↓CC →↓CO→↓BP.		Angiotensin II (end-product of RAAS) stimulates secretion of **aldosterone** → ↑reabsorption of Na and H_2O →↑BV→↑CO→↑BP.	**Atrial natriuretic peptide** (ANP) secreted by the heart. Causes vasodilation and ↑ renal excretion of H_2O →↓BP.
Vascular Effect （血管の役割）	**Sympathetic vasomotor nerves** innervate arterioles. Causes vasoconstriction →↑PR→↑BP.		Angiotensin II. Causes vasoconstriction →↑PR→ ↑BP.	**Nitric oxide** (NO)[*3]: A gas secreted by vascular endothelium. Causes vasodilation →↓BP.

Key: Na = sodium; CNS = central nervous system; PNS = peripheral nervous system; BP = blood pressure; BV = blood volume; CO = cardiac output; CC: Cardiac contractility; PR = peripheral resistance; ↑ increase; ↓decrease; → lead(s) to

[*1]In addition to information from baroreceptors, the cardiovascular center in the brainstem also receives information from higher parts of the brain such as the hypothalamus and cerebral cortex.

[*2]Norepinephrine is a hormone because it is released by a gland (the adrenal gland), but it is also a neurotransmitter because it is released by sympathetic nerve endings. In fact, about 80% of noradrenaline in the body is released by nerve endings.

[*3] It is debated whether NO should be classified as a hormone or a local signaling molecule.

6) *Prophylactic surgery* is surgery to prevent or reduce the risk of a harmful condition occurring. It is estimated that around 3% of the general population have an aneurysm in the brain (**intracerebral aneurysm**). Most of these people will live a normal life and die without ever knowing they had an aneurysm. However, in a small minority of people, an **aneurysm** will rupture, causing a very serious, often fatal, stroke. Due to the widespread use of imaging, including MRI scanning, more unruptured aneurysms are being found incidentally (**incidental discovery**). To prevent an unruptured aneurysm from rupturing in the future, some people choose to have an operation to clip the aneurysm. Such an operation is called **prophylactic aneurysm surgery**. Another example of prophylactic surgery is **prophylactic mastectomy**. This is surgery to remove one or both breasts in order to lower the chances of getting breast cancer. It is chosen by some women (and men) who have a mutation in the **BRCA1** or **BRCA2** gene and/or a strong family history of breast cancer.

Antibiotics are sometimes administered before surgery in order to reduce the risk of bacterial infection. This is called **antibiotic prophylaxis**. In 2012, the FDA in the USA approved a treatment for **HIV** called **pre-exposure prophylaxis** (PrEP). This treatment, which involves taking a daily oral medication, prevents a person at risk of contracting HIV (human immunodeficiency virus) from being infected with the virus.

WFE: The noun **prophylaxis** (adjective: **prophylactic**) is composed of the prefix *pro~* ("before") and *phylax*, meaning "guarded, protected." So, prophylaxis means "guard against."

Anaphylaxis is a serious allergic reaction. This word was **coined** by Charles Richet, a French doctor who won The Nobel Prize in Physiology or Medicine in 1913. It is said that Richet first used the prefix *an~* ("not") to form the word "anphylaxis," meaning "unguarded," but he later changed the prefix to *ana~* meaning "too much/over." In anaphylaxis, instead of being protected by the immune system, the body is made hypersensitive (or "over-guarded"). In such a hypersensitive state, an allergen such as a peanut can trigger an **anaphylactic reaction**, causing potentially life-threatening symptoms.

SD 4C: Narrow Japan; wide Europe

I started studying Japanese after arriving in Japan in the early 1990s. In one of my first Japanese lessons, I learnt the adjectives *hiroi* (広い) and *semai* (狭い). Translated into English they mean "wide" and "narrow," respectively, but my teacher taught me that *semai* has a greater range of meaning than just "narrow." She illustrated this with a famous traffic-safety slogan from the early 1970s: ***semai** nihon, sonna ni isoide doko he iku* (せまい日本、そんなに急いでどこへ行く). The teacher told us that in this slogan, *semai* did not mean "narrow," but "small": "Where are you going to in such a rush, in this *small* country of Japan? (It must be said that Japan is really not that small—the land mass of Japan's four main islands is around the same as that of Germany). What's this got to do with the topic of strokes? Be patient, please, I'm doing my best to get back on topic. Anyway, moving from "narrow" Japan to the continent of **Europe**. One of the theories on the origin of this continent's name is that it contains the Greek root *eurys*, meaning "wide." And *eurys* is also found in the medical word **aneurysm**, a permanent *widening*, or dilation, of a vein or artery.

7) ***Ruptured***: If something ruptures, it breaks or bursts suddenly. A man I knew suffered a **ruptured spleen** in a karate competition. The spleen stores a lot of blood, and, if it is ruptured, serious **internal bleeding** can occur. A ruptured spleen is a medical emergency.

WFE: In the word "rupture," the root *rupt* means "break." It is the root of many common words, including, **corrupt**, **erupt**, **interrupt**, and **disrupt**.

*& After taking the medicine, the girl had an allergic reaction and her skin **erupted in a rash**.*

*& Mount Fuji last **erupted** in 1707. (e~ → ex~ = "out")*

& If you need to talk to someone who is talking to someone else, it is polite to say "Sorry, for **interrupting***." (inter~ = "between")*

& Heavy snow always **disrupts** *public transport in London. (dis~ = "apart")*

& Dioxin is an **endocrine disruptor***, a chemical that can affect the function of the endocrine system. In Japan, most dioxins are produced by the burning of household and industrial waste.*

8) ***Ningendokku* is a regular, often annual, health check.** As well as blood and urine tests, a *ningendokku* (人間ドック) appointment often includes MRI, CT and PET scans, ultrasound to check the carotid artery for atherosclerosis, and procedures to examine the digestive system (gastroscopy and/or a colonoscopy). For many years, I assumed that *ningendokku* was a combination of "human" and "doctor"—*ningen* (人間) is the Japanese for "human." However, I later learnt that *dokku* is from the English "dock." A ship is regularly inspected and repaired in a **dry dock** to make it safe for the next sea journey. In the same way, people are checked to screen for any problems such as cancer, heart problems, kidney disease, or an aneurysm. Detecting diseases early can often improve the prognosis.

9) ***Subarachnoid hemorrhage* is bleeding in the space between the brain and the membranes that cover the brain.** The membranes that cover and protect the brain are called the **meninges**. There are three meninges. The membrane nearest the brain is called the **pia mater**, the middle membrane is the **arachnoid mater**, and the membrane nearest to the skull is the **dura mater**. The space between the pia mater and the arachnoid mater is called the **subarachnoid space**. Bleeding into the subarachnoid space is a subarachnoid hemorrhage. Partly because of its aging population and a high-salt diet contributing to hypertension, Japan's **incidence** of subarachnoid hemorrhage is particularly high (in Japan the incidence is 15-23 people per 10,000 compared to approximately 8 per 100,000 of population in the UK).

The meninges can become infected by a pathogen such as a bacteria or virus causing inflammation of the meninges, or **meningitis**. Especially dangerous is **bacterial meningitis**, which can kill in hours. A stiff neck is a common symptom of meningitis, but I recommend that you watch an online video about meningitis to familiarize yourself with the various symptoms of this life-threatening condition.

WFE: "Subarachnoid" is made of three WFEs: *sub~* (= "under"), *arachno* (= "spider") and *~oid* (= "similar to"). It is called the "arachnoid mater" because it resembles a spiderweb. **Arachnophobia**, an "irrational or disproportionate fear of spiders," is one of the most common phobias (*phobos* is Greek for "fear"). The meninges protect the brain like a mother protects a child, and the Latin word *mater* means "mother." The innermost layer, nearest the brain, is thin and delicate (*pia* means "soft" in Latin), while the outermost layer, nearest to the skull, is composed of dense tissue that makes it strong and thick (*dura* means "hard" in Latin).

The three layers of the meninges can be translated as "tough mother" (硬 膜), "spiderweb-like"(クモ膜), and "soft mother" (軟膜).

SD 4D: The brain is not only neurons

There are two main types of cells in the brain: **neurons** (nerve cells) and **glial cells**. There are three types of glial cell: **astrocytes, microglia,** and **oligodendrocytes**. The name "glial" is derived from the ancient Greek word *glia,* meaning "glue/cement." The scientist who coined this name in 1856 was Rudolf Virchow (he actually called them "neuro-glia"). Virchow and other scientists at the time hypothesized that glial cells functioned mainly to hold the brain cells together. However, it is now known that glial cells have a range of important functions. For example, astrocytes, which are star-shaped cells (the Greek word *astron* means "star"), regulate **synaptogenesis** (the formation of synapses between neurons), and oligodendrocytes assemble the **myelin sheath**, the fatty membrane that covers the axons of some nerve cells. The presence of a myelin sheath greatly speeds up the **propagation** of nerve impulses (check out **"saltatory conduction"** to find out more). Glial cells are numerous; in fact, they may actually outnumber neurons. It is only neurons, however, that can transmit signals, in the form of nerve impulses, to other cells.

All neurons have three parts: **dendrites** (receive signals from other neurons), **cell body** (the control center of the cell), and **axon** (transmit information to different neurons, muscles, and glands). Where neurons meet there is a gap called a **synapse**, and in order for messages to cross this gap a **neurotransmitter** (e.g., dopamine, serotonin) is needed. Many drugs that act on the nervous system work by affecting the balance of these neurotransmitters. After a stroke, axons that were not damaged make new branches that connect to other nerve cells. This sprouting of new nerve branches is called **collateral sprouting**, and it is thought to be stimulated by rehabilitation. Collateral sprouting is one way the brain recovers lost functions.

Finally, a short etymology lesson: "dendrite" is from *dendron,* the Greek word for "tree." This is because the dendrites are tree-like in that they have many branches. Oligodendrocytes are so called because they only have a *few* branch-like structure coming out of the cell body. The prefix *oligo~* means "a few." Dehydration is the most common cause of **oliguria,** production of only a *small amount* of urine. **Oligosaccharides** are a type of carbohydrate made up of only a few (i.e., between 3 to 10) glucose units linked together (in contrast, starches, a type of polysaccharide, contain between 300 to 1,000 of glucose units joined together in a long chain; "poly" means "many"). Oligosaccharides are contained in various foods and also in human milk, and they are said to have various health benefits. There are several types of government systems in the world, including democracy, communism, monarchy, and **oligarchy**. This final system is "rule by a few people" (*archon* = "to rule"; e.g., monarchy literally means "rule by one person"). The modern meaning of **oligarch** is "someone who is extremely rich and powerful, especially a person from Russia who became rich after the end of the former Soviet Union" (Cambridge Dictionary). After Russia's invasion of Ukraine in February, 2022, many Russian oligarchs had **sanctions** imposed on them by various governments.

10) *Systemic hypoperfusion stroke* **is a type of ischemic stroke caused by a reduction of blood flow to all parts of the body.** The reduction in cerebral blood flow is most often caused by a failure of the heart to pump sufficient blood around the body as a result of **myocardial infarction** (heart attack), or **ventricular fibrillation** (a type of **arrhythmia** that causes **cardiac arrest**). In a stroke caused by systemic hypoperfusion, the whole brain is affected, but most seriously affected are certain regions—known as **watershed areas**—that are located furthest from the brain's main arteries. If you imagine major highways as being the main cerebral arteries, watershed areas are those areas between the main roads that are supplied by only small minor roads. Watershed areas of the brain are supplied with blood by the smallest branches of blood vessels, meaning they are most vulnerable to tissue death resulting from low cerebral blood flow. Systemic hypoperfusion stroke is also called a **watershed stroke**.

WFE: In medicine, **systemic** means "affecting the whole body." For example, a scratch on the finger from a pet cat can cause as a **localized infection** limited to that one finger. But if the infection enters the bloodstream, it can cause a **systemic infection**. This word is often used to talk about social problems that are deeply rooted in society or in an institution.

*& Some people say that the police force in the USA is **systemically racist**.*

*& Japan has one of the highest levels of gender inequality out of the developed countries. One reason for this is **systemic inequality** that prevents women fulfilling their potential.*

The word "system" is made up *syn~* (= "together") and *stem* (*ste→sta* = "to stand"). So, system means "stand/place together."

The word **hypoperfusion** contains the prefix *hypo~* (= "low/less than normal") and perfusion. Perfusion is the movement of blood through blood vessels and delivery of blood to a part of the body. The prefix *per~* means "through," and *fusion* contains the WFE *fus*, meaning "to pour." So, perfusion means "pour through." Other words with the WFE *fus* are **refuse** (lit. "pour back"), **confuse** (lit. "pour together"), and **transfuse** (lit. "pour across").

*& When I started to learn the Japanese language, I used to **confuse** the words kawaii, meaning "cute" and kowai, meaning "scary."*

*& A small percentage of women require a **blood transfusion** after giving birth.*

11) *Thrombolytic drugs* **dissolve clots in blood vessels and so restore blood flow to tissues.**

WFE: The root *thrombo* means "clot of blood." **Thrombin** is a vital part of the clotting process. It is an enzyme that catalyzes the conversion of **fibrinogen** to **fibrin**, which forms the scaffold for a blood clot. The suffix *~ase* is often used to form the names of enzymes (e.g., amylase and lipase), although the suffix *~in* is also used (e.g., pepsin, renin). Thrombin, therefore, means "clotting enzyme." The word "clot" itself is from Old English meaning "lump." (A very delicious, but fattening, food is **clotted cream**, which is cream that has been made very thick by cooking. In England it is often eaten with scones and jam as part of a cream tea.) The WFE *lysis~* means to "break down or dissolve." **Autolysis** is the breakdown of a cell with enzymes released by the cell itself. Another name is "self-digestion." **Analysis** means to look at a complex issue by breaking it up into simpler parts.

The blood of some people may clot too easily. This condition is called **thrombophilia**, and it can increase the chances of stoke, deep vein thrombosis (DVT), and pulmonary embolism. The WFE *philia* means "a tendency to," but it can also mean "a liking for." An **Anglophile** is a person who likes and is interested in England and things English. **Lipophilicity** is the **affinity** of a drug for a lipid environment. It is an important property of a drug because a lipophilic drug diffuses readily across cell membranes and is more quickly absorbed into the body. A rare blood disorder is **hemophilia** (*hemo~* = "blood"). In people with hemophilia blood does not clot properly, so they have "an affinity, or tendency, to bleed."

Heparin induced thrombocytopenia is a very rare side effect of heparin, an anticoagulant drug. In people who get this side effect, the immune system reacts to heparin by producing antibodies against platelets, causing the blood platelet count to fall.

The word **thrombocytopenia** is composed of *thrombo* + *cyte* + *penia*. A **thrombocyte** is another name for **platelet**; (*cyte* = "cell") and *penia* is the Latin for "deficiency/lack of." The WFE *penia* originates from *Penia*, the ancient Greek goddess of poverty. A word meaning "being in a state of extreme poverty" is **penury**. An abnormally low level of white blood cells is known as **leukopenia** (*leuk* = "white"). **Neutropenia** is a low blood cell count of neutrophils, a type of white blood cell. Neutropenia, a common side effect of chemotherapy, results in lowered immunity and so increases the risk of infections. **Sarcopenia** is a loss of muscle mass that occurs in older people and in diseases such as cancer (*sarco* = "muscle/flesh"). The word **sarcasm** literally means to "tear off flesh."

4-3 Dozen in Detail (D) （12の話題を詳しく）

1) *Rehabilitation* **refers to various interventions that are designed to improve functioning and reduce disability in people with health conditions.** Stroke can cause severe disability. The main disability people associate with a stroke is **paralysis** and loss of movement. This is because neural connections that control movement are damaged by a stroke. But stroke can cause other types of problems such as **aphasia** (problems understanding or using language), **sensory disturbances** (loss or reduction in the ability to sense sensations such as temperature and pain), **cognitive disturbances** (problems with memory and thinking), and **emotional disturbances**, such as depression and anxiety. Fortunately, disabilities caused by a stroke can often improve. This is because a function

that was carried out by a part of the brain damaged by a stroke can be taken over by an undamaged part. This can occur because **neural pathways** (connections formed between neurons along which messages travel from one part of the nervous system to another) are not fixed, but they can be rewired through **neuroplasticity**. Neuroplasticity is the capacity of the brain to reorganize neurons in response to learning or experience. However, for the rewiring of neural pathways to occur, **rehabilitation** is vital.

In rehabilitation, the person who has had a stroke will practice movements many times. This practice stimulates the rewiring of the brain, helping a person to relearn skills lost due to the stroke. For example, imagine that a stroke has left a middle-aged woman unable to write. In rehabilitation sessions, this woman will need to relearn the letters of the alphabet like a five-year old child. Practicing writing letters and words hundreds of times should enable her to regain the ability to write. The brain is most susceptible to rewiring soon after the stroke (most improvement is often made in the first 6 months), which is why rehabilitation may begin in hospital the day after a stroke.

SD 4E: Can the brain regenerate?

While organs such as the liver and skin have a capacity to regenerate, the brain cannot regenerate new brain cells. At least this has been **conventional wisdom** for many years. However, research in recent decades suggests that the brain can create new cells by a process called **neurogenesis**. Neurogenesis in adult life seems to be limited to specific areas of the brain, but future medical techniques, perhaps using stem cells, may be developed to promote neurogenesis to repair parts of the brain damaged by a stroke.

2) *Antiplatelet and/or anticoagulant drugs:* **together with thrombolytics, these are drugs that affect blood clotting.** Let's just clarify the difference between these three drug classes. Both anticoagulants and antiplatelet drugs are **antithrombotic** drugs. This means that they prevent blood clotting (**thrombosis**). However, they do this through different mechanisms of action.

- **Anticoagulant medicines** work by inhibiting **clotting factors** in the blood. There are 12 clotting factors, which are proteins synthesized in the liver. The factors are involved in a series of reactions (called the **coagulation cascade**) that change liquid blood into a blood clot.
- **Antiplatelet medicines** work by inhibiting platelets (also called **thrombocytes**) from **clumping** together (**platelet aggregation**).
- **Thrombolytics** dissolve clots in blood vessels that have already formed, but they do not prevent clots forming in the first place. They are also called **fibrinolytics** because they act to break up the strands of fibrin that bind a clot together.

To understand how antiplatelet drugs work, we need to know a little bit more about blood clotting. When you cut your finger and blood comes out from the wound, this means you have broken a blood vessel. **Hemostasis**, or the stopping of bleeding from a blood vessel, has three components. Firstly, **vascular spasm** occurs. This is contraction of the wall of the blood vessels that supply blood to the broken vessel. This stops blood flow to the damaged area and so reduces blood loss. Next, is **platelet recruitment**. This is when platelets migrate to the site of a broken blood vessel. At the site of the broken vessel, platelets are activated to become "sticky," causing them to **clump** together. They also **adhere** (stick) to the blood vessel wall. The platelets make a plug that seals the broken blood vessel. However, the platelet plug is not that strong, so the clumped platelets release chemicals that activate clotting factors in the blood.

The last step in the coagulation cascade is the conversion of **fibrinogen**, one of the clotting factors, to **fibrin,** an insoluble, fibrous protein. This step is catalyzed by the enzyme **thrombin**. Strands of fibrin become caught in the platelet plug to forms a **mesh**, a bit like a fishing net. More platelets, red blood cells, and other components in the blood become trapped in the mesh and a strong blood clot is formed. Platelet activation and the coagulation cascade is very important for stopping bleeding when a blood vessel is broken from a cut or from some other injury. However, blood clotting can also occur inside blood vessels (**intravascular clotting**).

A well-known antiplatelet drug is **aspirin**, which works by inhibiting an enzyme called **COX-1** (cyclo-oxygenase). COX-1 is required to make a substance called **thromboxane**. Thromboxane is released by platelets and it stimulates the activation of other platelets, making platelets stick together. So, by inhibiting thromboxane, aspirin stops platelet activation and **platelet aggregation** (i.e., the sticking together of platelets).

The most well know anticoagulant drug is **warfarin**. It works by inhibiting an enzyme called $VKORC_1$ (vitamin K epoxide reductase) that is essential for activating vitamin K. Simply put, warfarin prevents the production of vitamin K, preventing the liver from producing certain clotting factors so that clots cannot be created. More specifically, vitamin K is a **cofactor** that is needed to activate 4 of the 12 clotting factors; therefore, the blocking of vitamin K by warfarin will reduce with synthesis of vitamin K-dependent clotting factors and stop the coagulation cascade. Warfarin has been used an anticoagulant since 1954, and in subsequent years it has prevented may early deaths from stroke, heart attack, and other conditions. It might surprise you, however, that before it started to be used as a human medicine, warfarin had been used since 1948 as a **rodenticide**, a **pesticide** to kill **rodents**. A famous American who took this "rat poison" soon after it was **authorized** was US president Dwight D. Eisenhower. He was prescribed the drug after a heart attack in 1955. That fact that warfarin had saved the life of an American president was widely reported in the press around the world and its use increased dramatically.

We have not talked about the discovery of warfarin, but it is an amazing story of cows dying in pools of their own blood, moldy hay, and a chance meeting one winter's night in 1933 between a **distraught** farmer and a **tenacious** biochemist named Karl Paul Link. It is a story of **serendipity**, together with methodical science, to **isolate** the compound that would become the active ingredient of warfarin. If you are curious to know more about this story, an internet search will reveal all.

SD 4F: After how long is novel no longer novel?

Shingata korona uirusu kansenshou (新型コロナウイルス感染症) is the Japanese for Covid-19, an infectious disease caused by the SARS-CoV-2 virus. The *shingata* part of the name means "novel [viral] strain." Even though several years have passed since the virus was identified, this name is still commonly used in the Japanese press. When will this "novel" virus no longer be novel? Using the word "novel" to name a new disease may be unwise because nothing is new for ever.

The same can be said for medicines. Until 2010, warfarin, approved in 1954, was the only oral anticoagulant widely available for use in humans. It has been used for a number of indications, including for the prevention of stroke in patients with atrial fibrillation, and as a prophylaxis and treatment of venous thrombosis. In 2010, the FDA in the USA approved a new type of oral anticoagulant, called **dabigatran**, that had a different mechanism of action from warfarin. Whereas warfarin reduces the production of clotting factors by blocking vitamin K, dabigatran binds directly to **thrombin** (clotting factor IIa) and inhibits it. This inhibition prevents the conversion of fibrinogen to fibrin by the enzyme thrombin, thus interfering with the clotting process.

Following the approval of dabigatran, several other drugs became available that directly inhibited clotting factors other than thrombin. These newly available drugs were called **NOACs (novel oral anticoagulants)**. However, after a few years, these drugs were no longer "novel," and there were calls by experts to rename this class of drugs. The acronym that is now most widely used is **DOAC**, which stands for "**direct oral anticoagulant**." The "D" explains the mechanism of these anticoagulants (i.e., they directly bind to specific clotting factors). Perhaps it would have been less confusing if DOAC, not NOAC, had been used from 2010. Although more expensive than warfarin, DOACs have several advantages over warfarin, including being easier to use and safer. For this reason, DOACs are replacing warfarin as the recommended anticoagulant for the prevention of **thromboembolic** events. Table 4.4 compares some pros and cons of warfarin and DOACs.

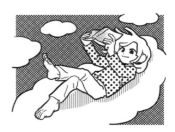

Table 4.3

Comparison of Warfarin and DOACs　（ワーファリンと直接経口抗凝固薬の比較）

	Warfarin　（ワーファリン）	**DOACs**　（直接経口抗凝固薬）
Need for routine blood testing （採血によるモニタリング）	Yes	No
Drug and food interactions （薬物と食事との相互作用）	Many	Few
Dietary restriction　（食事制限）	Restrictions on foods rich in vitamin K	Not necessary
Bleeding risk　（出血のリスク）	Higher	Reduced
Onset of action　（効果発現）	Slow	Rapid
Half-life*[1]　（半減期）	Longer (20-60 hours)	Shorter (14-17 hours for dabigatran; other DOACs are as short as 5 hours)
Dosing*[2]　（飲む量）	Variable	Fixed
Cost　（薬価）	Cheap	More expensive
Antidote*[3]　（解毒剤）	Yes (vitamin K)	Available only for certain types

*[1] A drug's half-life is the duration of action of a drug. It is the time required for the concentration of drug in the blood to be reduced by one-half by being metabolized or eliminated from the body. DOACs have a short half-life, meaning an antidote is not necessary in most cases (because the body will quickly metabolize the drug). A disadvantage of a short half-life is the higher risk of a blood clot if the patient forgets to take a dose.

*[2] For warfarin, the anticoagulation effect cannot be accurately predicted by dosage alone, which is why close monitoring is required. Also, there is great individual variation with warfarin; for example, one person may need a low dose of only 5 mg per week, while another person of the same weight may require 70 mg to achieve the same protective effect. For DOACs, the therapeutic effect is predictable meaning that the dose does not need to be constantly monitored.

*[3] An antidote is an agent that counteracts or reverses the effect of a substance (often a poison) An antidote to reverse the effect of dabigatran was approved in 2018 by the FDA, but not all DOACs have an antidote.

SD 4G: Drugs from pig guts and bat spit

While warfarin was the first oral anticoagulant medication, **heparin** was the first anticoagulant agent to be discovered, isolated, and used as a medicine. But unlike warfarin, heparin is not orally absorbed, and it must be injected directly into the body (this is called **parenteral administration**). Because heparin can only be administered by injection, it is mostly used for patients in hospital. One advantage of heparin over other anticoagulants is that it has a faster onset of action. Heparin was isolated in 1916 from dog liver cells (*hepar* is Greek for "liver"), but it was not used in humans until the late 1930s. Heparin works by preventing thrombin and fibrin from working correctly. It is synthesized and released by mast cells, a type of white blood cell, in many body tissues, including the lungs, liver, and intestine.

The source of heparin for medicine is the intestines of pigs that are killed for meat. China is the world's largest pork consumer, and it kills more pigs than any other country, so it is perhaps not surprising that China is also the world's top exporter of heparin. There are stories of vegans refusing treatment with heparin because it is made from animals, but Jewish and Islamic rules would permit its use, although eating pork is forbidden in both religions.

The function of naturally occurring heparin in the body is not fully understood, but it seems to play an important role in enhancing the body's mechanisms to dissolve (**lyse**) clots. For other animals, however, natural coagulants play a much clearer function. For animals that feed on blood (called **hematophagous** animals), it is important that blood does not coagulate while feeding (coagulated blood is difficult to suck—in the same way that it is difficult to suck up a very thick milkshake!). Blood sucking animals include **leeches** and mosquitoes. One of the anticoagulants contained in the saliva of leeches is called **hirudin**, a protein that inhibits the function of thrombin. Hirudin produced by recombinant DNA technologies has various indications, including the treatment of deep vein thrombosis. **Vampire bats**, found in Central and South American, are the only hematophagous mammal. The natural anticoagulant produced by vampire bats and contained in their **saliva** has the interesting name of **Draculin**. There has been research into Draculin's potential use as a drug to treat ischemic stroke.

3) *Thrombus*: Blood clotting is a vital process because without it we could bleed to death from a simple cut. However, blood clots are sometimes formed **inappropriately** on the wall of a blood vessels or in the heart. A thrombus is a blood clot that forms inside a blood vessel and remains **in situ** (i.e., it stays where it is formed). A thrombus can be dangerous because it can obstruct blood flow within a blood vessel. The condition in which a blood clot blocks a blood vessel is called **thrombosis**. Thrombi that form in arteries, called **arterial thrombi**, are different from those that form in veins. Arterial thrombi are composed mostly of platelets in a mesh of fibrin. Such thrombi are usually formed on the surface of atheroma. Thrombi in veins, called **venous thrombi**, usually form when blood flow is very slow or static, as can happen after major surgery when someone is unable to walk around. Venous thrombi contain relatively few platelets (instead, red blood cells and fibrin fibers are the major components). Because arterial thrombi are mostly composed of platelets, antiplatelet drugs such as aspirin are considered to be more effective for preventing arterial thrombi compared to fibrin-rich venous thrombi.

4) *Cardiogenic cerebral embolism*: A stroke caused by an embolism is called an **embolic stroke**. An embolic stroke occurs when a blood clot that forms in one place in the body is carried in the blood to the brain. Cardiogenic means "produced in the heart," and a cardiogenic cerebral embolism (or **cardiogenic stroke**) is when a blood clot that causes a stroke originates in the heart. In most cases, this type of stroke results from **atrial fibrillation**, a type of **arrhythmia** (abnormal heart rhythm) caused by a problem with the heart's electrical-conduction system.

Atrial fibrillation is when the two upper chambers of the heart, called the **atria**, beat irregularly and too rapidly, preventing blood in the atria from completely emptying into the ventricles with each beat. Instead, blood **pools** in the atria. Clots are more likely to form in such **stagnant** blood, and a stroke can occur if one or more of these clots is pumped out of the heart and carried to the brain. I first heard of this type of stroke in 2004, when **Shigeo Nagashima** (長嶋 茂雄), a former baseball player and baseball team manager, suffered a cardiogenic stroke aged 68. People with atrial fibrillation are often prescribed **antiarrhythmics**, medications to treat abnormal heart rhythms.

SD 4H: Emboli are not only blood clots

An embolus is any material inside a blood vessel that travels in the bloodstream from its original location to block a vessel in another location. Although an embolus is most often a blood clot (thrombus), it can be formed from a number of other things, including: a piece of an atherosclerotic plaque; fat (e.g., released from **bone marrow** due to a bone fracture); cancer (pieces of a tumor can break off from the main tumor causing a **tumor embolism**); and air/gas bubbles. Causes of **air/gas embolism** include air being injected into a vein accidentally by a syringe or an IV line, a traumatic injury to the lungs, or a scuba diving accident. (If you do a scuba diving course, you will learn about the danger of air embolism in scuba diving. To find out more, do an internet search for "**pulmonary barotrauma** and **decompression sickness**.")

Let's return to thrombi (blood clots), the main cause of emboli. In 1856, Rudolf Virchow put forward an explanation of clot formation in blood vessels. He **postulated** that in order for a clot to form, three conditions or factors are necessary: **hypercoagulability**, **stasis** (i.e., the pooling of blood), and injury to the vessel wall (**endothelial damage**). Because there are three factors, they have been named **Virchow's triad**. Each of the factors can have various causes; for example:

- hypercoagulability could be caused by dehydration, cancer (tumor cells secrete substances that promote thrombosis), **contraceptive medication**, and **inherited thrombophilia**.
- stasis could be due to prolonged **immobility** as can occur when a person is bedridden after a hip operation.
- endothelial damage could result from smoking, hypertension, atherosclerosis, and injury to blood vessels from surgery.

Rudolf Virchow is known as "the father of modern pathology." He studied cells in detail and stressed that all diseases involved some type of cell change. He was not only a medical doctor and pathologist, but also an anthropologist, historian, politician, and several other things as well. This German **polymath** also opposed the view that the "Aryan" or "German" race was superior to other races, a view that would lead to the rise of the Nazis around 30 years after his death (Virchow died in 1902). Surprisingly, Virchow opposed Charles Darwin's theory of evolution, and he called Charles Darwin an "**ignoramus**," which means an ignorant or stupid person.

5) *Deep vein thrombosis (DVT)* **occurs when a thrombus forms in a deep vein in the body, often in the lower leg.** Deep veins are those that are deep in the body, beneath the layers of tissue and muscle. **Superficial veins** are those below the skin's surface. If you look at the back of your hand or under your wrist, the bluish veins that are visible are superficial ones. (If you accidently cut one of these superficial veins, blue blood would

not flow out. Blood is always red, although blood that contains less oxygen is a darker shade of red. The reason veins appear bluish is primarily related to what happens to different wavelengths of light when they hit the skin. If you want a detailed explanation, type **"why are veins blue"** into a search engine.) While arteries carry blood away from the heart, veins carry it back to the heart (a good mnemonic: both "artery" and "away" begin with the letter "a"). Blood is pushed through arteries by the force of the beating heart, but blood in the veins is under low pressure. This means that the return of blood to the heart must be assisted by the action of the **skeletal-muscle pump**. As skeletal muscles contract and relax, they squeeze on the veins that pass through them. This squeezing action pushes blood forward. The veins also contain **valves** to stop **backflow**.

Being inactive for a prolonged period can cause blood in the veins to pool because the skeletal-muscle pump is unable to help blood return to the heart. Clots are more likely to form in blood that is **sluggish** (slow moving) or **static** (not moving). Such blood clots that form in the legs can cause swelling and leg pain, although they are often "silent" and cause no symptoms. But the real danger of DVT is that it can lead to a **pulmonary embolism**, caused by a blood clot in the lungs.

How does a pulmonary embolism occur? Suppose that a blood clot has formed in a vein in the lower leg. If this clot breaks off, it can be carried in the blood through a large vein called the **inferior vena cava** and to the **right atrium** of the heart. From the right atrium, the clot moves into the **right ventricle**, which then pumps the deoxygenated blood, together with the clot, to the lungs. The clot can block an artery in the lungs, thus restricting pulmonary blood flow and leading to the death of lung tissue (**pulmonary infarction**). A blood clot in the lungs is a medical emergency that can be fatal.

Apart from not moving around much (as can happen during a long plane flight, or during a stay in hospital), there are various other risk factors for DVT. These include being overweight, being pregnant, smoking, and taking the contraceptive pill (estrogen, which is contained in "the pill," is **prothrombotic**). People can reduce the risk of DVT by taking regular exercise (e.g., walking up and down the aisle of an airplane every few hours during a flight), drinking lots of water (keeping **hydrated**), and losing weight if overweight. People in hospital, or who are immobilized in other ways, are often instructed to wear **compression stockings** that improve blood flow.

After the **Great East Japan Earthquake** in 2011, the incidence of DVT in the disaster area increased. This was because many people were in **cramped** disaster shelters. Elderly people in particular were unable to move around. Also, many people became **dehydrated** because of diarrhea, lack of drinking water, or not drinking water on purpose in order to avoid having to use the inadequate toilet facilities. Dehydration increases the risk of DVT because it makes the blood more viscous and slows circulation.

6) *Diabetes* (or **diabetes mellitus**, as it is more accurately called) is one of the main risk factors for stroke. In fact, taking two people of the same sex and age, the person with diabetes is around twice as likely to have a stroke as someone who doesn't have the condition. Diabetes is characterized by high blood sugar levels, or **hyperglycemia**. The exact mechanism by which diabetes leads to stroke is still being researched, but high blood sugar levels are thought to increase **systemic inflammation**, thereby contributing to the development of atherosclerosis. Hyperglycemia is also thought to cause dysfunction of endothelial cells lining blood vessels, contributing to a **prothrombotic state** (or **hypercoagulability**)—a tendency of the blood to clot. Common **comorbidities** of diabetes are **obesity**, **hypertension**, and **hypercholesterolemia** (high levels of blood lipids) and/or **dyslipidemia** (an unhealthy balance of different lipid types). Each of these comorbidities is also a major stroke risk factor.

7) FAST: The **acronym** FAST (Facial drooping, Arm weakness, Speech, Time) was first developed in the UK in 1998 for training ambulance personnel, but it became widely known after 2009, when it was used by the British Government in a **public awareness campaign**. FAST is now used in many countries, including Japan, to educate people on detecting symptoms of a stroke. It must be emphasized that there are other signs of stroke apart from those expressed by FAST. One organization in the USA has come up with **FASTER**, which stands for Face, Arms, **Stability**, Talking, **Eyes**, and React. "Stability" refers to the fact that a stroke sometimes causes a loss of balance, and "eyes" refers to problems with eyesight such as **blurred vision** or **double vision** that stroke can bring on. "React" is telling you to call the ambulance if you see any single one of these symptoms. Another version is **NOWFAST**: "N" is for "new symptoms" (symptoms which are of sudden onset) and "nausea" (with or without vomiting); "O" is for "**ocular**," which means "eyes/vision" (changes in vision); and "W" is for "walking" (suddenly unable to walk properly, or a loss of balance).

SD 4I: Time is brain, so bring the CT scanner to the patient

When it comes to ischemic stroke, the sooner that a blocked blood vessel can be unblocked and blood flow restored, the better the prognosis. Quick treatment can minimize the damage to the brain and greatly improve a person's chances of leaving hospital with fewer complications. Prompt treatment can sometimes even be the difference between life and death. In Melbourne, Australia, there is a specialized ambulance called a **mobile stroke unit** (MSU). This ambulance is equipped with a CT scanner, enabling a person with a suspected stroke to have a head CT on the way to the hospital. As well as two **paramedics**, the team on this specialized ambulance consists of an expert stroke nurse, and a **radiographer** to operate the CT scanner. A neurologist is also either on board the ambulance or in contact with the ambulance team via **telemedicine**. The CT scan and other data is shared with the hospital by Wi-Fi. In this way, stroke type can be diagnosed, and the patient's condition assessed, *before* he or she reaches the hospital. With the mobile stroke unit, about 20% of patients begin treatment within the first 60 minutes after a stroke. This is almost impossible when the patient is bought to hospital in a regular ambulance and is scanned after arriving at the hospital. The Melbourne MSU does cost a lot of money, but **health economists** say it is **cost effective** because it can save people from severe disability. Providing long-term care for people with severe disability costs the Melbourne healthcare system much more than the investment needed to run a MSU.

8) *Hematologic disorders* **are disorders of the blood cells or the organs that form the blood**. A number of hematologic disorders are associated with stroke. One example is **thrombocythemia**. In this rare disorder, which is often inherited, the bone marrow makes too many platelets, increasing the **propensity** of the blood to clot. **Sickle cell disease** (also called sickle cell anemia) is a blood disorder that can cause ischemic stroke. People with this condition have sickle-shaped red blood cells that are sticky and are not flexible like normal red blood cells, so they tend to stick to each other, to other cells, and also to the walls of blood vessels. This can cause blockage of blood vessels, leading to stroke. **Hemophilia** is a bleeding disorder in which the blood does not clot properly. People with hemophilia lack certain clotting factors that are vital for coagulation. Not having enough of these clotting factors can cause bleeding into joints or muscles, or external bleeding after a minor injury. A rare, but very serious bleeding event in a person with hemophilia is bleeding in the brain (**intracranial hemorrhage**), causing a hemorrhagic stroke. In people, with severe hemophilia, even heading a soccer ball could cause a bleed in the brain. A brain bleed may also occur **spontaneously** (i.e., without any trauma).

9) *Lacunar stroke* **happens when blood flow to one of the small arteries deep within the brain becomes blocked.** There are various symptoms of lacunar stokes (also called lacunar **infarcts**), such as hand numbness and **dysarthria** (slow or slurred speech). But lacunar stroke can be **clinically silent,** meaning there are no obvious symptoms. Recurrent lacunar strokes is associated with the development of **vascular dementia**, the most common cause of dementia after Alzheimer's disease. Vascular dementia is defined as changes to memory, thinking, and behavior that result from conditions affecting cerebral blood vessels. Blockage of small blood vessels in the brain that occurs in lacuna stroke is usually caused by atherosclerosis. The small arteries in the brain are particularly vulnerable to the buildup of atherosclerotic plaques because they are under very high blood pressure (this blood pressure exerts great force against the walls of blood vessels, damaging them; and atherosclerosis develops readily on such damaged walls).

Small blood vessels in the brain are exposed to high blood pressure because such vessels branch directly off from a main artery carrying blood high under pressure. As an analogy, imagine thousands of people running very fast down a street that is 30 meters wide to escape a tsunami, but due to collapsed buildings on both sides of the street, its width suddenly narrows to 5 meters. As thousands of people squeeze into this narrowed street, they push against the collapsed walls on either side of the street. In a similar way, blood under high pressure in a large cerebral artery that flows into a much narrower artery will exert a sideways force (called **shear stress**) on the inner walls of the small blood vessel. Over years, this shear stress damages the walls of the blood vessels, and, as mentioned above, this vascular wall damage promotes the development of atherosclerosis.

When a small artery is occluded, a little area of brain dies, leaving empty spaces of destroyed brain tissue. The word **lacunar** means "blank or empty space." A hole is an empty, or hollow, space, and if a large hollow area of land fills with water it can form a lake. In fact, "lake" is derived from *lacuna*, the Latin word for "hole."

10) Secondary prevention: Disease prevention involves a range of actions, called **interventions**, that aim to reduce risks to health. Prevention can be divided into primary, secondary, and tertiary prevention. **Primary prevention** aims to prevent disease before it occurs. Rolling out a population-wide vaccination program, for example, vaccination against measles, is an easy-to-understand example. Other examples of primary prevention include condom use to prevent **STD**s (sexually transmitted diseases), going to the dentist regularly to maintain **oral hygiene**, and educating school children about a healthy diet. **Secondary prevention** is detecting a disease early and trying to prevent the disease and its symptoms from getting worse. An example is an annual health check that screens employees for different conditions. During the annual health checkup at the university where I work, **faculty members** and staff give a urine sample, and this urine is tested for the presence of glucose. In this way, people with diabetes can be picked up early before the disease progresses. Another example is taking a low-dose aspirin after a TIA (transient ischemic attack) to reduce the chance of having a major stroke later. **Tertiary prevention** is aimed at people who are already affected by a disease. It aims to prevent or slow down the progression of the disease, reduce the severity of disease, improve the quality of life, and increase life expectancy. Examples include chemotherapy for people diagnosed with cancer and rehabilitation programs for people who have suffered a stroke.

11) *Tissue plasminogen activator* **(tPA) is a thrombolytic drug known by the generic name alteplase.** Alteplase is manufactured by **recombinant DNA technology** and is sold under the brand name of Activase. Thrombolytic drugs dissolve a blood clot that has already formed (compared to anticoagulant and antiplatelet drugs, whose main effect is to inhibit a blood clot from forming in the first place). Because tPA is administered intravenously (IV), it must be given at hospital. It works by converting **plasminogen**, a protein in the blood, to **plasmin**, an enzyme that is capable of "cutting" the links between fibrin molecules. (Plasmin is a **proteolytic enzyme**, meaning it breaks down proteins such as fibrin). Fibrin holds a blood clot together, so once the fibrin mesh is cut into pieces (in a process known as **fibrinolysis**), the clot dissolves. Dissolving the blood clot restores blood flow to brain tissue.

You may have heard of a Hollywood movie called *Ghostbusters*. Released in 1984, the movie is about a team of four people who get rid of, or bust, ghosts. Well, alteplase, approved for the treatment of ischemic stroke in the USA in 1996 (and in 2005 in Japan), has been called a "**clot buster**" in the media because it "busts" blood clots.

"Time is brain" is an expression that stresses the importance of starting treatment as soon as possible after stroke symptoms are noticed. It is estimated that during an ischemic stroke two million neurons die each minute. If too much time passes between the start of a stroke and arrival at hospital, it might be too late to start tPA treatment. In fact, when tPA started to be used in 1996, it was **indicated** only for patients who had arrived at hospital and could start treatment within 3 hours of stroke **onset**. In other words, the **therapeutic time window** for thrombolytic therapy following stroke was 3 hours. This window is now considered to be 4.5 hours. Because tPA breaks down fibrin, it increases the risk of bleeding in the body, including in the brain. For this reason, certain people are **excluded** from treatment. An **absolute contraindication** for thrombolytic treatment is a recent intracranial hemorrhage, while **relative contraindications** are having a peptic ulcer and being pregnant.

12) Unstable plaques: Atherosclerosis develops when cholesterol, cellular waste products, and other substances build up in the inner lining of an artery. This cholesterol buildup forms a **plaque (atheroma)**. As the plaque grows, a cap of hard calcium forms over the lipid core of the plaque. This **calcified** cap is a bit like the hard chocolate coating on top of an ice cream. The word "**unstable**" generally has a negative meaning. Would you prefer to be employed in a "stable job" or an "unstable job", to be in a "stable relationship" or an "unstable relationship", or to live in a country with a "stable government" or an "unstable government"? For atheroma too, the word "unstable" is also negative. This is because unstable plaques are more susceptible to rupturing. Rupturing of a plaque exposes the lipid core of the atheroma, and this core is highly **thrombogenic** (i.e., it promotes the formation of a blood clot). What makes an unstable plaque unstable is the way it is formed with a large lipid core and a thin cap. On the other hand, a **stable plaque** has much less lipid in the core and a much thicker cap (imagine a small amount of ice cream and a thick covering of chocolate). They are called "stable" because they are less prone to rupturing.

SD 4J: Controversial issue: Should statins be used for primary prevention?

I have been interested in statins for several years and devote one whole lesson to this medication. Here are just three reasons for my interest. Firstly, although I have never used them, of few of my relatives in England do, which is not surprising since they are one of the world's most commonly prescribed drugs (in the USA, over a quarter of adults 40 years of age or over are on a statin). Secondly, they were discovered by a Japanese biochemist, **Akira Endo** (遠藤 章), who was inspired as a child by Alexander Fleming's research on fungi that led to the development of penicillin. Thirdly, statins may have saved the lives of hundreds of thousands, or even millions of people, but there has been a lot of controversy around their use. Here are some of the key points I include in my lesson on statins.

a) Because lipids, such as cholesterol and triglycerides, are **hydrophobic** (insoluble in water), they must be transported in the bloodstream by being combined with a soluble protein. The cholesterol-protein complex is called a **lipoprotein**. Lipoproteins are classified into several groups according to their density. The two lipoproteins that are most important for this discussion are **low-density lipoproteins (LDL)** and **high-density lipoproteins (HDL)**. Particles of LDL are very small (diameter <70 nm), allowing them to easily penetrate the walls of arteries. If the bloodstream contains an excess of LDL, they cross into the innermost layer of the artery wall, where they accumulate and promote atherosclerosis (the exact way LDL does this is complex, but it is partly related to the **oxidization** of accumulated lipids triggering structural and metabolic changes in the arterial wall). Because LDL is **atherogenic**—it causes atherosclerosis—it is known as "bad" cholesterol. In contrast, HDL accepts excess cholesterol from cells in artery walls and returns it to the liver. In this way, HDL is protective against atherosclerosis. This is why HDL is known as "good" cholesterol.

b) Epidemiological studies have shown a strong positive correlation between **dyslipidemia** and cardiovascular diseases. However, it is important to remember that cholesterol is also vital for life. For example, cholesterol is an essential component of cell membranes, the structures that surround every cell in the body. Cholesterol is also needed to manufacture **steroid-based hormones** such as sex hormones (e.g., testosterone and estrogen), aldosterone, and cortisol. Cholesterol enables the body to form **bile acids** (needed for fat breakdown in digestion), and it is also required for the skin to manufacture **vitamin D**. Cholesterol is so important that the body manufactures it to ensure there is a constant supply. Indeed, around 85% of cholesterol is manufactured *de novo* (from new) in the liver, and the rest comes from dietary sources (cholesterol obtained in the diet is known as **exogenous cholesterol**).

c) HMG-CoA reductase inhibitors, or statins as they are commonly called, are the most important lipid-lowering drug. There are many drugs that work by blocking enzymes, and statins also work in this way. Statins inhibit an enzyme called 3-hydroxy-3-methyl-glutaryl-CoA reductase, usually shorted to **HMG-CoA reductase**. This enzyme catalyzes a vital step in the pathway of cholesterol synthesis (called the **mevalonate pathway**) in the liver. By inhibiting this enzyme, statins reduce hepatic (liver) cholesterol synthesis, leading to a reduction of cholesterol in the blood. Another effect of statins is to increase the expression of LDL receptors on hepatocytes (liver cells). These receptors "grab" onto LDL and remove it from the bloodstream. The LDL is then broken down by hepatocytes. By reducing hepatic cholesterol synthesis and increasing LDL clearance from the blood, statins lower blood cholesterol levels, and particularly that of LDL cholesterol. Interestingly, statins actually raise levels of HDL cholesterol, the "good" cholesterol. The cholesterol-lowering effect of cholesterol can slow the progression of atherosclerosis and reduce the risk of developing cardiovascular diseases.

d) It was the research by a Japan biochemist called **Akira Endo** that led to the first statin. Endo was born in 1933 in a rural area of Akita Prefecture in northern Japan. His passion for **mycology** (the scientific study of fungi) eventually led Endo to begin a search for compounds from **fungi** that could interfere with cholesterol production. Much of Endo's research was conducted while he was employed at a big **pharmaceutical company** in Tokyo, but he also spent two years as a researcher at the Albert Einstein College of Medicine in New York City. After screening thousands of **fungal cultures**, Endo **isolated** a compound from a mold called *Penicillium citrinum* (*P. citrinum*). This is a mold often found on oranges and other **citrus fruit** that have been in the fruit bowl for too long, but Endo's sample of *P. citrinum* was collected from a rice sample found in a grain shop in Kyoto. The active compound that Endo purified from *P. citrinum* was named **mevastatin**, signifying a substance that stops **mevalonic acid** synthesis. Mevalonic acid is crucial in the pathway that synthesizes cholesterol; indeed, the synthesis of cholesterol in cells is also called the **mevalonic acid pathway**. This pathway can be summarized as follows:

$$\text{acetylCoA} \rightarrow \text{HMG-CoA} \xrightarrow{\text{E}*} \text{mevalonic acid} \rightarrow \text{cholesterol}$$

*The ^{E} represents the step dependent on the enzyme HMG-CoA reductase; it is this enzyme that statins inhibit

Mevastatin is structurally very similar to HMG-CoA (it is **structural analogue** of HMG-CoA). HMG-CoA is a **reaction intermediate**, a substance formed as a middle step in a reaction. In cholesterol synthesis, HMG-CoA reductase catalyzes the reaction that converts HMG-CoA into mevalonic acid. This is a vital step in the chemical reactions to produce cholesterol. As a structural analogue of HMG-CoA, mevastatin binds to the **active site** of HMG-CoA reductase. This interferes with the conversion of HMG-CoA into mevalonic acid and blocks the synthesis of cholesterol. Mevastatin, discovered in 1976, was the first statin drug, although it was never marketed. Further research and clinical trials followed, and in 1987, **lovastatin** became the first statin to be approved for commercial use by the FDA in the USA. Today, there are several types of statins, including **atorvastatin** and **simvastatin**. They are called "statins" because their generic names end with the suffix ~*statin*. This suffix indicates a compound (~*in*) that stops (~*stat*), or inhibits, cholesterol synthesis.

e) An important course in all pharmacy degrees is **pharmacokinetics**. This is a branch of pharmacology that, simply put, studies what the body does to a drug. Early on in a pharmacokinetic course, students are taught the acronym **ADME**, which stands for absorption, distribution, metabolism and excretion. The body absorbs a drug, distributes it around the body, metabolizes it, and then excretes it to remove it from the body. Drug metabolism mainly occurs in the liver (but also in other tissues, particularly in the wall of the small intestine), and it is predominantly carried out by a group of enzymes called **cytochrome P450** (**CYP450**). These CYP450 enzymes (of which there are over 30) alter (or **biotransform**) a drug into a more **hydrophilic** form, so that it can be more easily excreted from the body by the kidneys.

Metabolism of a drug by CYP450 enzymes means that not all of the drug that is administered enters the **systemic circulation.** For example, simvastatin, a commonly prescribed statin, undergoes extensive metabolism in the liver resulting in only about 5% of the orally administered drug actually entering the systemic circulation (in other words, 95% of drug is lost, mainly due to it being metabolized in the liver). Here it is appropriate to introduce two important terms used in pharmacology:

- **Bioavailability** is the proportion of an administered dose of a drug that reaches the systemic circulation. If a drug is injected into the body, bioavailability is assumed to 100% because the drug is delivered directly into the blood stream. For orally administered drugs it can be much less, mainly because of first pass metabolism.
- **First-pass metabolism** (also called the **first-pass effect**) is the metabolic breakdown of a drug, mainly in the liver, that results in a reduced concentration of the active drug.

Knowing about liver enzymes, bioavailability, and first-pass metabolism is important for understanding about **drug interactions**. For example, I take a daily dose of carbamazepine, a drug for epilepsy. If I were also prescribed simvastatin, the metabolism of the statin could be affected by the epilepsy drug. This is because carbamazepine is an **enzyme inducer**, meaning it stimulates the activity of enzymes. One of the enzymes carbamazepine induces is CYP3A4 (one of the CYP450 group of enzymes), and CYP3A4 is involved in metabolizing simvastatin. Because carbamazepine stimulates CYP3A4, it will metabolize even more of the simvastatin than usual. This will result in less simvastatin entering the systemic circulation from the liver, and lead to a lower blood concentration of simvastatin. As a result, the cholesterol-lowering effect of the statin would be reduced.

On the other hand, let's suppose that someone, let's call her Maki, who is taking a simvastatin was also prescribed **erythromycin** (a common antibiotic), for a skin infection. Erythromycin in a potent **enzyme inhibitor**. This means that it reduces the activity of CYP3A4. This enzyme inhibition by erythromycin results in simvastatin undergoing less breakdown by CYP3A4, leading to more non-metabolized drug reaching Maki's circulation (i.e., erythromycin increases the systemic bioavailability of statins). This can increase Maki's risk of suffering side effects from simvastatin. Another well-known inhibitor of CYP3A4 is **grapefruit juice** (and also fresh grapefruit). The compounds in grapefruit juice responsible for the inhibition of CYP3A4 are called **furanocoumarins**, a class of **phytochemicals** (substances found in plants; *phyto* comes from the Greek word meaning "plant"). The furanocoumarins in grapefruit inhibit CYP3A4 mostly in the small intestine rather than in the liver (as mentioned above, the liver is not the only location of drug metabolism). Not all people are equally affected by this grapefruit juice-statin interaction. This individual variation partly depends on inherited differences in the levels of **enteric** (intestinal) CYP3A4.

f) In general, statins are **well tolerated**, but some people taking them do experience side effects. Minor, but troublesome, side effects include diarrhea, nausea, and headache; however, the most commonly reported side effects are muscle related, most often muscle pain (**myalgia**) or weakness. A number of studies have found that muscle pain and other statin symptoms can be caused by the **nocebo effect** (this is when side effects occur because of a person's negative expectations of the drug), but there is no doubt that in some cases muscle pain, aches, and similar symptoms are due to the effect of the statin itself. Statins can also trigger **rhabdomyolysis**, the breakdown of skeletal muscle that leads to the contents of muscle fibers such as myoglobin being released into the blood. In high concentrations, this "free" myoglobin can cause acute kidney damage. Rhabdomyolysis is very rare, affecting fewer than 2 out of every 100,000 people taking statins, although the risk is increased with **concurrent** use of medications that inhibit CYP3A4. Some studies have also found that statin use is asscoiated with an increased risk of developing diabetes mellitus and dementia. On the other hand, other studies have not found any association between statin use and these conditions. Different studies on side effects and complications of statins have **conflicting results**, making it difficult to correctly evaluate the risk of this medicine.

g) The side effects of statins are generally **dose dependant**, with the risk of more severe side effects increasing at higher doses. Side effects are also influenced by whether a statin is **lipophilc** or **hydrophilic**. Lipophilic statins (e.g., atorvastatin and simvastatin) readily dissolve in lipids, while hydrophilic statins (e.g., pravastatin) are easily soluble in water. Lipophilic statins are more easily absorbed into muscle and brain tissue, which may be why they are associated with a higher incidence of muscle-related side effects compared to hydrophilic statins. Because cholesterol is vital for the formation of cell membranes, it is needed for normal fetal development. And since statins interfere with cholesterol synthesis, it has been thought that they could harm the developing fetus in the womb. In animal studies, statins have been shown to have **teratogenic** effects (i.e., cause birth defects), so it is not surprising that they have been contraindicated in pregnancy. However, more recent studies suggest that statins may be safe to take during pregnancy.

h) While we must bear in mind the possiblity of side effects from taking statins, many doctors will stress that, for most people, the benefits of lowering LDL with statins **outweighs** the risk of serious side effects. In addition, statins may have some "extra" benefits apart from lowering cholesterol. For example, there is evidence that statins improve endothelial function in blood vessels, reduce inflammation, inhibit the growth of cancer cells, and have antiviral effects. There is much research into statin's **pleiotropic effects** (i.e., the effects of a drug other than those for which the drug was originally developed).

i) Statins are most often associated with the prevention of heart disease, but they are also considered important in stroke prevention. Here we will look only at stroke prevention. Statins are often prescribed to people who have had a previous ischemic stroke or TIA in order to reduce the risk of another stroke. This is **secondary stroke prevention**. It is generally accepted that statins are important in secondary prevention. However, the use of statins for **primary stroke prevention** (i.e., in people with no history of TIA or stroke) is much more **contentious**. In the UK, USA and other countries, statins are prescribed to millions of people with certain risk factors for developing cardiovascular disease (e.g., having hypertension, being overweight, or being a smoker), but who are otherwise healthy. Critics of prescribing statins for primary prevention say that it is exposes people to the risk of serious side effects with little or no benefit. To understand the concerns of such critics it is helpful to understand the concept of **number needed to treat** (**NNT**). NNT is the number of people who would have to receive a treatment in order for one person to benefit. One study found that the number needed to treat for primary prevention of stroke was 260. This means that 260 people who had never had a stroke would need to take a daily statin for 5 years in order to prevent one person from having a stroke. Is it worth this many people taking a medicine every day for 5 years in order to prevent just one person from having a stroke? Whenever a drug is prescribed, the prescriber and patient must weigh up the risk of side effects (and perhaps the financial cost) of taking a drug with its benefits. "BRAN" is an acronym that may be useful when considering the value of a medicine or some other intervention:

B: What are the **Benefits**? (e.g., statins lower LDL cholesterol)

R: What are the **Risks**? (e.g., side effects, including muscle pain)

A: What are the **Alternatives**? (e.g., lifestyle changes to reduce cholesterol levels.)

N: What if I do **Nothing**? (What is my chance of a stroke or heart attack if I don't take a statin?)

Regarding "A" above, it needs to be stressed that lifestyle changes are not only an alternative to statins, but they are also important for people who take statins. Lifestyle changes include lowering LDL cholesterol by doing regular exercise and eating a healthy diet with lots of fresh fruit and vegetables. A high consumption of only fish is associated with increased HDL cholesterol concentrations.

j) Although some cholesterol comes from the diet, a significant amount is **endogenous** (i.e., produced inside the body), mostly in the liver. In humans, most cholesterol synthesis in the body takes place at night. It would, therefore, make sense to take a statin before going to bed at night, when it will interfere most effectively with endogenous cholesterol production. This, indeed, is the case for statins that have a short half-life (are short-acting). For such statins bedtime dosing allows the greatest statin concentration to be present in the body when endogenous cholesterol synthesis is at its highest. On the other hand, a statin with a longer half-life can maintain a therapeutic drug concentration over the whole day, meaning it can be taken at any time. For example, simvastatin has a half-life of under 3 hours, so it is best taken at night. On the other hand, atorvastatin, with a half-life of 14 hours can be taken at any time.

In common with almost every other organism on earth, humans have an **internal clock** that regulates our physiology and behavior. Our internal clock follows 24-hour cycles called **circadian rhythms** (*circadian* is from the Latin words *circa*, meaning "around" and *diem*, meaning "day"). Circadian rhythms can affect the best timing for taking a drug, as the above example of statins show. Many other body processes are also driven by circadian rhythms; for example, blood pressure drops at night when sleeping and undergoes a steep increase in the morning (which could affect the best time to take an **antihypertensive medicine**), and the secretion of **human growth hormone** from the pituitary gland peaks at night during sleep (so my daughter, who needs to take synthetic growth hormone, is given her injection at night to mimic the natural secretion of growth hormone). A field of research called **chronopharmacology** looks at how circadian rhythms and the timing—*chrono* means "time"—of drug administration affects the effectiveness of drugs. (On the topic of time, it is interesting that stroke, both ischemic and hemorrhagic, occur most frequently in the morning. Two possible reasons for this are the circadian-driven increase in blood pressure and the fact that in the morning the blood is most **prothrombotic**, that is, it has a greater tendency to clot).

k) Statins are the **first-line drugs** for lowering LDL cholesterol, but another type of cholesterol-lowering drug may be required when a person's blood cholesterol remains high even after trying a statin, or when a person cannot tolerate a statin's side effects. One alternative to statins that has been used for many years is a class of medicines called **fibrates**. In 2021, a new cholesterol-lowering drug called **inclisiran** become available on the NHS (National Health Service) in the UK. Unlike statins, which are an oral medication taken daily, inclisiran is given as a twice-yearly injection. It has a mechanism of action that is completely different from that of statins. Inclisiran inhibits or "silences" a particular gene called PCSK9. This gene provides instructions to make a protein that regulates the expression of LDL receptors on the surface of cells. Silencing of the PCSK9 gene results in more LDL receptors on the surface of liver cells, leading to an increase in the amount of LDL being removed from the blood. Inclisiran has been shown to cut LDL levels in the blood by around 50%. Clinical trials of inclisiran have started in Japan, but it may take a number of years before it is approved in this country because there tends to be a delay in drug-approval time in Japan compared to the United States and Europe (this delay is known as a "**drug lag**").

4-4 Well, what do you know?

（どのくらいわかるようになったか試してみよう）

Are the following statements true (T) or false (F)?

1. Low-dose aspirin is used as an antiplatelet treatment.
2. Hemiparesis is weakness of both sides of the body.
3. A subarachnoid hemorrhage is sometimes preceded by a severe headache.
4. A lacuna stroke is caused by occlusion of large blood vessels in the brain.
5. Alteplase is a powerful drug that is used to prevent blood clots from forming.

What is the meaning of the underlined WFE?

1. A **lipoma** is a fatty lump that grows under your skin. It is harmless and does not usually need treatment.
2. Krakatoa, a huge volcano in Indonesia, **erupted** in 1883. The eruption triggered huge tsunamis that caused the death of over 36,000 people.
3. A **sarcoma** is a type of cancer that starts in bone or muscle.
4. Because hormones regulate so many activities in our bodies, the endocrine system plays an integral role in **homeostasis**
5. I once met a Japanese woman who was a real **Francophile**. She loved everything French, such as French wine, French cheese, and French movies.
6. Insulin secretion follows a **circadian** rhythm, with insulin secretion rates rising during the day and falling at night. Epidemiological studies show that people who work night shifts have an increased risk of developing type 2 diabetes mellitus, and this could be partly due to disruption of circadian regulation of insulin secretion.

Choose the correct word for the gap

a) eligible   b) thrombocyte   c) resolve   d) fear   e) permission
f) propensity

1. A study found that rainfall can affect our mood, how hungry we feel, and even our ☐ to commit crime.

2. Platelets are made in the bone marrow. Platelets lack a nucleus and so are not classed as true cells. Rather, they are cell fragments produced by cells in the bone marrow called megakaryocytes. Another name for a platelet is ☐.

3. In Japan, foreigners who were born in Japan or have been in Japan for decades are not ☐ to vote in any election, whether local or national. However, in New Zealand and Sweden, and some other countries, non-citizens can vote in certain elections.

4. A sore throat will often ☐ on its own, but you should go to the doctor if a sore throat is severe or persists for longer than a week.

5. A relatively new word to appear in the dictionary is "nomophobia," which is short for "no mobile phone phobia." It is a ☐ of being without a mobile device that is so severe it affects a person's life.

4-5 May Jo's Health-Podcast

（メイ・ジョーの健康ポッドキャスト）

Podcast presenter May Jo (MJ) and Dr Jason Cohen (Dr) are discussing "mini strokes."

MJ: Many listeners may have heard that the famous Hollywood actor Mark Rebel had a mini stroke while filming his new movie. A mini stroke is also known as a TIA, and to talk about TIAs is Jason Cohen, Professor of clinical neurology at the Royal Tree hospital in London. First of all, Professor Cohen, what is a TIA?

Dr: It stands for transient ischemic attack. Ischemic means that there is a blockage in a blood vessel that interrupts blood flow. But unlike in a full-blown stroke where a blockage is permanent, in a TIA the blocked blood vessel somehow becomes cleared and blood flow is restored.

MJ: So, the blockage and the symptoms are transient rather than permanent.

Dr: That's right. The symptoms typically last for around 10 minutes.

MJ: And what kind of symptoms should we look out for?

Dr: Things like weakness or numbness on one side of the body, slurred speech, and confusion.

MJ: Many regular listeners will be familiar with the FAST, an acronym that helps us to remember the main signs of a stroke. If you're not familiar with it, enter the keywords "FAST" and "stroke" into your internet search engine. Professor, why is a TIA transient?

Dr: Well, it's thought that the clot dissolves on its own or gets dislodged by blood flow.

MJ: A TIA is often called a "mini stroke." Is this an accurate description?

Dr: I don't really like the term "mini stroke" because it suggests that a TIA is not serious. I think a more appropriate name is "warning stroke."

MJ: You mean it can be a warning of a bigger stroke?

Dr: That's right. Research shows that between 9% to 17% of patients who've experienced a TIA will go on to have a full-blown stroke within 90 days. This means it's really important to get medical treatment if you suspect that you or someone else has had a TIA.

MJ: Is it possible to distinguish between a TIA and a full stroke in the initial stages?

Dr: That's an excellent question. The answer is no. You can't differentiate a TIA from a full stroke until the symptoms have resolved.

MJ: So, you only know the transience of a TIA with hindsight.

Dr: That's a good way to put it.

MJ: Can anything be done to prevent a stroke after a TIA?

Dr: Yes. Taking low-dose aspirin within a few hours of a TIA can reduce the risk of a major stroke by about 80% over the following few days.

MJ: How does aspirin do this? What's the mechanism?

Dr: The mechanism is a little complicated, but basically, aspirin blocks an enzyme called cyclooxygenase-1, or COX-1. Inhibiting COX-1 prevents the production of a substance called thromboxane, and thromboxane is necessary for platelet aggregation.

MJ: So, aspirin prevents platelets from sticking together and forming a blood clot.

Dr: Exactly.

MJ: Aspirin is well known for some serious side effects such as gastric bleeding, so it's important for people on aspirin to be monitored by a doctor.

Dr: That's right. But for most people who've had a TIA, the risk of side effects is outweighed by the protection against a stroke that aspirin gives.

MJ: Dr Cohen, thanks so much for joining us today.

Dr: You're welcome, it was great to talk to you.

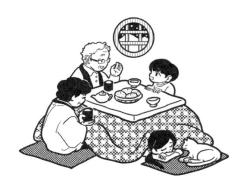

Chapter 5 **Pneumonia**
（肺炎）

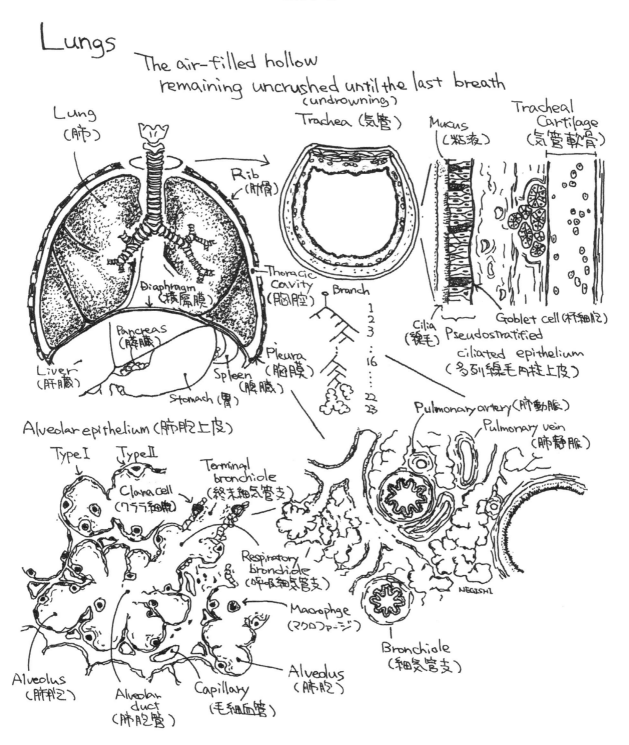

Lungs

The air-filled hollow remaining uncrushed until the last breath (undrowning)

NAVvocab 60 （案内役の単語 60）

1. alveoli・肺胞
2. antibiotic resistance・抗生物質耐性
3. antimicrobial peptide・抗菌ペプチド
4. antitussive・鎮咳剤
5. aspiration pneumonia・誤嚥性肺炎
6. atypical pneumonia・非定型肺炎
7. auscultation・聴診
8. brainstem・脳幹
9. bronchiolitis・細気管支炎
10. bronchoconstriction・気管支収縮
11. bronchodilation・気管支拡張
12. case fatality rate・致命率
13. caustic・腐食性の
14. cellular respiration・細胞呼吸
15. cilia・繊毛
16. ciliated columnar epithelium・線毛円柱上皮
17. comorbidity・併存疾患
18. compromise・損なう
19. contagious・伝染性の
20. cyanosis・チアノーゼ
21. differential diagnosis・鑑別診断
22. epiglottis・喉頭蓋
23. exudate・滲出液
24. genus・属
25. geriatric・老年者
26. goblet cells・杯細胞
27. hemoptysis・喀血
28. hypoxemia・低酸素血症
29. hypoxia・低酸素症
30. impede・妨げる
31. infant mortality・乳児死亡率
32. innate immune system・自然免疫
33. lobe・（肺）葉
34. lower respiratory tract・下気道
35. lung consolidation・コンソリデーション（浸潤影）
36. mucociliary escalator・粘膜繊毛体のエスカレータ
37. mucous membrane・粘膜
38. neonate・新生児
39. neutrophile・好中球
40. passive immunity・受動免疫
41. phonation・発声
42. pleura・胸膜
43. pneumococcal pneumonia・肺炎球菌性肺炎
44. pulmonary capillary・肺毛細管
45. pulmonary circulation・肺循環
46. pulmonary edema・肺水腫
47. respiratory center・呼吸中枢
48. respiratory droplets・飛沫
49. route of transmission・感染経路
50. sanitation・公衆衛生
51. sepsis・敗血症
52. stethoscope・聴診器
53. tachypnea・頻呼吸
54. thoracic cavity・胸腔
55. tidal volume・一回換気量
56. trachea・気管
57. trimester・妊娠第 3 期
58. tuberculosis・結核
59. ventilation・換気（肺におけるガス交換）
60. zoonosis・ズーノーシス(人獣共通感染症)

5-1 Essay — Pneumonia: Fluid-Filled Air Sacs

（肺炎：肺胞がおぼれてしまう病気）

[1]I was shocked when the doctor gave the **prognosis**. She had said that my father "probably had around twelve months." But three months later his health seemed to be improving. After many weeks in hospital, he had finally been moved to a care home in a leafy suburb of London. The care home had a big garden where my father would often sit, enjoying the summer sun. My father was a talented artist, and an exhibition of his paintings was to be held at the care home on August 20, 2019. He was really looking forward to the exhibition, but on the morning of the twentieth he felt unwell, and he was unable to leave his room to attend his exhibition. That evening my father was taken to hospital, where he was diagnosed with **pneumonia**[E8]. Doctors administered **antibiotics**, and for a time he seemed to be getting better. Soon after, however, his condition **deteriorated**, and he died on August 24, nine days after his ninety-first birthday.

[2]Pneumonia, inflammation of the lungs caused by an infection, was once known as "**the old man's friend**" because it was regarded as bringing a quick death to old people, often those who had been suffering with other illnesses. My father was old, **frail,** and he had several **comorbidities**, most serious of which was **heart failure**[D7], that made him more **susceptible** to getting pneumonia. However, I wish that "the old man's friend" had not come so soon. Just a few more days would have let dad enjoy a final chance to chat with people about art at his exhibition.

[3]"The old man's friend" was an appropriate description of pneumonia in the early 20th century. Doctors were more **fatalistic** then because there was often little they could do for patients with severe pneumonia. Nowadays, however, thanks to various medical advances, a person hospitalized with pneumonia has a much better chance of recovering. One of these advances is **antibiotics**. The discovery that led to the development of **penicillin**[D9], the first modern antibiotic, was made by **Alexander Fleming** on September 3, 1928 (less than a month after my father's birth on August 10, 1928).

[4]Penicillin and other antibiotics have helped to drastically reduce **mortality** from pneumonia. Nevertheless, even with antibiotics, pneumonia still ends the lives of many people. In fact, pneumonia was the fourth leading cause of death globally in 2020, and in Japan it was the third most common cause, after cancer and cardiovascular disease. The number of deaths from pneumonia in Japan has been increasing since the 1980s, in large part due to the aging of the Japanese population. While in developed countries pneumonia mainly kills elderly people, in many developing countries it is children under 5 years who

are its main victims. In **Sub-Saharan Africa**, for example, pneumonia is the second most common cause of **infant mortality**[E6]. Later, we shall find out why the very young and the elderly are more **susceptible** to developing pneumonia.

[5]Pneumonia is an infection of the **lungs**, a pair of air-filled organs in the **thoracic cavity** that are the main part of the **respiratory system**. The right lung is larger and is divided into three sections, or **lobes**; the left lung is divided into two lobes and is smaller because it needs to make room for the heart. The principal function of the respiratory system is to provide oxygen to the cells of the body and to eliminate carbon dioxide. Oxygen is essential for **cellular respiration**—the metabolic process that transforms food into the energy we need to function and stay alive. Carbon dioxide is a **byproduct** of cellular respiration. The respiratory system consists of a series of tubes that conduct air from outside of the body into the lungs. It is in **alveoli**, tiny air sacs deep in the lungs, that air from the outside atmosphere is exchanged with the blood. The exchange of gases between the lungs and the blood is called **external respiration**[E9]. The **circulatory system** then carries blood to the cells of the body, where gases are again exchanged (the exchange of gases between the blood and the cells is called **internal respiration**).

[6]To better understand the **pathogenesis** of pneumonia, it is useful to know the basic structure of the respiratory system. The respiratory tract can be divided into the **upper respiratory tract (URT)**—made up of the **nose**[D8], **pharynx**, and **larynx**—and the **lower respiratory tract (LRT)**, which consists of the **trachea** and the **lungs**. The lungs are composed of **bronchi, bronchioles**, and the **alveoli**. The respiratory tract is lined with **respiratory mucosa**, a type of **mucous membrane**. Mucous membranes line cavities and passageways in the body that are exposed to the external environment. The outer layer of the mucosa is composed of **epithelium**, a type of tissue made up of **epithelial cells**. There are various types of epithelial tissue in the body, but the type that lines most the respiratory tract is called **ciliated columnar epithelium**. "Ciliated" refers to microscopic hair-like structures called **cilia** that project from the surface of cells. There are between 200 to 300 cilia on each cell in most parts of the respiratory tract. **Interspersed** among the columnar cells are **goblet cells**, which secrete mucus. This mucus forms a layer that covers and protects the epithelial cells.

[7]**Breathing**[D3], or to use the medical terminology, **pulmonary ventilation**[E11], is the flow of air into and out of the lungs. It is usually an automatic process that is controlled **subconsciously** by the **respiratory center** in the **brainstem**. Air flows into the lungs during **inspiration** and out of the lungs during **expiration.** The **tidal volume**, the amount of **air**[E1] breathed into the lungs with each breath, is around 0.5 liters, and the average breathing rate (**respiration rate**) of an adult at rest is around 12 times a minute. This means that the total volume of air entering the lungs is about 6 liters per minute, or 8,640 liters a day. The huge volume of air that is continuously taken into the lungs from the outside atmosphere is full of **microbes,** some of which may be **pathogenic**, pollen grains, dust, pollutants, and a lot more besides. Therefore, there needs to be a

way to trap and remove airborne microbes and particles from the respiratory tract in order to protect the lungs.

[8]Fortunately, the respiratory tract has a mechanism to clean itself, and it involves the mucus and cilia mentioned above. It works like this: the mucus in the mucus layer is composed of proteins called **mucins**, which make the mucus sticky and very good at trapping things. The mucus layer also contains **antimicrobial peptides**, which are molecules that can kill microbes. The cilia are **motile**, and they beat in a coordinated way at over 1,000 times a minute. The **synchronized**, wave-like movement of cilia transports the mucus, together with the trapped microbes and particles, upwards like an upgoing escalator. In fact, this mechanism is known as the **mucociliary escalator**, or **mucociliary clearance** (**MCC**). The mucus is transported by MCC to the throat where it is eliminated from the respiratory tract through the mouth, or swallowed into the stomach via the esophagus (people swallow around 1.5 liters of mucus each day—in the stomach, microbes are destroyed by gastric acid and digestive enzymes). Mucus brought up from the LRS by coughing is called **sputum** or **phlegm**. That the MCC is a crucial part of the respiratory tract's defense mechanism is shown by the fact that people with **ciliopathy** (defective cilia) are **prone** to serious respiratory infections, as are people with **cystic fibrosis**, a condition in which abnormally **viscous** mucus is produced, impairing the MCC.

[9]Let's follow inhaled air on its journey along the URT and LRT. Air is taken in through the **nostrils** into the **nasal cavity**. Next, the air enters the **pharynx**, also called the **throat**. The pharynx is also part of the digestive system—it carries ingested food to the **esophagus**. From the pharynx air moves into the **larynx**, commonly called the voice box. The larynx contains the **vocal cords**, which are vital for **phonation** (the production of speech). The wall of the larynx is made up of nine **cartilage** plates connected together by **ligaments**. The largest of these plates, the **thyroid cartilage**, becomes more prominent during puberty, especially in males, forming what is known as the **Adam's apple**. At the entrance to the larynx is a structure called the **epiglottis**.

[10]The epiglottis is open when we talk or laugh, but it that acts like a lid that closes off the larynx when we swallow. This prevents food from entering the respiratory tract. If the epiglottis does not shut properly when eating, swallowed food may enter the trachea, leading to **chocking**, a partial or complete obstruction of the airway. The epiglottis can also become inflamed, a condition called **epiglottitis**. This inflammation causes swelling of the epiglottis that, if severe, may interfere with breathing. The most common cause of epiglottitis is a viral or bacterial infection, but it can also result from injury to the throat from, for example, swallowing a very hot liquid (**thermal injury**) or a **caustic**[E2] chemical.

[11]From the larynx, air enters the **trachea**, commonly called the **windpipe**, which is the first part of the LRT. (The lungs contain all the parts of the LRT excluding the trachea, meaning that the lungs are composed of the bronchi, bronchioles, and alveoli.) In adults, the trachea is about 10 cm long and 2 cm in diameter. Along the length of the trachea, there are between 16 to 20 rings of

cartilage, known as **tracheal cartilages**, that support the trachea and prevent it from collapsing. Tracheal cartilages are not complete rings (like onion rings), but are C-shaped. This shape makes the trachea more flexible and allows it to collapse a bit to allow food to pass down the esophagus, which is located just behind the trachea. The **distal** (bottom) end of the trachea divides into two branches, called the **left and right primary bronchi**, which lead into each of the lungs. In the two lungs, each primary bronchus divides to form further branches called secondary and tertiary bronchi. The branches of the bronchi divide many times, becoming increasingly narrower until they form very small passageways called **bronchioles**. The very smallest bronchioles, **terminal bronchioles**, have a diameter of around 0.5 mm.

[12]As the diameter of the bronchi decreases, the amount of cartilage in the airway wall decreases, until it becomes absent in the bronchioles. Another important point about the structure of the wall of the airways, from the trachea to the bronchioles, is that they contain **smooth muscle**. The smooth muscle helps to regulate the diameter of the airways; for example, during exercise, the bronchi and bronchioles **dilate** (increase in diameter). While **bronchodilation** improves oxygen delivery to the lungs, a narrowing of the airways, called **bronchoconstriction**, will decrease the amount of oxygen reaching the lungs. Acute bronchoconstriction, as occurs during an **asthma attack**, makes it harder to breathe. Inflammation of the bronchi (**bronchitis**) and bronchioles (**bronchiolitis**) can also cause breathing difficulties.

[13]The journey of air so far, from the nose to the terminal bronchioles, has been along the **conducting zone** of the respiratory tract. The basic function of this zone is to move air in and out of the lungs. The terminal bronchioles lead to microscopic **air sacs**, called **alveoli**. The alveoli form clusters, called **alveolar sacs**, that are often compared to bunches of grapes. The alveoli constitute the main part of the **respiratory zone**, the part of the respiratory tract where gas exchange occurs between the blood and the lungs. The alveoli make up around 90 percent of total lung volume.

[14]There are approximately 400 million alveoli in each lung. The huge number of alveoli provides a huge **surface area** to maximize the exchange of gases. The wall of each alveolus is very thin, being made up of a single layer of epithelial cells. Each alveolus is surrounded by a network of **pulmonary capillaries**. The barrier between the air in the alveoli and the blood in the capillaries, known as the **respiratory membrane**, is extremely thin. Being thin facilitates rapid and effective gas exchange (remember that gas exchange is the **diffusion**[E5] of oxygen from the alveoli to the blood and of carbon dioxide from the blood into the alveoli). For effective gas exchange to occur, the lungs must be well **perfused** with blood, and it is the **pulmonary circulation** that transports blood between the heart and the lungs. After picking up oxygen and giving off carbon dioxide in the alveoli, the oxygen-rich blood flows through the **pulmonary veins** back to the left side of the heart, from where it is pumped to the whole body.

[15]While in most of the rest of the respiratory tract, MCC helps clear the lungs, the epithelium in the alveoli does not have cilia or mucus-producing cells (if mucus lined the epithelium of the alveoli, its thickness would **impede** gas exchange). Instead, the alveoli are mainly protected by **alveolar macrophages**, a type of white blood cell located within the alveoli. Alveolar macrophages remove inhaled particles that have avoided the MCC and they ingest and destroy pathogens. Alveolar macrophages are key players in the lungs' **innate immune system**. Despite the respiratory system's effective defense mechanisms, bacteria and other pathogenic microbes that are inhaled with the air are sometimes able to **breach** its defenses. This can happen for many reasons; for example, due to MCC becoming **impaired** by cigarette smoke, or the immune system being **compromised** by a disease such as **AIDS**. Even when the defenses are not impaired, pathogens can get into the lungs and rapidly multiply if they are highly **virulent**.

[16]Alveolar macrophages protect the lungs by engulfing microbes and by initiating inflammation in response to an invasion by pathogens. However, it is actually this **inflammatory response** that causes pneumonia. The inflammatory response involves macrophages releasing **cytokines** (signaling molecules) that attract **neutrophiles** and other white blood cells to the site of infection. One effect of these cytokines is to increase the **permeability** of the alveolar capillaries. When the capillaries become too permeable (or "leaky"), the alveoli get filled with **pus** (dead white blood cells) and **exudate** (fluid that leaks out of blood vessels into nearby tissues). So, instead of air, the alveoli become filled with fluids, a situation known as **lung consolidation**. Lung consolidation interferes with gas exchange between the lungs and the blood at the respiratory membrane.

[17]Severe pneumonia can kill when it leads to **respiratory failure**. This is when gas exchange is impaired to such a degree that **hypoxia,** a deficiency in the amount of oxygen reaching the tissues, results. If the vital organs are deprived of sufficient oxygen for too long, they will stop working. The brain is very vulnerable to a lack of oxygen, and **cerebral hypoxia** can quickly result in death. Respiratory failure is not the only life-threatening **complication** of pneumonia. Another is **sepsis**[D10], which is when infection triggers a **hyperinflammatory** response of the immune system.

[18]The **signs and symptoms** of pneumonia depend on the severity, but some typical ones include fever (**pyrexia**), chills, **feeling run down**, and a **loss of appetite**. People may also experience a sharp chest pain when breathing or coughing that is caused by inflammation of the **pleura**, the membranes that surround the lungs. An important sign for recognizing pneumonia is **tachypnea**, an increased respiratory rate. **Shortness of breath**, sometimes called "air hunger," and known medically as **dyspnea**, is probably pneumonia's most frightening symptom. Pneumonia often causes coughing that is **productive**, meaning that phlegm is coughed up. Occasionally people with pneumonia may cough up phlegm

that is stained with blood, a symptom termed **hemoptysis**. A sign of **hypoxemia** (an inadequate amount of oxygen in the blood) is **cyanosis**[E4], an abnormal blue discoloration of the skin and mucous membranes. Cyanosis is commonly seen in the lips, tongue, and nail beds. It is important to note that elderly people with pneumonia do not always have typical symptoms such as fever and coughing; instead, **altered mental status** (e.g., confusion), and refusing to eat may be the main signs that something is not right.

[19]The symptoms of pneumonia can resemble those of other conditions, including **tuberculosis,** or **pulmonary edema** (fluid filling the lungs that is often a sign of a heart condition). It is the job of the doctor to make a **differential diagnosis** (i.e., to distinguish which condition is most likely to be the cause of a person's symptoms). To diagnose pneumonia, a doctor will first take a medical history from the patient or a family member. Next the doctor will perform a **physical examination**, the most important part of which is **auscultation,** or listening to the chest using a **stethoscope**. Following a physical examination, a chest X-ray and other **diagnostic tests**[D5] are usually carried out.

[20]Pneumonia can be classified in several ways, including by **etiology** (how it was caused), **where it was acquired**[D11], and the location and pattern of infection in the lungs. Here, we will look at classification based on etiology. Pneumonia is usually caused by an infection with **bacteria**, **fungi**[D6], or **virusus**. The most common type of bacterial pneumonia is called **pneumococcal pneumonia**, the causative organism of which is *Streptococcus pneumoniae* (*S. pneumoniae*), a bacterium that normally lives as a **commensal** in the upper respiratory tract. Commensal bacteria are those that do no harm to the host. However, these usually harmless bacteria can become pathogenic if they enter the lungs of people with a weakened immune system or those who are susceptible for other reasons. The most common **route of transmission** of *S. pneumoniae* is by **respiratory droplets** (small droplets of saliva or mucus) that are generated when a person sneezes or coughs (even normal talking can produce these droplets). The bacteria expelled in respiratory droplets may be inhaled by another person.

[21]Another common cause of bacterial pneumonia is *Mycoplasma pneumoniae* (*M. pneumoniae*). The **genus** Mycoplasma, to which this bacterium belongs, are the smallest known bacteria. In fact, Mycoplasma are the smallest living cell (viruses are much smaller than the smallest bacteria, but viruses are not cells). This bacterium often causes "walking pneumonia" (also called **atypical pneumonia**). This is pneumonia that is relatively mild, or at least not serious enough to require bedrest or hospitalization. One common symptom of *M. pneumoniae* is a **chronic cough**, a cough that **lingers** for over two weeks or so.

[22]In contrast to the relatively mild disease caused by Mycoplasma, a bacterium called *Legionella pneumophila* (*L. pneumophila*) is responsible for a potentially fatal form of pneumonia called **Legionnaires' disease**. In the USA, this disease has a **case fatality rate**

of around 10% (this means that around 10% of people who get Legionnaire's disease die from it). It is called Legionnaires' disease because it was first identified in 1976 among members of the American Legion (an organization that supports ex-soldiers, or veterans). Unlike *S. pneumoniae*, *L. pneumophila* is not **contagious** (i.e., it does not pass from person to person). People most often **contract** the disease by inhaling contaminated **aerosols** containing the bacteria. These aerosols are produced by, for example, water sprays or mists from shower heads and air conditioning units. In Japan, there have been several outbreaks of Legionnaires' disease at hot springs (*onsen*), often related to poor cleaning and **disinfection**.

[23]Legionnaire's disease is relatively uncommon, but its incidence is increasing, perhaps partly because of climate change (warmer and more humid temperatures increase the risk of spreading bacteria). Much rarer than Legionnaires' disease, is **psittacosis**. This is a disease caused by exposure to birds infected by a bacteria called *Chlamydia psittaci*. Psittacosis comes from the Greek *psittakos*, which means "parrot," although other birds can transmit this bacterium, including chickens. Psittacosis is an example of a **zoonosis**[D12], a disease that is transmitted from animals to humans. The pneumonia caused by psittacosis can be fatal, especially in older people. Diagnosing a rare disease such as psittacosis involves a doctor taking a detailed **patient history**. Asking a patient "Do you have a pet bird?", or a similar question, could help reach a diagnosis more quickly.

[24]Around seven months after my father died, the first death from **COVID-19** (an **acronym** for **coronavirus disease of 2019**) was reported in England. Caused by a virus named **SARS-CoV-2 (severe acute respiratory syndrome coronavirus)**, this infectious disease would go on to kill many more people in the UK and around the world. In the first year of the pandemic (until January 2021), the **death toll** in the UK was over 100,000. Respiratory symptoms of Covid-19 range from a mild cough to severe pneumonia. SARS-CoV-2 is one of many viruses that can lead to pneumonia. **Influenza**[E7] viruses are a common cause of viral pneumonia, and even **rhinoviruses**[E10], most often associated with the common cold, can also lead to it. The most common cause of lower respiratory infection in children is **RSV (respiratory syncytial virus)**. Spread by coughing and sneezing, RSV is a highly **contagious**. Every year, it kills an estimated 100,000 children under the age of five worldwide. It was this virus that put my eldest son, Eugene, in hospital for two weeks when he was two months old. Bacterial, viral, and fungal pneumonia do not necessarily occur in isolation. For example, viral pneumonia can leave a person vulnerable to **secondary infection** by bacteria. Secondary bacterial infection was likely responsible for many deaths during the **Spanish flu pandemic** (1918-1920).

[25]Various factors increase the risk of getting pneumonia. One important **risk factor** is **age**. The age groups most at risk are young children (2 years of age and younger) and

older adults (over 65 years of age). Antibodies are passed to the **fetus** through the **placenta** during the final **trimester** of pregnancy, which is why, following birth, a baby is protected to some extent from infection (this is an example of **passive immunity**). Despite this gift of immunity by antibodies from the mother, the immune system of **neonates** and young children is **immature**, leaving them more vulnerable to pneumonia. While in high-income countries with well-developed healthcare systems, death from pneumonia in children is relatively uncommon, in low-income countries (e.g., yemen), and in poor communities of middle-income countries (e.g., India), pneumonia takes the lives of many children. In such communities, the immature immune system of children is further weakened by **undernutrition** and **malnutrition**. Poor **sanitation** and a lack of clean drinking water greatly increase the risk of contracting pneumonia, as does exposure to **indoor air pollution**, caused by wood burning for cooking. These and other factors are **compounded**[E3] by a lack of access to medical care. Globally, childhood pneumonia is to a great extent a disease of poverty and inequality.

[26]From the very young, let's turn to pneumonia in the elderly (or as doctors might say "the **geriatric** population"). In higher-income countries such as the UK and Japan, the incidence of pneumonia is highest in people over 70 years of age. Here are just a few of the many reasons for this. Firstly, from about the sixth decade of life, the immune system becomes less effective at protecting against infections. Secondly, underlying conditions that **predispose** people to pneumonia are more prevalent in older people. These conditions include cardiovascular disease, type 2 diabetes, and **malignancy** (cancer). Being **hospitalized** is also a key risk factor for pneumonia, and hospitalization rates increase with age. There are many stories of elderly people going into hospital for a minor operation and ending up developing pneumonia. Another reason for elderly people's higher incidence of pneumonia is that they are more likely to inhale oral contents (e.g., food, drink, and saliva) into the lungs. This breathing into the lungs of oral contents can lead to **aspiration pneumonia**[D2].

[27]Factors that increase the risk of pneumonia at any age include **air pollution** and **tobacco smoking**. Both air pollution and tobacco smoking are also involved in the pathogenesis of **lung cancer**, **asthma**[D1] and **COPD**[D4]. Having a weakened immune system also leaves people susceptible to pneumonia. **HIV** (**human immunodeficiency virus**) causes a decline in the number of T cells (white blood cells that fight infection). This makes people with HIV/AIDS susceptible to infection from pathogens such as *Mycobacterium tuberculosis*, the bacterium that causes **TB** (**tuberculosis**), a disease that primarily attacks the lungs. A person's immune system can also be impaired a lack of sleep and a poor diet. Pneumonia cannot be completely prevented, but getting enough sleep, eating a nutritious diet, exercising, and following a healthy lifestyle helps to keep the immune system strong and reduce the risk of contracting respiratory infections.

²⁸Mild pneumonia does not usually require hospitalization and can be treated at home with rest, by keeping **hydrated** in order to replace fluids that have been lost by sweating, and by using medicine to ease symptoms. For example, taking an **NSAID (Non-Steroidal Anti-Inflammatory Drug)** or another **antipyretic**, should help to relieve the discomfort of a high fever. Although persistent coughing can disturb sleep, coughing is an important defense mechanism for the lungs. Therefore, people with pneumonia should not take cough medicines (also called **antitussives**) without checking with a doctor or pharmacist first. If the pneumonia is caused by bacteria, an **antibiotic** may be prescribed. Although people often feel better after taking an antibiotic for a few days, doctors emphasize the importance of finishing a whole course of antibiotics, because not doing so increases the risk of the infection returning and may lead to **antibiotic resistance**.

²⁹People with severe pneumonia will need to be treated in hospital, where they will usually be administered **intravenous** (IV) fluids and may be given oxygen therapy. Patients who suffer **respiratory failure**, a serious complication of pneumonia, will often need to be put on a **ventilator**, a machine that helps a patient breathe, or connected to an **extracorporeal membrane oxygenation (ECMO)** machine, which takes over the function of the heart and lungs.

³⁰In the mother's **womb**, a baby's lungs are filled with fluid, so fetal gas exchange occurs in the **placenta**. But within seconds of being born, the baby takes its first breath, and its lungs fill with air. From that point on, the millions of alveoli always contain air (which is why the lungs are the only internal organ that can float on water). So, from the moment we are born, our lungs are constantly connected with the outside environment. Despite this intimate connection to the outside air, human activity is threatening the **lungs of the Earth**, the world's rainforests and oceans (marine plants, plankton, and algae produce around 70% of the atmosphere's oxygen). As individuals, we can take care of our lungs by doing things such as not smoking, exercising, and taking measures to avoid infections. But as a species, our long-term respiratory health may depend on whether or not we stop our destruction of the "Earth's lungs."

5-2 Eleven Etymologies (E) 〈11 の単語を詳しく〉

1) *Air is the mixture of gases that surrounds the Earth and makes up its atmosphere.* The main gases in air are nitrogen (78%), and oxygen (21%). Air also has small amounts of other gases, including carbon dioxide (0.04%), neon, and hydrogen. Pure air has no color and no smell, but in the environment, air typically contains dust, pollen from plants, and fungi spores.

WFE: The word "air" is from the Latin *aer*. Words with this root include **aeroplane** (or "airplane," as it is often spelled in British English), **aerobic** (*bic* → *bios* = "life"; so, requiring oxygen from the air for life), **aerosol**, and the verb **aerate**:

℮ *Earthworms are very important for helping to **aerate** (add air) to the soil.*

The words "air" and "oxygen" are often used interchangeably, but they have different meanings. While oxygen is a pure gaseous element, air is a mixture of different gases. Oxygen literally means "acid producer" (the suffix ~*gen* means "produce/generate"). It has been estimated that rainforests are responsible for around 28% of the oxygen in the air and 70% comes from marine plants (e.g., phytoplankton). Plants on land and in the sea produce oxygen as a by-product of **photosynthesis**, the process by which plants use, or "put together," sunlight, water, and carbon dioxide to create energy in the form of sugar (*syn~* = "together" + *thesis* = "put"). The Greek WFE, *oxys*, meaning "oxygen," is found in a number of medical words, including the following:

- **Hypoxia**: low oxygen content in the tissues (*hypo~* = "low" + *ox* = "oxygen" + ~*ia* = a suffix for nouns, including names of diseases).
- **Hypoxemia**: low oxygen content in the blood (*em* = "blood"). Because the blood transports oxygen to the tissues, the presence of hypoxemia usually indicates the presence of hypoxia.
- **Oximeter**: A device to measure oxygen in the air or dissolved oxygen (*oxi* = "oxygen" + *meter* = "measure"). A **pulse oximeter** is a medical device for measuring a person's **oxygen saturation**.

An **artery** is a blood vessel that carries blood from the heart to other parts of the body. Arteries usually carry oxygen-rich blood (one is exception is the **pulmonary artery**, which carries deoxygenated blood from the heart to the lungs). The word "artery" is derived from a Greek word meaning "to keep or hold air" (*ar* = "air" + *ter* = "to keep"). People used to believe that arteries were pipes for carrying air, not blood, around the body. One reason for this belief is that, after death, the arteries of humans and other mammals tend to be empty of blood. Early anatomists noticed this and assumed that in living animals, too, the arteries were "wind pipes." The etymology of **trachea**, the actual wind pipe, is the Greek word *trachea arteria*. Trachea means "rough," so "trachea arteria" literally means "rough airpipe." It is so called because the rings of cartilage around the trachea give it a rough appearance and feel.

SD 5A: High-Altitude Hypoxia

A few years after arriving in Japan, I got a job working as a bell boy in a luxury hotel in Shizuoka Prefecture. The hotel was on a small island called Awashima (淡島), in Suruga Bay (駿河湾). Across the bay was Mt Fuji, the highest mountain in Japan, whose summit is around 3776 meters above sea level. A **perk** of the job was having amazing views of Mt Fuji every day. One early summer morning, I climbed Mt Fuji, together with a few other staff from the hotel. The climb up the mountain was much harder than I expected, and by the time I reached the top I was out of breath and felt a bit giddy. I realize now that I was probably experiencing mild symptoms of high-altitude hypoxia. The composition of air remains constant, regardless of the altitude (so air contains 20.9% oxygen at sea level and on top of Mt Fuji). However, as altitude increases, air pressure decreases, which causes the number of oxygen molecules in a given volume of air to also decrease. At the top of a high mountain oxygen molecules in the air are further apart because there is less pressure pushing them together. The air is "thinner" at high altitudes, meaning there are fewer oxygen molecules inhaled with each breath. At altitudes above around 3,000 people can suffer hypoxia, symptoms of which include headaches, vomiting, inability to sleep, impaired thinking, and extreme fatigue. At altitudes above around 7,600 meters, acute high-altitude hypoxia (also called **mountain sickness**) can kill.

Some groups of people who have lived at high altitudes for generations have evolved various **physiological adaptations**. For example, Tibetan highlanders who live in the mountains of Tibet have a higher rate of breathing, allowing more air to be taken into the lungs. Also, the blood vessels of Tibetans expand, or **vasodilate**, more than the blood vessels of people who live at sea level. This vasodilation facilitates the rapid delivery of oxygen to the muscles and organs of the body. Tibetan highlanders are "super vasodilators" because the lining of their blood vessels produces more **nitric oxide** than people not adapted to mountain living (nitric oxide is a potent vasodilator).

2) *Caustic* **substances are able to burn or corrode living tissue.** Caustic substances are highly acidic (low pH) or highly basic (high pH) ("pH" stands for "potential of hydrogen"; pH is a measure of the concentration of hydrogen ions in a substance.) Some common household products, such as drain and toilet bowl cleaners, contain caustic substances such as **sodium hydroxide** and **sulfuric acid**.

WFE: Caustic comes from the Greek *kaustikos*, meaning "to burn," and it forms part of the word **holocaust**. The original meaning of holocaust was an animal sacrifice, in which the whole animal was burnt and offered to God, but the word came to describe something, often a war, that causes mass destruction and the death of many people.

℮ There are now enough nuclear weapons in the world to cause a "nuclear holocaust."

Used with a definite article ("the") and a capital letter, **"The Holocaust"** usually refers to the systematic extermination of around 6 million Jews by Nazi Germany during World War II. The prefix *holo~*, meaning "entire or whole," is in the words **Cat<u>holic</u>**, **<u>holo</u>gram**, and **<u>holi</u>stic**:

*℮ When treating a person with depression, anxiety, or other mental health issues, it is important to take a **holistic** approach, considering not only symptoms, but also the person's home and work-life balance, diet, amount of exercise, and the like.*

3) *Compound*: **Used as a verb, "to compound" means to make something worse by adding something to it.**

*℮ For John, work gave him his meaning in life, and when he was made redundant, he became anxious and depressed. These feelings were **compounded** by the death of his father a week after losing his job.*

In chemistry, a compound is a substance formed when two or more WFEs combine chemically. Water (H_2O), for example, is a **chemical compound**, with each water molecule consisting of two atoms of hydrogen and one atom of oxygen.

WFE: The Latin root *pone* means "to place/put". So, compound means "put together/add to" (*com~* = "together"). In the above sentence about John, his depression from losing his job was made worse by adding a death of a parent. In the past, one of the main jobs of a pharmacist was the compounding of medicine. **Drug compounding** is the process of combining ("putting together") two or more different ingredients to create a medication that is tailored to the needs of an individual patient. The rapid growth of mass drug manufacturing by the pharmaceutical industry after the Second World War means that many pharmacists are now no longer required to compound medicines.

Other words with *pone* or variations of this root (*pose, posit*) include **component**, **opponent** ("put against"), **impose** ("put from above"), **dispose** ("put apart"), and **postpone** ("put after"). If your hobby is gardening, you have no doubt used **compost**, a mixture of leaves, food waste, manure, and other things all "put together."

4) *Cyanosis* **is an** *abnormal bluish discoloration of the skin and mucous membranes.* It is caused by high levels of deoxygenated blood circulating in the capillaries near the skin. Cyanosis is most obvious in parts of the body where the skin is thin and there are many capillaries, such as the lips, ears, and the mucous membranes in the mouth. It is often caused by diseases of the heart or lungs. **Peripheral cyanosis**, when the tissues in the hands or feet turn blue, can be caused by vasoconstriction due to exposure to the cold.

WFE: The Latin *cyan* means "blue." This WFE is in **cyanobacteria**, a microbe with a blue-green color. Billions of years ago, oxygen generated by cyanobacteria is thought to have helped the development of complex life on earth. **Cyanide**, a potentially lethal poison, is so called because a blue iron pigment, named Prussian blue, was used to **isolate** it (**hydrogen cyanide** was first isolated in 1782). Certain invertebrates such the crabs and octopuses have blood that is blue. This is because the respiratory pigment that carries oxygen in the blood of such animals contains a copper pigment called **hemocyanin**. When hemocyanin binds to oxygen, it absorbs mostly red light, making crab blood appear blue. (On the other hand, hemoglobin is an iron-containing respiratory pigment. When iron binds to oxygen, it is mostly blue light that is absorbed, causing the blood in humans and all other vertebrate animals to appear bright red). The suffix ~*osis* indicates a process or a state, usually a state of disease. For example, **phagocytosis** is a process by which certain cells engulf and ingest other cells or particles. **Atherosclerosis** is a disease of the arteries. Two infectious diseases with this suffix are **psittacosis**, a viral pneumonia transmitted to humans by contact with birds (it is a zoonotic disease, or **zoonosis**), and **tuberculosis (TB)**, an infectious disease caused by *Mycobacterium tuberculosis*.

Around 80% of TB infections are in the lungs (**pulmonary tuberculosis**), but TB can affect other organs, including the bones and brain. Tuberculosis gets its name from **tuber**, a stem of a plant that grows underground. Tubers, such as potatoes, are often small and round, and TB causes small swellings or **tubercules** in the lungs that resemble plant tubers. TB used to be known as **consumption** because people suffering from it became very thin—it was as if the disease was consuming the body.

Until 1950, TB was the leading cause of death in Japan, but after the World War II the number of TB cases in Japan declined rapidly. A key reason that the prevalence of TB fell in Japan in the 1950s was due to the widespread use of **streptomycin**, the first antibiotic that was effective against TB. In 2021, the incidence of TB in Japan was around 10 people per 100,000, so TB is still not a disease of the past in this country.

SD 5B: Don't eat raw bamboo shoots!

Cyanide is so lethal because it blocks cellular respiration in the mitochondria, and so prevents cells from using oxygen and producing energy. Without energy, muscle cells, including the those in the diaphragm and heart, cannot contract. In relation to E2 above, about the etymology of the word "Holocaust," it was hydrogen cyanide (HCN)—known by the trade name of Zyklon B—that was the poisonous gas used to kill Jewish people and others in the Nazi gas chambers. Also, it was a "suicide pill," a capsule containing potassium cyanide (KCN), that Adolf Hitler used to commit suicide on April 30, 1945.

I am writing this in April, and spring in Japan is when bamboo shoots are in season. Several hours ago, I ate two portions of seasoned steamed rice with bamboo shoot (炊き込み御飯) and a bowl of miso soup with bamboo shoot that my wife made. The two bamboo-shoot dishes were delicious, but if I had eaten that amount of raw bamboo shoot, I would now be very sick. This is because bamboo contains a type of **cyanogenic glycoside** named taxiphyllin. A cyanogenic glycoside is a chemical compound that releases **hydrogen cyanide** when digested. Fortunately, taxiphyllin is quickly destroyed by boiling in water ("cyanogenic" means "cyanide producing").

5) *Diffusion* **is the movement of molecules from an area of higher concentration to an area of lower concentration.** When we breathe, inhaled oxygen moves from the alveoli (higher concentration of oxygen) into the blood flowing through the capillaries (lower concentration of oxygen) by diffusion, and carbon dioxide moves from the blood (higher concentration) into the alveoli (lower concentration). The gas diffusion that occurs in the alveoli is an example of **passive diffusion** (i.e., diffusion that does not use energy for the transport of molecules). For passive diffusion to occur, there must be a **concentration gradient** (i.e., the concentration of molecules is higher in one region than in another region). If a person's breathing stopped, for example due to chocking, no new air would enter the lungs, and the concentration gradient of oxygen between the alveoli and the blood would eventually be lost. Another situation in which this could occur is in a morphine overdose because **opioids** inhibit a part of the brainstem involved in breathing, causing respiratory depression. In people with pneumonia, the diffusion of oxygen into the capillaries is **impeded** by a physical barrier (i.e., fluid and pus) inside the alveoli that lowers the **permeability** of the alveoli membrane. And membrane permeability is an important factor affecting passive diffusion.

WFE: "Diffuse" is composed of the prefix *dis~* ("apart") and *fuse* ("to pour"). The literal meaning of diffusion is "spread out." Other words with this root are **refuse, confuse** ("pour

together"), **transfuse** ("pour across"), and **perfuse** ("spread all through"; *per~* = "through").
*Ɛ In order for gas exchange to occur efficiently, there has to be adequate ventilation of the lungs and good **perfusion** of blood in the alveolar capillaries.*

6) *Infant mortality* is the death of a child before their first birthday. Infant mortality has declined in western countries; for example, in the United Kingdom, in 1800, there were over 300 deaths per 1000 births in children under five years of age; in 2022, this was 3.4 deaths per 1000 births. Fewer children dying from infectious diseases, including pneumonia, is the main reason for this decline.
WFE: The root *fa* (*fat, fam*) means "speak/say," so **infant** is a child "unable to speak" (*in ~* = "not"). Other words with this root include **famous** (lit. "someone or something everyone speaks about") and **preface**. The word **fate** originally meant a prophecy spoken by god. From fate we get the words **fatalistic** (a belief or feeling that an event cannot be avoided whatever is done) and **fatal**, which means "causing death" (in ancient Rome, people thought that death was decided by what was "spoken" by the gods). The noun **fatality** means "a death caused by an accident or by violence," and the **fatality rate** is the number of deaths from a specific cause in a population over period of time.

A term with a similar meaning to fertility rate is "**mortality rate**." The root of the word mortality is *mort*, meaning "death." Words with this root include **mortuary**, **postmortem**, and **immortal**. A surprising word with this root is **mortgage**, a loan from a bank that helps a borrower buy a house. The "gage" part of this word means "a **pledge**," so mortgage literally means "death pledge" (the pledge, or agreement, between the borrower and lender would end, or "die," either when the borrower paid off the loan or when the borrower failed to pay in time and the lender could take the house). There are three death-related words in the following sentence:
*Ɛ During the Ukraine war, many of the **fatalities** were civilians. The bodies of some of those who were killed were taken to hospital **mortuaries**, but many **corpses** lay in the streets for days.*

The word **corpse** means "a dead human body." It is from the Latin *corpus* ("body"). During the COVID-19 pandemic some of the very sickest patients were put on **ECMO** machines. An ECMO machine pumps blood from the patient's body to an oxygenator (an "artificial lung") that adds oxygen to it and removes carbon dioxide. The acronym ECMO stands for **extracorporeal membrane oxygenation**. "Extracorporeal" means "outside the body." **Corporal punishment** is the physical punishment of people, especially of children.
*Ɛ In 1958, Sweden became the first country in the world to ban **corporal** punishment in schools.*

7) *Influenza*, commonly known as "the flu," is an infectious disease caused by influenza viruses. The symptoms of influenza include fever, aches, and fatigue. Influenza sometimes leads to life-threatening complications. Serious flu complications include pneumonia, inflammation of the heart (**myocarditis**), inflammation of the brain (**encephalitis**), and **sepsis**. There are 3 types of influenza virus, but influenza types A and B are the types responsible for seasonal flu epidemics. While influenza

A viruses can infect humans, birds, pigs, and other animals, influenza B viruses are only found in humans. Influenza A viruses are divided into subtypes according to the structure of two protein on the surface of the virus. These two proteins are **hemagglutinin** and **neuraminidase**. The 1918 influenza pandemic, commonly called the **Spanish flu**, was caused by an H1N1 virus of **avian** (bird) origin. The "H1" stands for **hemagglutinin** type 1 and the "N1" for **neuraminidase** type 1. At present, there are 18 known subtypes of hemagglutinin (H1–18) and 11 known subtypes of neuraminidase (N1–11). However, only H1N1, H3N2, and H3N3, currently cause widespread disease in humans. Although the common cold and the flu are both respiratory illnesses and they can have similar symptoms, they are certainly not the same. Table 5.1 compares these two conditions.

Table 5.1

Comparison of Influenza (flu) and Cold Symptoms　(風邪とインフルエンザとの症状比較)

Signs and symptoms (徴候と症状)	Influenza　(インフルエンザ)	Cold　(風邪)
Onset of symptoms	Sudden	Gradual
Fever	Usual (including high fever)	No, or mild fever
Muscle aches	Usual, often severe	No, or mild
Chills	Uncommon	Common
Fatigue	Usual, often severe. Can last for weeks	Mild and brief
Headache	Common	Rare
Sneezing	Sometimes	Typical
Nasal congestion	Sometimes	Common

WFE: Influenza is from the Latin *influentia*, meaning "to flow into." Until about 500 years, it was believed that the stars gave off a kind of fluid that affected humans, including causing disease. Influenza referred to an outbreak of a disease that was thought to be "influenced" by the stars. Other words with the root *flu* (to flow") are **fluent** and **affluent** (*af~* → *ad~* = "to"; so, "wealth flows to someone"). **Influx** means "to flow in," and **reflux** means "to flow back."

℮ *Wars often cause an **influx** of refugees into neighboring countries.*

℮ *Gastroesophageal **reflux** disease (GERD) occurs when acidic stomach juices flow back up from the stomach into the esophagus. This can cause various unpleasant symptoms, including a pain in the middle of the chest called "heartburn." In some people, the stomach acid can flow back to the throat from where it can be inhaled into the lungs. This could cause aspiration pneumonia.*

Flux is also a word meaning "change":

℮ *The COVID-19 pandemic and the Russian invasion of Ukraine highlight how the world is in a **state of flux**. When you read this, the future may be even less predictable than it is now.*

SD 5C: Disease names can stigmatize

The influenza pandemic of 1918 to 1919 was caused by an H1N1 influenza that infected an estimated 500 million people around the world (over 30% of the global population at that time). It is estimated that the pandemic killed over 50 million people. In contrast to COVID-19, which tends to be most severe in elderly people and people with underlying conditions, the influenza pandemic of 1918 also killed many healthy adults, aged between 20 to 40 years. The 1918 pandemic was given the name of the "Spanish flu." You may assume that the pandemic started in Spain, but this was not the case. In fact, evidence suggests that the first people infected with the virus were soldiers on an army base in Kansas, USA.

So, why was it named the "Spanish flu"? It was because the spread of the influenza around the world started while the First World War was still raging (the war ended on November 11, 1918). Nations fighting in the war had strict **censorship** of the press, and governments in these countries suppressed the news of the influenza. On the other hand, because Spain remained neutral during the war, it did not have war-time censorship and its newspapers freely reported the true number of influenza cases. This is why people assumed that the infection had originated in Spain. Calling the 1918 influenza pandemic the "Spanish flu" was not only inaccurate, but it also stigmatized Spain and Spanish people (**stigmatize** is to label something or someone in a negative way). In 2015, the WHO issued guidelines for naming diseases. The WHO strongly recommended that the following should not be used when naming diseases:

- Geographic locations (e.g., Spanish flu, Japanese encephalitis, Marburg virus disease)
- People's names (e.g., Kawasaki disease)
- Species of animals (e.g., swine flu, monkeypox [mpox])
- Groups in society and occupations (e.g., Legionnaires' disease; GRID an acronym for "Gay Related Immune Deficiency"—this was later renamed AIDS).

8) *Pneumonia*: In the opening paragraph of this article, I defined pneumonia as "inflammation of the lungs," but to be more exact pneumonia is primarily inflammation of the alveoli. You would expect a term for "inflammation of the lungs" to have the suffix ~*itis*, which denotes inflammation. The word "**pneumonitis**" does, in fact, exist. The difference between pneumonia and pneumonitis is this: pneumonitis is a general term for lung inflammation, but pneumonia is used specifically to refer to lung inflammation caused by an infection. So, pneumonia is a type of pneumonitis. Although pneumonitis can be used to refer to lung inflammation of any cause, it usually refers to inflammation with **noninfectious etiologies**. For example, if gasoline is aspirated into the lungs, it can cause **chemical pneumonitis**. Other causes of pneumonitis are inhalation of smoke (e.g., from a house fire) or chlorine gas (e.g., from chlorine bleach used for cleaning). Radiation therapy to the chest area (e.g., for cancer treatment) can result in lung inflammation, a condition known as **radiation pneumonitis**.

WFE: The root **pneumo** means "lungs" or "air." In the term "pneumonia," the suffix ~*ia* makes various words into nouns. It is often used in the names of diseases (e.g., **dementia**, **schizophrenia**), and countries (e.g., Australia, Algeria). If you want a challenge, you can learn the spelling of **<u>pneumo</u>noultramicroscopicsilicovolcanoconiosis**, which is one of the longest words in English and a lung condition caused by inhaling silica dust from a volcano.

The Greek word *pneumon* became *pulmo* in Latin. Examples of words with this Latin root are **pulmonary** ("relating to the lungs"; e.g., **pulmonary artery**), **cardiopulmonary** ("relating to the heart and lungs") and **pulmonologist** ("a doctor who specializes in lung conditions").

As stated above, the suffix *~itis* indicates inflammation of a tissue or organ. The verb "inflame" literally means "to set on fire." In addition to inflammation, **fever** is another natural response to an infection and is a common symptom of pneumonia. Medicines that are used to lower a fever are called **antipyretics**. The root *pyra* means "fire." There is a mental illness called **pyromania**, sufferers of which feel a strong urge to start fires. In India people are often **cremated** outside on a pile of wood called a **funeral pyre** (from the Latin *pyra*). Cremating the dead on a funeral pyre is a part of Hindu tradition, but it has an impact on the environment because it uses a lot of wood, contributing to deforestation, and it is also a source of air pollution. Air pollution is a risk factor for pneumonia and other respiratory illnesses. So, burning dead people can lead to health problems for the living.

SD 5D: What is sleep apnea?

Sleep apnea is a potentially serious sleep disorder that occurs when a person's breathing stops and starts during sleep. This interruption of breathing typically lasts for between 10 to 30 seconds. In people with serious sleep apnea, breathing can stop more than 30 times in an hour. The most common type of sleep apnea is called **obstructive sleep apnea** (OSA). This type of sleep apnea occurs when the airway in the throat (**pharyngeal airway**) collapses periodically. The causes of OSA are complex, but being overweight is a risk factor. Also, some people are susceptible to OSA because they are born with an upper airway that is narrower than normal. Two symptoms of OSA are loud snoring and excessive daytime sleepiness. Feeling sleepy during the day occurs because a person wakes up briefly each time the throat collapses. Waking up dozens or even hundreds of times each night seriously disrupts sleep. There have been numerous traffic accidents caused by people with OSA who **doze off** while driving. In the UK, drivers diagnosed with OSA and who suffer from excessive sleepiness may have to give up their driving license until their condition improves. The root *pnea* means "breathing" and the prefix *a~* means without, so apnea is "without breathing." **Dyspnea** is the medical term for "shortness of breath," a common symptom of pneumonia, but the literal meaning is "disordered breathing" (*dys~* = "abnormal/disordered"). The medical term for normal breathing is **eupnea** (*eu~* = "good").

9) *Respiration* **is the action of breathing (external respiration), or the production of energy in cells (cellular respiration).** Cellular respiration is a complicated metabolic process, but here is a simple equation for **aerobic respiration,** respiration that uses oxygen to turn food into chemical energy: *sugar (from food) + oxygen (from inspired air) → carbon dioxide + water + energy.*

Carbon dioxide and water are **byproducts** of aerobic respiration. Much of the carbon dioxide is exhaled into the environment.

WFE: The Latin *spiritus* means "breath," and the prefix *re~* means "again," so **respiration** is to "breathe in and out."

*ℰ Because canaries have a rapid **respiratory rate** (60-80 breaths/minute) and a high metabolism, they are very sensitive to carbon monoxide and other toxic gases. This is why these small birds were once used by miners to detect dangerous gases in coal and other mines.*

People with asthma may be given a <u>**spirometry test**</u>. A **spirometer** is a medical device that measures the volume of air flowing in and out of the lungs when breathing. The root *spiritus* is in several frequently used words, including **aspire**, **conspiracy**, and **expire**:

*ℰ Young adults in the UK generally **aspire** to become homeowners, but property prices are so high that many cannot afford to buy a house. (a~ → ad~ = "towards"; so "breath desire towards [buying a house]")*

*ℰ Some people believe that the failure of the English education system in Japan is because of a secret policy made by "power holders" in Japan. According to this **conspiracy theory**, these power holders actually want people to finish their English education with a very low level of English proficiency. If Japanese people had a high level of English, they would be encouraged to leave the country. And the people in power want to prevent a brain drain of ambitious young people from Japan. (con~ → com = "together"; lit. "to breathe together")*

"Expire" literally means "to breathe out," but it can also mean "to die." A more common use of this word is for when a passport, credit card, or the like comes to an end.

*ℰ My bus pass **expires** next week, so I need to renew it.*

Perspire is the medical word for "to sweat." The prefix *per~* means "through," so perspire means to "give out sweat through the pores in the skin." The prefix *per~* is in many other words, including **persistent**:

*ℰ A <u>**persistent**</u> cough can be a symptom of lung cancer.*

The root of "per<u>sist</u>ent" is from the Latin *sister*, meaning "to stand firm," and is in words such as **resist**, **assist**, and **armistice** (*arm* = "weapon"; so, "stand with your weapon and not fight").

*ℰ The **armistice** that ended WWI came into force at 11am on the 11ᵗʰ day of the 11ᵗʰ month of 1918.*

The word **spirit** comes from *spiritus*. Spirit has several meanings, including religious ones, but one meaning is "life force/essence."

*ℰ When I draw my last breath, will my **spirit** leave my body and become a ghost?*

If a person disappears without anyone noticing, we can say he or she was "spirited away." It is as if they were taken by a ghost. "Spirited Away" is the English title for the 1999 Japanese anime movie *"Sen to Chihiro no Kamikakushi"* (千と千尋の神隠し).

10) Rhinovirus: It is estimated that around half of all common colds, a highly contagious viral infection, are caused by **rhinoviruses**, while around 15% are caused by coronaviruses. Human rhinoviruses generally cause infections of the upper respiratory tract, but in infants, the elderly, and immunocompromised people, they can also lead to lower respiratory tract infections.

WFE: The prefix *rhin* means "nose." **Rhinoceros** is from the Greek *rhinokeros*, meaning "nose-horned." The WFE *keros* is in the word **keratin**, the substance forming animal horns, feathers, finger and toe nails, and hair. One symptom of the common cold is **rhinorrhea**, the medical term for a **runny nose**. The WFE ~*rrhea* means "flow/discharge" (e.g., **diarrhea**, **amenorrhea**). **Rhinitis**, inflammation of the mucous membrane inside the nose, is often caused by an allergen. **Allergic rhinitis** is commonly known as **hay fever**.

11) *Ventilation* is the movement of air around a room or other closed space.
ℰ *Before I start my lesson, I always open the classroom windows as well as the doors in order to ensure good **ventilation** of the classroom with outside air. This helps to reduce the concentration of any respiratory pathogens that may be in the classroom air.*
Pulmonary ventilation is the movement of air into and out of the lungs, and is commonly known as "breathing."
WFE: The Latin *ventus* means "wind." The noun **vent** is an opening through which air, smoke, or the like enters or leaves (e.g., a **volcanic vent**). As a verb, "to vent" can mean to express an emotion, often anger, that has been bottled up.
ℰ *In my experience, Japanese people don't tend to become aggressive or violent when drunk, but they sometimes **vent** their dissatisfaction about work, homelife, the state of the economy, and such things.*
   While *ventus* means wind, the WFE *flare* means "to blow." It is part of **inflate** and **deflate**:
ℰ *Air moves into the lungs when they **inflate** and moves out of the lung when they **deflate**.*
The words **inflation** and **deflation** are commonly used in economics to describe an increase or decrease in the price of goods and services. The medical term for "gas generated in the digestive system" is **flatus** (although most people use the word **fart** or the euphemistic term "**to pass wind**"). The word **flavor** also derived from *flare*. It is interesting that the Japanese word for flavor, *fūmi* (風味), contains the Chinese character for "wind," a natural phenomenon that *blows*.

5-3   Dozen in Detail (D)   （12の話題を詳しく）

1) *Asthma* is a chronic inflammatory condition that affects the airways in the lungs. It is classified as an **obstructive lung disorder**. These disorders, which also include COPD, are characterized by difficulties in breathing, especially in **exhalation** (breathing out), due to an obstruction of airflow for some reason. (Other conditions cause **restrictive lung disease**, in which the lungs are restricted from expanding, causing inhalation of air to be restricted. This can happen when a disease such as **asbestosis** damages the lung tissue itself, or due to **extra-pulmonary** causes such as weakness of respiratory muscles, as happens in **ALS**, also known as **motor neuron disease**.) Asthma is most common in children, but it can occur at any age. In UK around 10% of children have asthma. The prevalence of asthma is highest in developed countries such as the United States, the United Kingdom, and Australia. The etiology of asthma is complex with both genetic and environmental risk factors. There are several types of asthma, but the most common type is **atopic asthma** (also called **allergic asthma**), which is triggered by **allergens** like pollen, pets, and **dust mites**. Many people with allergic asthma have a related immune condition such as hay fever, **eczema** (also called **atopic dermatitis**), or food allergies. Asthma is characterized by **airway hyperresponsiveness.** This means the airways of people with asthma tend to narrow excessively in response to certain stimuli (or **triggers**) that would have little or no effect in people without asthma. This airway narrowing, called **bronchoconstriction**, is caused by the sudden contraction of **smooth muscle** in the walls of the bronchi. The triggers that cause bronchoconstriction vary from person to person, but common ones include:

- Environmental allergens such as pollen and animal hair
- Environmental **irritants** such as tobacco smoke and perfumes
- Exercise (**exercise-induced asthma**)
- Cold air
- Air pollution
- Respiratory infections such as colds and **sinus** infections
- Emotional stress
- Ingestion of aspirin (in some people with asthma, aspirin can bring on an attack of asthma, a condition known as **aspirin-induced asthma**).

In addition to narrowing of the airways, another characteristic of many people with asthma is **mucus hypersecretion**. Airway mucus is essential for lung defense, but excessive mucus can further narrow the airways (mucus can form plugs in the airway that completely obstructs them). This airway narrowing increases the resistance to air flow as air is inspired and expired. What underlies asthma is **chronic inflammation of the bronchi**. It is this chronic inflammation that makes airways **predisposed** to bronchoconstriction in response to a trigger. Inflammation also causes the inner lining of the airways to swell and produce the mucus mentioned above.

Typical symptoms experienced by people with asthma include coughing that is often worse at night, breathlessness, and chest tightness (which has been described as "feeling like an elephant sitting on your chest"). Another key symptom is **wheezing**, a high-pitched whistling noise that most often occurs during expiration (a whistle makes a whistling noise when we blow it because air is quickly forced out through the narrow opening—similarly, expiration out of a narrowed airway causes the whistling sound of wheezing).

When asthma symptoms suddenly become worse it called an **asthma attack**, or asthma **exacerbation**. Asthma attacks are often mild and short-lived, and with treatment the constricted airways will open up again within a few minutes to a few hours. But severe asthma attacks require immediate medical help. During a severe asthma attack, breathing becomes **labored** and wheezing becomes worse due to extreme airway narrowing. An **ominous** sign that the asthma attack is leading to respiratory failure is when the wheezing stops, a situation called **silent chest**. It occurs when the airway narrowing is so severe that air cannot pass through the airways. Fortunately, there are medications that help prevent asthma attacks and medications to stop an asthma attack in progress. Even so, asthma still kills. In Japan, for example, there were around 1,700 deaths from asthma in 2017 (compared to over 7000 people during the 1970s). The majority of those who died were elderly people over 70 years of age.

SD 5E: Treating asthma and its environmental costs

As explained above, in asthma, an environmental allergen such as dust or some other trigger results in narrowing of the airways. This narrowing occurs due to airway swelling resulting from inflammation and **edema** (accumulation of fluid in the tissues of the airways due to leakage of fluid from the surrounding blood vessels), excess mucus secretion, and bronchoconstriction (contraction of smooth muscles around the airways).There are many drugs that target these causes of airway narrowing, but asthma medicines can be broadly divided into **controller medicines** that help control asthma by suppressing inflammation (and thereby reducing swelling and excess mucus secretion); and **rescue medicines** that give quick relief during an asthma attack. Controller medicines, which are taken daily for long periods, help to prevent an asthma attack. These medications can also prevent or reduce **airway remodeling**, which is when chronic inflammation leads to damaging changes in the structure of the airway wall. Corticosteroids, drugs that have **potent** anti-inflammatory and **immunosuppressant** effects, are the most effective controller medication.

The first-choice drug for the quick relief of asthma symptoms are short-acting β_2 (Beta-2) receptor agonists. The preferred **route of administration** of asthma drugs is **inhalation**. This is because inhalation delivers the drug directly to the lungs, enabling the drug to work more rapidly, allowing smaller doses to be used, and reducing the risk of systemic (whole-body) side effects compared to oral medications. People with asthma use a medical device called an **inhaler** to deliver medicines into the lungs. There are two main kinds of inhalers: **metered dose inhalers** (MDIs) and **dry powder inhalers** (DPIs). The MDIs use a **propellant** to deliver the medicine into the airways. Dry power inhalers do not use a propellant; instead, the inhaler releases the medicine, which is in a dry powder form, when a person sucks in the medication.

From an environmental perspective, MDIs are a problem because the gases used as propellants are powerful **greenhouse gases**. In the UK, over 60 million inhalers are prescribed each year. Of these, over 70% are MDIs. The propellants in MDIs account for around 4% of the entire **carbon footprint** of the **NHS** (the National Health Service). The NHS is encouraging more people with asthma to switch to DPIs as a way to reduce the carbon footprint of the NHS. Asthma inhalers are just one example of the many environmental impacts of health care.

SD 5F: Why "fussy" drugs are better

I enjoy cooking dishes from different countries and using many interesting ingredients. While my daughter eats anything that I cook, my son is quite a **fussy eater** who only eats a limited number of Japanese dishes that my wife makes. Eating a wide variety of foods is usually better for the health and, I think, makes life more enjoyable. However, **pharmaceutical scientists**, the people specialize in drug development, seek to make extremely "fussy" drugs. Scientists, however, don't use the word "fussiness," but "selectivity." **Drug selectivity** is the degree to which a drug acts on a given receptor relative to other receptors. To illustrate drug selectivity, let's look at why drugs called **β-blockers** (beta blockers) are often **contraindicated** in people with asthma. Receptors are molecules, usually proteins, on the surface of a cell (although steroids receptors are inside a cell). A receptor recognizes a certain chemical signalling molecule, for example, a hormone or neurotransmiter, and binds to it with a chemical bond. This chemical binding leads to a change in cell function. There are three subtypes of beta receptors, known as beta 1 (β1), beta 2 (β2) and beta 3 (β3), but only β1 and β2 receptors are important for this discussion. These two receptor subtypes are located in various tissues of the body, but the key point is this: β1 receptors are dominant on **cardiac myocytes** (heart muscle cells), while β2 receptors are dominant in the airways. (A **mnemonic**: 1 heart = β1; 2 lungs = β2).

The full name of β receptor is **β-adrenergic receptor**. "Adrenegic" indicates that the receptor is stimulated by **adrenaline** (a hormone) and **noradrenaline** (a neurotransmitter and hormone) and other adrenergic substances. When adrenaline or noradrenaline bind to β1 receptors in cardiac myocytes, it increases the heart rate, and makes the heart contract with more force. This will increase the **cardiac output** (the volume of blood pumped per minute by the heart). An increase in cardiac output causes a rise in blood pressure. In the airways, binding of adrenaline or noradrenaline to β2 receptors causes smooth muscle relaxation, resulting in **bronchodilation** (and an increase in the diameter of the airways). These receptors are targets for two commonly used drugs:

- **Beta-blockers**: This class of drugs is often used to treat **hypertension**. They bind to beta-receptors, thereby blocking adrenaline and noradrenaline from binding to β1 receptors on heart muscle cells. This slows the heart rate and reduces the heart's strength of contraction, causing a reduction in cardiac output and a lowering of blood pressure. Beta-blockers are an example of an **antagonist** drug (i.e., one that acts against and stops the action of another substance).
- **Beta 2-agonists**: An agonist drug is one that binds to a receptor and stimulates it. When a beta-2 agonist drug binds to β2 receptors in the lungs, it causes bronchodilation. This reverses the bronchoconstriction seen in asthma.

Back to drug selectivity: I wrote above that β1 receptors are dominant in the heart and β2 receptors are dominant in the lungs. But "dominant" just means that there are more of one receptor in one location compared to another. The reality is that β2 receptors also exist on cells in the heart and β1 receptors are also present on airway smooth muscle. For example, one study found that lung tissue of mice contains β2 and β1 receptors in the proportion of around 70:30.

When beta blockers were first used in the 1960s, there were many reports of the drug causing asthma attacks. This was due to beta-blockers binding to β2 receptors in the airways, thereby blocking the action of noradrenaline and adrenaline. This blocking results in **bronchoconstriction**, which is the last thing a person with asthma needs! Another problem with beta-blockers is that because they block β2 receptors in the airways, they prevent beta 2-agonists (drugs important in treating asthma attacks) from binding to β2 receptors. From the mid-1970s, beta-blocker drugs that were selective for β1 receptors became available. These **cardioselective beta-blockers** are much less likely to cause respiratory side effects in asthmatics who also require a beta-blocker to treat hypertension. However, **absolute selectivity** is very difficult for pharmaceutical scientists to achieve, and even cardioselective beta-blockers may also have some action on β2 receptors, **precipitating** an asthma attack in susceptible people. For this reason, asthmatics should avoid cardioselective beta blockers or use them with caution. Similarly, Beta 2-agonists used in asthma treatment are not completlely specific for β2 receptors, so they also bind to β1 receptors on cardiac muscle, causing side effects such as **tachycardia** (an increase in heart rate).

2) *Aspiration pneumonia:* When swallowed, food, drink, and saliva should enter the esophagus, the "food pipe" that leads to the stomach. However, if such things are inhaled into the trachea, they can carry bacteria from the mouth into the lungs. These bacteria can then multiply in the lungs, causing a lung infection known as aspiration pneumonia. In Japan, it is estimated that 30% of those who die of pneumonia had been diagnosed with aspiration pneumonia. Elderly people are at increased risk of aspiration pneumonia because they are more likely to have **dysphagia** (difficulty in swallowing). Swallowing problems are particularly common in people with **Alzheimer's disease**. Other common causes of dysphagia in elderly people are Parkinson's disease and stroke. Elderly people sometimes have an impaired **cough reflex**, making them vulnerable to aspiration pneumonia. Aspiration pneumonia is more common in elderly people, but it can happen at any age; for example, it has been the cause of death of young people who inhaled vomit after **binge drinking** on alcohol.

Certain medications, including **opioids**, inhibit the cough reflex and increase the likelihood of aspiration pneumonia. On the other hand, medications that increase cough sensitivity may help prevent aspiration pneumonia. A dry cough is a well-known side effect of **ACE inhibitors**, drugs that are commonly used to treat hypertension. This side effect occurs because ACE inhibitors cause an increase in the levels of **bradykinin**, a peptide produce by the body, and bradykinin enhances the cough reflex. A few studies have found that elderly people taking ACE inhibitors had a lower incidence of pneumonia. This is example of a **therapeutic side effect**.

SD 5G: Brushing your teeth can also be good for your lungs!

Good **oral hygiene** is important at any age for preventing **dental caries**, but tooth brushing is also a prevention against aspiration pneumonia, especially in elderly people. Bacteria, including those that could cause pneumonia, find a home in the mouth. These populations of mouth bacteria feed on the food that remains in the mouth. Brushing the teeth properly at least twice a day reduces the population of harmful mouth bacteria, and so reduces the risk of pneumonia if saliva is aspirated into the lungs.

3) *Breathing* **(also called external respiration or ventilation) is the process of taking air into the lungs (inhalation) from the outside environment and expelling air from the lungs into the outside environment (exhalation).** The lungs contain no **skeletal muscle**, so they are unable to expand by themselves. Instead, the work of breathing requires the **diaphragm** and other **respiratory muscles**. The diaphragm, a dome-shaped muscle between the lungs and abdominal cavity, is the most important muscle for breathing, but it is assisted by muscles between the ribs (**intercostal muscles**), muscles in the neck, and abdominal muscles. The contraction and relaxation of muscles acts to change the volume of the thoracic cavity, which in turn changes the lung volume and, as a result, the pressure within the lungs. A number of diseases, including ALS, and poisons such as **tetrodotoxin**—a potent neurotoxin found in various organs of the pufferfish (*fugu*)—can stop breathing by **paralyzing** the respiratory muscles.

A more common reason for a person to stop breathing is **choking**, which happens if the airway becomes blocked. Coughing is an important defense mechanism of the respiratory system that can often dislodge a piece of food stuck in the airway if the obstruction is partial; however, if the airway is completely obstructed, coughing will not be possible. Because the airway is blocked, new air will not be able to reach the lungs, and the brain will become deprived of oxygen. One way to save a person who is chocking is if someone performs the **Heimlich maneuver (abdominal thrusts)**, a choking-rescue technique. To find out how to do the Heimlich maneuver, watch a video on the Internet, or, better still, do a **first-aid course** (in Japan, many fire departments offer such courses). The Heimlich maneuver was invented by an American doctor called Henry Heimlich, who died in 2016, at the age of 96. Several months before he died, Dr Heimlich performed the maneuver that he invented on an 87-year-old woman, a fellow resident in the retirement home where Dr Heimlich lived. The woman had choked on a piece of meat during dinner at the home, but she was fortunate enough to be sitting next to the inventor of the Heimlich maneuver.

SD 5H: Another vital function of breathing

In addition to bringing air into and out of the lungs for gas exchange, another vital function of breathing is to help regulate the body's balance between acidity and alkalinity, referred to as the **acid-base balance**. The normal function of the body's physiological processes depends on the balance of acids and bases in the blood being maintained within a narrow range. Blood is normally slightly basic (alkaline) at close to pH 7.40, but the pH* may range from about 7.35 to 7.45. Even a minor deviation from the normal range can have fatal consequences (e.g., a pH above 7.8 and less than 6.8 is usually fatal). The kidneys, lungs, and liver work together to control the blood's acid-base balance. It is a complex process. Here we will briefly look at the role of the lungs.

Carbon dioxide (CO_2) is a waste product of cellular respiration (when oxygen is combined with molecules from food to produce energy). This CO_2 passes from cells into the blood. One way CO_2 is carried in the blood is by being converted to **carbonic acid** (H_2CO_3), which is formed when CO_2 reacts with water. When the level of CO_2 in the blood rises, as it does if you hold your breath for as long as you can, more carbonic acid is formed. This causes the blood pH to drop (carbonic acid rapidly splits apart to produce bicarbonate ions and **hydrogen ions**, the latter lowering the pH of the blood). When you can no longer hold your breath and you start breathing again, you will breathe faster and/or deeper, so that you exhale more CO_2. Reducing the amount of CO_2 will reduce the level of carbonic acid in the blood, thereby raising blood pH to the normal level.

Because of narrowed airways, a person having an asthma attack may not be able exhale enough CO_2, resulting in too much CO_2 accumulating the blood (a condition known as **hypercapnia**), and leading to a fall in blood pH. This condition is called **respiratory acidosis**. Acute respiratory acidosis, when carbon dioxide builds up very quickly, can be fatal. The opposite of holding your breath is **hyperventilation**—excessively deep and rapid breathing—as can happen during a panic attack. Hyperventilation greatly increases how much carbon dioxide is exhaled. This loss of too much carbon dioxide from the blood will raise the pH level of the blood, a condition known as **respiratory alkalosis**. This condition can cause symptoms such as dizziness and **fainting**.

* The pH of a solution indicates the concentration of **hydrogen ions** in that solution. The higher the concentration of hydrogen ions in the blood, the lower its pH and the more acidic it is; and the lower the number of hydrogen ions, the higher the pH and the more alkaline it is.

SD 5I: How long can you hold your breath underwater?

Breathing is usually automatic, regulated through the **respiratory center** in the **brainstem**. The main stimulus to increase the rate and depth of breathing is a high level of CO_2 in the blood. An increase in blood CO_2 is detected by the respiratory center, stimulating an increase in the rate and depth of breathing. More CO_2 is thus exhaled from the body, returning CO_2 levels to a normal range.

The other day, I went swimming with my son. We had a competition to see who could stay underwater for longer. I only managed 60 seconds. One way to increase the time I could hold my breath is by hyperventilating (breathing in and out quickly and deeply). Hyperventilating for a number of minutes before I put my head underwater will blow off (remove) most of the CO_2 from my blood (an abnormally low level of CO_2 in the blood is called **hypocapnia**). Removing CO_2 from the blood removes the desire to breath. While going underwater with a very low blood CO_2 would enable me to hold my head under water for longer, the lack of oxygen in my blood could also cause me to **pass out** (lose consciousness). And, as you can imagine, passing out underwater could cause me to drown. Hyperventilating as a way to stay underwater for longer is definitely not recommended for most people. In 2021, a man called Budimir Buda Sobat broke the record for underwater breath-holding. His record was 24 minutes 37.36 seconds! He was able to do this after many years of training and by hyperventilating on pure oxygen before he put his head underwater.

4) *COPD*, which stands for chronic obstructive pulmonary disease, is a lung disease characterized by airflow obstruction that makes it hard to breathe. It is one of the top three causes of death worldwide, and 90% of COPD deaths occur in low-and middle-income countries. Around 80% of COPD cases are caused by smoking tobacco, and the remaining 20% is due occupational exposure to dust, outdoor air pollution, and indoor air pollution from cooking and heating. It is likely that some people have a genetic predisposition to COPD because only around 15% of lifelong smokers develop the condition.

COPD is comprised of two main conditions: **emphysema** and **chronic bronchitis**. Chronic bronchitis is inflammation of the bronchial tubes, leading to swelling and narrowing of the bronchial tubes. A key feature of COPD is excessive production of **mucus (sputum)**, also the result of airway inflammation. A buildup of mucus is difficult to clear from the airways and causes chronic coughing and breathing difficulties. People with COPD often use **mucolytics**, medications that break down mucus and reduce its **viscosity** (thickness), making it easier to cough out.

In emphysema, the walls of the alveoli become damaged and lose their **elastic recoil** (the tendency to deflate following inflation). Over time, the walls between many of the alveoli break down, and the alveoli merge into each other. So, instead of tiny air sacs, air spaces develop in the lung. In lungs with extensive damage from emphysema, these air spaces can be over than 1 cm in diameter. These airspaces trap old air and are useless for gas exchange. The more alveoli that are damaged in this way, the greater the reduction in total surface area available for the exchange of oxygen and carbon dioxide between the lungs and the blood. Apart from a productive cough, typical symptoms of COPD include **exertional breathlessness** (shortness of breath when making a physical effort), trouble taking a deep breath, and wheezing. These symptoms often get worse in winter. The symptoms of COPD can be similar to asthma, but, as shown in Table 5.2, the two conditions have important differences.

Table 5.2

Differences Between COPD and Asthma   （慢性閉塞性肺疾患 (COPD)と喘息との違い）

	COPD （慢性閉塞性肺疾患）	**Asthma** （喘息）
Family history	Uncommon	Common
Smoking as a risk factor	Around 90% of patients are smokers or ex-smokers	Increasing evidence that it is*
Symptoms under age 30	Rare	Often
Breathlessness	Persistent and progressive	Episodic (may have long periods with no symptoms)
Progressive disease	Yes. It gets worse over time, although medication and lifestyle changes can slow the progression	Not usually. Symptoms come and go
Reversible	No. Lung damage cannot be reversed	Yes. Airway-narrowing is reversible
Changes to lung tissue	Destruction of alveoli	Airway remodeling in severe and uncontrolled asthma
Effect of bronchodilators	Often limited effect	Often good response
Spirometry	Never normalizes	Often normalizes

* Children raised in households in which one or both parents smoke are more likely to develop asthma. Also, the offspring of women who smoked during pregnancy have a higher risk of both childhood asthma and **adult-onset asthma**. In 2022, a paper in the *European Respiratory Journal* reported that children are at higher risk of asthma if their father was exposed to tobacco smoke when he was growing up. In other words, even if a child's father has never smoked, if the child's paternal grandfather smoked, the child's risk of asthma increases. For details, search the internet for this article:
Pre-pubertal smoke exposure of fathers and increased risk of offspring asthma: a possible transgenerational effect

5) *Diagnostic tests* **are medical tests used to help diagnose a disease or condition.**

Different medical tests are used to diagnose pneumonia, including blood tests and **sputum culture**. Blood tests are most often used to determine the presence and extent of inflammation. A patient with pneumonia will often have a raised white blood cell count and an elevated **C-reactive protein** (**CRP**). CRP is a protein produced by the liver in response to inflammation and is present in the blood. Sputum is a thick type of mucus produced in the lower respiratory tract. A sample of sputum, coughed up by the patient, is placed in a **Petri dish** (also called a **cell-culture dish**). The dish contains a **culture medium** that encourages the growth of bacteria. If no bacteria are present after two or three days, the culture is negative; if bacteria are present the culture is positive. A pathologist can identify the specific bacteria using a microscope, and this information is then used to determine the best antibiotic to treat the infection. Because it takes a few days to get the results of the sputum culture, doctors often need to start antibiotic treatment before the results come back from the pathologist. Treating patients with an infection before the microbe causing the infection has been identified is called **empiric antibiotic therapy**. Empiric therapy depends on the doctor making educated guesses, and thus depends on clinical experience (the word "empiric" derives from a Greek word for "experience").

A **chest X-ray** is often used to diagnose pneumonia and to find out the extent and location of the infection. Healthy lungs will show up as black on an X-ray because they are filled with air. Air has a low density and will not absorb any radiation from the X-ray. It thus allows the X-rays to pass through easily. On the other hand, the rib cage, which protects the lungs, appears white on an X-ray because bone is dense and absorbs much of the radiation. In pneumonia, lung tissue that should be filled with air becomes replaced by **inflammatory exudate** (i.e., fluid and pus)—a pathological process known as **consolidation**. On a chest X-ray, areas of consolidation appear as white or gray because inflammatory exudate does not allow the passage of X-rays. Substances that do not permit X-rays or other radiation to pass through are said to be **radiopaque**.

Doctors often classify pneumonia based on the pattern of infection (i.e., the areas of the lung infected by the pathogen) as shown on an X-ray. Two main patterns of infection are **lobar pneumonia** and **bronchopneumonia**. The lungs are divided into sections called **lobes** (the right lung has three lobes and the left lung has two). In lobar pneumonia, all or part of a lobe is affected. While lobar pneumonia affects a continuous area of the lung, in bronchopneumonia the infection is **patchy**. Bronchopneumonia is so called because the infection involves not only the alveoli, but also the terminal bronchioles. Bronchopneumonia is common in children under 5 years of age.

SD 5J: A French doctor's motivation for inventing the stethoscope

Auscultation is using a **stethoscope** to listen (*aus* means "ear") to the sounds inside the body as a way to help diagnosis and treatment. Before the invention of the stethoscope, a doctor had to put his ear directly on the patient's chest (I say "his" because in France and other countries woman were not allowed to become doctors in the early 19th century). For René

Laennec (1781-1826), a doctor in Paris, putting his ear to the chests of young women was quite embarrassing, which is one of the reasons he invented the stethoscope in 1816. The original stethoscope that was designed by Laennec was just a hollow tube about 25 cm long. Laennec not only invented the stethoscope, but he also greatly advanced the diagnosis of pulmonary diseases by **correlating** chest sounds in living patients to changes in the lungs found on **post-mortem** examination. For example, suppose that Laennec, using his stethoscope, heard short cracking or bubbling noises in a female patient with the symptoms of pneumonia. When this patient died, Laennec would cut open her body and examine her lungs. If he found that her alveoli were filled with fluid, this would suggest that the presence of cracking or bubbling sounds on auscultation was a sign of pneumonia. In his 1819 book, Laennec reported on the relationship between various lung sounds and post-mortem findings. One of the diseases he described in detail was tuberculosis (TB), the disease that Laennec himself died of at the age of 45.

6) Fungi are a kingdom of organisms that are neither animals nor plants. Fungi are **eukaryotic** organisms (i.e., their cells have a clearly defined nucleus that is bound within a nuclear membrane) and are **heterotrophs** (i.e., unable to make their own food). Examples of fungi include mushrooms and yeasts. Most fungi are **decomposers**, which means they feed on decaying organic matter such as leaves, wood, and dead animals, and return nutrients to the soil. Fungi play many vital roles in ecosystems. (As someone who is fascinated by the natural world and has watched the destruction of it by humans, I would say this: The disappearance of fungi would *kill* the Earth, but the disappearance of humans would *heal* it.)

Fungi are beneficial to humans in so many ways. For example, we eat mushrooms, and **fermentation** by yeasts and molds (types of fungi) is needed in the production of bread, cheese, beer and wine. Many medicines are made using fungi, including antibiotics (e.g., penicillin), **statins** (cholesterol-lowering drugs), and **immunosuppressives** (e.g., cyclosporine, which is used to treat autoimmune conditions and to help prevent rejection after an organ transplant).

On the other hand, certain types of fungi are **pathogenic**, causing diseases in humans, including pneumonia. While bacteria and viruses are often spread through the air in respiratory droplets, fungal pneumonia most often starts by inhaling fungal **spores**. Compared to bacteria and viruses, fungi account for only a small portion of pneumonia in the general population. However, in people who are **immunocompromised**, fungal pneumonia is a common cause of **morbidity** and **mortality**. Immunocompromised is having a weakened immune system due disease (e.g., AIDS) or medical treatment (e.g., chemotherapy).

Fungal infections that cause pneumonia are often **opportunistic**. Opportunistic fungal infections are caused by fungi that are non-pathogenic or have low pathogenicity in **immunocompetent** people (i.e., people with a normal immune response), but become pathogenic in immunocompromised people. An example of an opportunistic infection is

aspergillosis, caused by a **mold** called **aspergillus**. The spores of this mold are in the air, and most people probably inhale many hundreds of them each day. In most people, these spores do not cause any health problems, but in people whose immune system is impaired, they can result in a serious lung infection. If the infection spreads from the lungs into the bloodstream, it can lead to **invasive pulmonary aspergillosis**, a systemic infection with a high mortality rate. During the COVID-19 pandemic, there were reports from India of opportunistic fungal infections in people with severe COVID-19. Such people were vulnerable to fungal infection partly because of the **corticosteroid therapy** that was used to treat COVID-19 pneumonia. Corticosteroids such as **dexamethasone** proved to be a **double-edged sword** in the treatment of COVID-19 patients. Although corticosteroid therapy is effective in reducing inflammation, it inhibits the immune system and so predisposes patients to secondary infections.

7) *Heart failure* **is a chronic, progressive condition in which the heart is unable to pump enough blood to meet the body's requirements.** The body of humans and other multicellular organisms can be seen as having four levels of organization: **cells**; **tissue** (groups of similar cells working together); **organ** (two or more tissues working to accomplish a specific function); and **organ system** (groups of organs working together to perform one or more functions). The human body has 11 different organ systems, including the topic of this chapter, the **respiratory system** (made up of the organs such as the nose, trachea, bronchi, and lungs). The various organ systems are not islands within the human body, but are interdependent, working and communicating with one another to keep us alive. The symptoms of heart failure illustrate well the close connection between the **cardiovascular system** (heart, blood vessels, blood) and the respiratory system. Heart failure can affect the left or right side of the heart, but it often affects both sides. One of the main symptoms of heart failure is shortness of breath, or **dyspnea**, especially during physical effort (exertion). Dyspnea occurs due to **left-sided heart failure**, the most common type of heart failure. Left-side heart failure is when the heart's **left ventricle** is longer able to pump enough blood to the body (the function of the left ventricle is to pump oxygenated blood around the body). This causes blood to build up in the pulmonary veins, the blood vessels that carry oxygenated blood from the lungs back to the left side of the heart. The pulmonary veins become so full of blood that pressure increases in these blood vessels, causing fluid to be pushed out from the blood vessels and into the alveoli. The alveoli fill with fluid, a condition called **pulmonary edema** (also called **pulmonary congestion**). Pulmonary edema impedes the diffusion of gases between the alveoli and the blood. One reason that heart failure increases the risk of getting pneumonia is that pulmonary edema impairs clearance of pathogens from the lungs.

8) *Nose:* The two openings in the nose, called **nostrils**, allow air to enter the respiratory system. The nostrils continue into a space called the **nasal cavity**, which is divided down the middle by a thin cartilage wall called the **nasal septum**. The mucous membrane inside the nose is covered in hairs that help trap dust, pollen, and other larger particles in the air before they can enter deeper into the respiratory tract (it is an interesting paradox that as men get older and lose head hair, nasal hair grows more vigorously!). The mucus in the nose is not only good for trapping things, but, because it is wet, it adds moisture to the air as it moves through the nasal cavity. In addition, the nasal cavity has a rich blood supply, which warms the inspired air. (**Epistaxis**, commonly called a nosebleed, is caused by the rupture of capillaries in the mucous membrane.) So, as well as being filtered and cleaned, air is also conditioned (warmed and moistened) by the nasal cavity.

In addition to its respiratory functions, the **olfactory system** (sense of smell) is in nasal cavity. Olfaction is not only important for checking if we have **BO** (body odor), or to alert us to a fire, but it is also vital for the **perception of flavor**. Problems with the sense of smell include **anosmia** (loss of smell), **olfactory dysfunction** (changes in the ability to smell), and **parosmia** (a distortion in the sense of smell). Research has shown that problems with smell can be an early sign of dementia and Parkinson's disease.

SD 5K: Mouth breathing or nose breathing. Is one better?

The mouth is not considered part of the URT, but we can and do breathe through it, especially during exercise or when the nose is blocked up. However, nose breathing is considered healthier than mouth breathing because the nasal cavity filters, warms and humidifies air in a way that the mouth cannot. In most people, the majority of inspiration is through the nose, so wearing a mask without covering the nose—something that was a common sight in Japan during the COVID-19 pandemic—does not make much sense. In addition, SARS-CoV-2, the virus that causes COVID-19, typically infects people through the nasal cavity. This is why scientists have developed COVID-19 vaccines that are sprayed up the nose **(intranasal vaccines)**. Inhaling a vaccine stimulates the production of antibodies in mucous membranes that line the nose, mouth and lungs. This could produce **sterilizing immunity** (i.e., immunity that stops a pathogen from replicating in the body and prevents someone getting infected).

9) *Penicillin* is the first naturally occurring antibiotic to be discovered. It was discovered in 1928 by Sir Alexander Fleming, a Scottish medical doctor and bacteriologist, in his laboratory at St Mary's Hospital in London. Penicillin is a chemical released by a **mold** called *Penicillium notatum* (this mold got its name from its brush-like structure; the original meaning of "pencil" was "a fine brush for painting"). Why and how Fleming noticed that this mold stopped the growth of bacteria is a great example of **serendipity**, an unplanned fortunate discovery, and is probably the most famous discovery story in science (do an internet search for "Fleming+serendipity," and see how many hits you get).

The discovery of penicillin was a major medical breakthrough that revolutionized medicine, and it earned Fleming, and two other scientists, Ernst Chain and Howard Florey, the Nobel Prize in Physiology or Medicine in 1945. These two other scientists and their research team in Oxford University developed a system of **purifying** and growing penicillin, and they also tested penicillin on humans for the first time. The very first person in the world to be injected with penicillin was Albert Alexander, in February 1941. He was a 43-year-old policeman who had developed a life-threatening infection after scratching his face on a rose bush. Mass production of penicillin began in the USA during the Second World War. In the last few years of the war, penicillin helped save many thousands of **Allied soldiers**.

Now you know a little about the discovery of penicillin, let's look at **antibiotics** more generally. First of all, what are antibiotics? In a general sense, antibiotics are substances produced by microorganisms that act against the growth of other microorganisms; however, in medicine, an antibiotic is a drug derived from fungi or bacteria that is used to treat infections caused by bacteria. A similar term is **antibacterial**. Strictly speaking, an antibacterial refers both to drugs derived from fungi or bacteria (i.e., from natural sources) and also to drugs synthesized in the laboratory. However, usually the terms antibiotic and antibacterial are used **interchangeably**. Here are some key points on antibiotics that I cover in my university lesson on the topic.

- Many of the antibiotic drugs used today were discovered from around 1950 to 1960. This period could be called the "**golden age**" of antibiotic discovery. Many of these antibiotics were derived from microbes in the soil. Because penicillin, which is derived from a mold, is the most well-known antibiotic, people may assume that all antibiotics are from fungi. In fact, the majority of the antibiotics used today are from bacteria. The group of bacteria that have yielded most antibiotics are filamentous bacteria called **Actinomycetes**. A question that you may be asking is why do bacteria and fungi produce antibiotics in the first place? Well, the substances produced by soil microbes that humans use to make antibiotic drugs are **secondary metabolites**. Secondary metabolites are not directly involved in growth or development, but they are important in other ways for the survival of the producing organism. Secondary metabolites have many functions, including for signaling between microbes, and as chemical weapons against other soil organisms. Secondary metabolites are vital for soil microbes in the competition for resources.

- Penicillin kills bacteria by disrupting the synthesis of the bacterial cell wall. The cell wall of most types of bacteria is made of **peptidoglycan**, a substance forming **cross-links** that not only strengthens the cell wall, but also prevents the content of the bacterial **cytoplasm** from leaking out. Penicillin works by preventing the cross-linking of the peptide chains in peptidoglycan, resulting in the bacterial cell wall becoming fragile and full of holes. The process of **osmosis** then causes water from the outside environment to quickly pass through the leaky cell wall and enter the bacterium. This inflow of water causes the bacterium to swell and burst, like a balloon filled with too much water. This bursting, which kills the bacterium, is known as **osmotic lysis**.

- If administering penicillin to a person with a bacterial infection kills bacteria by osmotic lysis, you may be wondering, "Doesn't penicillin also cause human cells to burst?" The answer is "No." This is because antibiotics exploit the differences between bacterial and human cell structure. Human cells and bacterial cells have many differences, the most obvious of which is that human cells are **eukaryotic**, meaning DNA is stored in a membrane-bound nucleus, while bacterial cells are **prokaryotic**, meaning there is no nucleus. Although both human cells and bacterial cells have a **phospholipid cell membrane**, almost all bacteria also have rigid **cell wall** outside the cell membrane. Because the cells of humans do not have a cell wall, penicillin does not target human cells. We can say that penicillin has **selective toxicity** against bacteria—it kills the infecting bacteria without harming human cells. Does this sound too good to be true? It is. Penicillin can cause side effects, some of them serious. Moreover, it does not kill all types of bacteria.

- No one knows how many species of bacteria there are on Earth, but it has been estimated that just in 30 grams of soil from a forest, there are a million species of bacteria. Scientists have different ways to classify these single-cell organisms; for example, according to the bacterium's basic shape, or its oxygen requirements (e.g., **obligate aerobic bacteria** cannot survive without oxygen, while **obligate anaerobic bacteria** grow only in the absence of oxygen). But the classification that is most important when considering antibiotic treatment is whether the bacteria causing an infection are **Gram-positive** or **Gram-negative**. The word "Gram" refers to Hans Christian Gram, a Danish bacteriologist who, in 1884, devised a method for differentiating bacteria according to the composition of their cell wall. He applied a certain **dye** to a colony of bacteria, and found that if the bacteria had a thick peptidoglycan layer in the cell wall, they **stained** purple. On the other hand, bacteria that did not turn purple had only a thin peptidoglycan layer. Simply put, Gram-positive bacteria have a thick cell wall, while Gram-negative bacteria have a thin cell wall. The method of **"Gram staining"** is still widely used today in **microbiology** ("staining" means using dyes to highlight structures in microbes and other cells and tissues, so that they can be more easily distinguished under a microscope). You may think that, with their thick cell wall, Gram-positive bacteria would be more difficult to treat with penicillin, but in fact the opposite is true. Gram-positive bacteria are easier to kill with penicillin because their thick peptidoglycan layer more easily absorbs antibiotics. In contrast, penicillin is not effective on Gram-negative bacteria because they have an additional lipid membrane outside their thin peptidoglycan layer (Gram-positive bacteria do not have this outside lipid membrane). It is the presence of this extra lipid membrane that impedes the entry of penicillin into Gram-negative bacteria.

- Penicillin was found to be ineffective against Gram-negative bacteria. Fortunately, other antibiotics were discovered in nature, or synthesized in the laboratory, that have different modes of actions from penicillin and are able to target Gram-negative bacteria. Some antibiotics work by affecting bacteria protein synthesis. Proteins in bacteria are made in intracellular structures called **ribosomes**. Tetracycline, which was isolated from soil bacteria in 1948, binds to bacterial ribosomes and disrupts a specific step in bacterial protein synthesis. Human cells also rely on ribosomes for protein synthesis, but because ribosomes in human cells are shaped differently from bacterial ribosomes, antibiotics cannot bind to ribosomes in human cells. Another mechanism of action employed by some antibiotics is blocking the synthesis of **folic acid** within the bacterium. Folic acid is a B-vitamin that is vital for the synthesis of DNA. Some antibiotics inhibit an enzyme called **dihydrofolate reductase**, preventing the formation of folic acid. Without folic acid, DNA synthesis is also prevented. DNA synthesis in human cells is not affected by such antibiotics because humans obtain their folic acid from the diet rather than having to make it themselves.

- Synthetic antibacterial drugs are created by chemical procedures in the laboratory. Semi-synthetic antibiotics are derived from natural antibiotics, but they have been altered in the laboratory to give them advantageous characteristics. An important example of a semi-synthetic antibiotic is **ampicillin**. This antibiotic has the basic structure of penicillin, but differs from penicillin by the presence of an **amino group**. Adding this amino group enables ampicillin to pass through small pores in the outer lipid membrane of Gram-negative bacteria, something that penicillin cannot do. Having passed through the outer lipid membrane of Gram-negative bacteria, it then inhibits cell wall synthesis in the same way as penicillin. Ampicillin is a **first-line** antibiotic for children with community-acquired pneumonia.

- The most common side effects of antibiotics are **gastrointestinal** (GI) problems such as **diarrhea**, **nausea**, and **vomiting**. These GI side effects occur mainly because the antibiotic damages the beneficial bacteria in the gut (the **microbiome)**. Certain antibiotics cause more serious side effects than others. For example, **aminoglycosides**, a class of antibiotic often used to treat serious infections such as pneumonia and sepsis, are sometimes toxic to the ear (**ototoxicity**) and can cause deafness. Around 1 in 15 people have an **allergic reaction** to antibiotics. In most cases, the allergic reaction is mild to moderate, with symptoms such as a skin **rash**, itching, and runny nose. But in some people, antibiotics, particularly penicillin, can cause **anaphylaxis**.

- Some antibiotic drugs, including penicillin, are **bactericidal**, meaning they kill bacteria. Other antibiotics are **bacteriostatic**, which means that do not directly cause bacterial death, but they stop the growth or reproduction of bacteria. An antibiotic can also be classified as being **narrow-spectrum** or **broad-spectrum**. Narrow-spectrum antibiotics target a few types of bacteria, while broad-spectrum antibiotics target many types. A narrow spectrum antibiotic is usually chosen if the bacteria causing an infection is known. Broad-spectrum antibiotics are useful when the causative bacterium has not been identified; however, these antibiotics are more likely to disrupt the gut microbiome and more likely to lead to antibiotic-resistant bacteria.

- Antibiotics are not effective against viruses, which are responsible for colds, influenza, and many other respiratory illnesses. Although both viruses and bacteria are classed as microbes, viruses and bacteria have a completely different structure and way of existence from each other. Here are just a few of the many differences. Viruses are around 100 times smaller than bacteria; bacteria are unicellular organisms with a well-defined cell wall, while viruses are non-cellular organisms without a cell wall (instead they have a protein shell called a **capsid**, containing the virus' genetic material); bacteria contain ribosomes and other **cellular machinery**, but viruses do not have any cytoplasmic organelles; and bacteria are able to reproduce independently, but viruses cannot (instead, viruses have to enter a host's cell and "hijack" its cellular machinery in order to replicate; this is why viruses are called **obligate intracellular parasites**). Because viruses are unable to replicate independently and they do not meet most of the other **characteristics of life**, some microbiologists consider viruses to be non-living. Antibiotics are highly specific in targeting the cell wall or the cellular machinery that bacteria, and only bacteria, use to grow and replicate. Viruses have no cell wall nor any cellular machinery, so we should not be surprised that antibiotics do not work on viruses.

SD 5L: A huge threat to human health: Antibiotic resistance

Antibiotic resistance is the ability of bacteria to resist the effects of antibiotics. Like all organisms, bacteria undergo random mutations of their genetic material (RNA or DNA). Rarely, a mutation results in a change in a bacterium that makes it capable of defending itself against an antibiotic. Although a mutation that **confers** antibiotic resistance probably only occurs in fewer than one in a million bacteria, bacteria replicate by **asexual reproduction** very frequently (often once every 20 minutes), so a single resistant bacterium could generate over two million offspring in 7 hours. In addition, bacteria without the advantageous mutation are susceptible to the antibiotic and are eliminated by it. So, by the process of **natural selection**, bacteria that are better suited to the environment (i.e., able to resist the antibiotic) survive and pass on this **adaptive trait** (a characteristic that gives some advantage) to the next generations. Antibiotic resistance is not only passed on to the **descendants** of the original mutant bacterium, but it can also be passed to non-resistant bacteria by a process called **bacterial conjugation**.

In bacterial conjugation, pieces of DNA (called **plasmids**) are transferred from one bacterium to another through a **tubule** that temporarily connects the two bacteria. Bacterial conjugation enables the rapid spread of antibiotic resistance through a bacterial population. Resistance to not just one, but multiple antibiotics, can be transferred between bacteria. When a bacterium is resistant to more than one antibiotic it is said to be **multidrug-resistant**. An example is **methicillin-resistant *Staphylococcus aureus*** (**MRSA**). Methicillin, a semisynthetic derivative of penicillin, is an antibiotic developed in the late 1950s that is no longer used, but the *Staphylococcus aureus* that became resistant to it is now resistant to several classes of antibiotics. The resistant genes generated by random mutation alter the bacterium in ways that enables it to counteract antibiotics. These **mechanisms of antibiotic resistance** include:

- Enzyme inactivation: bacteria produce enzymes that inactivate the antibiotic before it enters the bacterial cell; for example, the resistance of staphylococcus bacteria to penicillin is due to its ability to secrete **beta-lactamase**. This enzyme breaks open the **beta-lactam ring**, a key part of penicillin's chemical structure, thereby splitting the penicillin molecule.
- Pump mechanism: bacteria actively "pump out" the antibiotic from themselves.
- Altered target: bacteria change the site to which the antibiotic usually binds so that the antibiotic no longer recognizes the binding site.

Resistance to antibiotics is a natural phenomenon that occurs in the natural world, and in his

1945 Nobel lecture, Alexander Fleming warned against the risk of bacteria developing resistance to penicillin. However, the problem of antibiotic resistance has accelerated greatly in recent decades, and it is now one of the biggest health threats facing humankind. In 2019, it was estimated that antibiotic resistance killed over 1 million people worldwide, and it is estimated that by 2050 this number will grow to over 10 million.

The WHO has warned we are entering a "post-antibiotic era." In a world where antibiotics don't work, pneumonia, sepsis, diarrhea, urinary tract infections, gonorrhea, and many other bacterial infections are untreatable; and simple surgery or chemotherapy is too dangerous because there are no antibiotics to prevent or treat bacterial infections. In such an era, even a small cut that becomes infected could be fatal. Some regions of the world are already in a "post-antibiotic era" because even the **last-resort antibiotics** are no longer effective (a "last-resort antibiotic" is used to treat infections with bacteria that are resistant to all other common antibiotics).

Some of the main reasons that antibiotic resistance has become such a serious problem include:

- Over-prescription of antibiotics: doctors are prescribing antibiotics for viral infections such as colds and influenza. Antibiotics cannot kill viruses, so, with a few exceptions, they should not be prescribed for viral infections. There is no doubt that some doctors prescribe antibiotics when they are not needed in order to make money, but sometimes patients demand doctors to prescribe them antibiotics, even when they are not needed.
- Obtaining antibiotics without a prescription: in some countries, antibiotics can be bought from a pharmacy without a doctor's prescription. Powerful antibiotics can also be easily obtained on the internet.
- Patients not finishing the whole antibiotic course: for many years doctors and pharmacists have told patients that stopping an antibiotic course too early will encourage antibiotic resistance. However, recent research suggests that this advice may not always be correct.
- Overuse of antibiotics in agriculture: antibiotics are used therapeutically to treat animals that become sick and **prophylactically** (to prevent disease). Antibiotics are also given to chickens, pigs, and cows to make them grow faster. Bacteria that become resistant to antibiotics inside animals can then spread to humans.
- Poor infection control in hospitals.
- Lack of new antibiotics being discovered: Since the 1980s there has been no new class of antibiotics (all the new antibiotics that have come to market are variations on existing drugs discovered in the 20th century). There are several reasons for this, one of which is that big pharmaceutical companies have reduced their research and development into new antibiotics. This is partly because antibiotics are not very profitable since they are generally used for only a short period of time (a course of antibiotics for an infection is usually taken for a week or so, but medications for chronic diseases such as diabetes and hypertension are often taken by a patient for many years). Bacteria are acquiring resistance to antibiotics faster than humans can develop new types of antibiotics. Unless, we continuously create new antibiotics, humans will lose the **arms race** with the microbes.

SD 5M: Secondary bacterial infections

While antibiotics are not effective against viruses, they are sometimes administered to people with a viral infection to prevent or treat a **secondary infection** by bacteria. A secondary infection occurs when an initial infection, known as a primary infection, makes a person more **susceptible** to disease. For example, a viral infection may damage the epithelium of the respiratory tract, making it easier for bacteria to infect it. Also, the viral infection weakens the immune system, leaving a person less able to fight off a bacterial infection. Researchers in the USA examined lung tissue that had been preserved from victims of the 1918 influenza pandemic. In their 2011 study, the researchers reported that most people had died not as a direct result of the influenza virus, but from secondary bacterial pneumonia. If antibiotics had been available in 1918, the **death toll** from the pandemic may not have been so high.

10) *Sepsis* **is the dysregulated immune response to an infection that causes organ dysfunction**. Instead of the immune system just attacking the pathogen causing a local infection, in sepsis the immune system overreacts and attacks the whole body. Sepsis is a life-threatening condition, especially if it leads to **septic shock**. This is when the blood pressure drops so low that blood flow to the vital organs decreases drastically causing damage to, and then failure of, multiple organs. The drastic drop in blood pressure occurs mainly due to **systemic vasodilation** (i.e., the dilation of blood vessels all over the body). This systemic vasodilation is caused by a dysregulated immune response that triggers an excessive release of small proteins called **cytokines** and other inflammatory regulators. Inflammatory cytokines not only cause vasodilation, but they also make blood capillaries leaky, causing fluid to be lost from the blood and blood volume to decrease. The most common cause of sepsis is a bacterial infection, but it can also be due to infections caused by viruses and fungi. Infection in any part of the body can lead to sepsis, but common sites include the lungs—pneumonia is one of the most frequent causes—and the urinary tract (people using a **urinary catheter** are particularly susceptible to urinary tract infections caused by bacteria). Even a small skin infection can lead to sepsis. Some signs of sepsis include a fever, **lethargy**, mental confusion, a rapid heart rate, increase in respiratory rate, and passing less urine than usual. Sepsis can progress very quickly—from the appearance of the first symptoms to death can take under 12 hours. If you suspect that you or someone else has sepsis, quickly get medical help. I strongly suggest that you watch a few online videos on sepsis to familarize yourself with the signs and symptoms of this potentially deadly condition.

SD 5N: When the immune system causes a storm

It is not the infection-causing pathogen itself that is responsible for sepsis, but the way the body's immune system overreacts to the infection. The extreme, or **hyperinflammatory**, response of sepsis is driven by cytokines, a large group of proteins made by **macrophages** and other immune cells that act to transmit signals between cells. There are different types of cytokines, but the ones involved in sepsis are **proinflammatory cytokines**, which alert the immune system to the presence of infection and trigger immune cells to rush to the site of the infection. During the COVID-19 pandemic, the term "**cytokine storm**" was widely used in both medical journals and the popular media. The cytokine storm is when elevated levels of immune cells release an excessive number of cytokines into the blood, and these cytokines recruit even more immune cells that secrete even more cytokines. You can see that how this **vicious cycle** could cause the uncontrolled production of inflammation-causing (proinflammatory) cytokines that damage the body's own tissues. Many of the victims of COVID-19 died due to **multi-organ failure** resulting from a cytokine storm.

11) *Where it was acquired*: Pneumonia can be classified according to where the infection was acquired. My father got the pneumonia that ended his life while in a care home. Pneumonia that develops in a care home falls under the heading of **health care-associated pneumonia**. It is not surprising that pneumonia is common in care homes. Frail and elderly people, usually with **comorbidities**, often living in close contact with each other, and in daily contact with nurses and other staff, is **a perfect recipe** for the spread of infections. A person who develops pneumonia while in the hospital is said to have **hospital-acquired pneumonia** (also called **nosocomial** pneumonia). Nosocomial pneumonia includes **ventilator-associated pneumonia**, occurring in patients on a **mechanical ventilator** (a machine that takes over the job of breathing in people who are unable to breathe on their own). If pneumonia is acquired outside a hospital or other healthcare facility, it is called **community-acquired pneumonia**. It is important to know where a person developed pneumonia because certain bacteria are more common in certain settings. For example, infections caused by **MRSA** (Methicillin-resistant *Staphylococcus aureus*) and other **antibiotic-resistant bacteria** are more prevalent in hospitals, while *Streptococcus pneumoniae* is responsible for over 60% of community-acquired infections.

12) Zoonosis is a disease transmitted from animals to humans (since humans are, of course, animals it is more accurate to say from "non-human animals"). It is often said that zoonotic diseases "jump" the species barrier. Zoonotic pathogens may be viral, bacterial, fungal, or parasitic. A few examples of viral zoonoses include: avian influenza (from birds), Ebola (often from bats), **MERS** (Middle East Respiratory Syndrome; often from camels), **monkeypox** (often from **rodents**), **rabies** (mammals, particularly dogs). Of these examples, rabies is perhaps the scariest because once the symptoms of rabies appear, the case fatality rate is virtually 100%. A person's life can be saved if a rabies vaccine is given after being bitten by an infected animal (because the vaccine is given after exposure to the virus, it is called **postexposure prophylaxis**). But the vaccine must be given before any symptoms appear.

Bacterial zoonoses include the **bubonic plague**, caused by *Yersinia pestis*, a bacterium that is spread by fleas on rats and other animals. Tuberculosis (TB) in humans is primarily caused by *Mycobacterium* *tuberculosis*, the human form of TB, but it may also be caused by the *Mycobacterium bovis*, a bacterium that infects cows. Milk is **pasteurized** (heated to a specified temperature for a certain amount of time) in order to kill pathogens, including *Mycobacterium bovis*. Drinking unpasteurized cow's milk is dangerous because you could get TB from it.

It is estimated that over 60% of all known infectious diseases are zoonotic and around 75% of **emerging diseases** are transmitted from animals (emerging diseases are diseases that appear for the first time in a population, or that have existed before, but then rapidly increase in the number of cases and/or geographical range). The number of zoonotic diseases has increased in recent decades for several interrelated reasons; for example:

- Destruction of jungle and other natural habitat for agriculture and human settlements. This environmental destruction is driven partly by rapid human population growth. Such destruction brings animals and humans closer together, increasing the risk of a **zoonotic spillover**.
- Hunting **bushmeat** increases the risk of zoonotic pathogen transmission and threatens biodiversity. It is thought that **HIV** jumped the species barrier in the 1920s when a hunter in central Africa became infected from a chimpanzee carrying the **Simian Immunodeficiency Virus** (SIV).
- The exploitation by humans of wild species (e.g., the trade in wildlife for pets).
- Factory farming (**intensive farming**), involving the rearing of animals on an industrial scale. Having many animals packed closely together indoors is a perfect environment for pathogens to infect many animals, mutate, and then jump to humans.
- Global air travel has made the world interconnected, but it has also made it much easier for diseases to quickly spread across borders.

According to some **epidemiologists**, we are now in the "era of pandemics." As humanity continues to destroy the remaining natural environment, it is highly likely that COVID-19 will not be the only pandemic in your lifetime.

SD 50: The origin of SARS-CoV-2: Bats?

It has been reported that bats are the **animal reservoir** of SARS-CoV-2, the virus responsible for COVID-19 (the animal reservoir of an infectious pathogen is the animal in which the pathogen normally exists). Bats are carriers of a whole variety of viruses, including many types of coronaviruses. Some of the viruses that bats carry can cause serious, even fatal, infections in humans. However, bats seem to be unaffected by the viruses in their bodies (one exception is rabies—bats are also susceptible to the rabies viruses, which makes them sick and kills them). One reason bats carry many viruses is because they live in large colonies, which promotes the transmission of pathogens from animal to animal. There is a lot of research into why bats can carry so many viruses but be resistant to getting sick. One **hypothesis** is related to the fact that bats are the only mammal that can fly (a few mammals can glide, but only bats are capable of true flight). For bats, flying is very metabolically demanding, and it results in a rapid increase in the bat's body temperature—when a bat is flying, its metabolic rate increases by around 15-fold (in comparison with a 2-fold increase in the metabolic rate of birds when flying). This rapid rise in temperature is likely to result in cell damage in the bat's body. Usually cell damage triggers inflammation, but bats may have evolved a way to suppress the inflammatory response in order not to suffer from inflammation after every flight. This ability to control inflammation could allow bats to tolerate viruses without falling sick.

Bats do carry many viruses, some of which have jumped to humans and caused disease. But it is human activity, such as the destruction of the bat's natural habitat, that is the underlying cause of most zoonoses. Bats play a key role in many ecosystems, and they benefit humans in various ways; for example, insect-eating (**insectivorous**) bats eat large quantities of insects, which helps to suppress crop pests. Bats also eat many mosquitoes that are **vectors** for a number of human diseases (e.g., malaria). Moreover, many plants (e.g., banana, mango) rely on fruit bats for **pollination**.

SD 5P: Why I am not allowed to donate blood in Japan

I am unable to donate blood in Japan because I lived in the UK during the 1980s (I was at high school in London during that decade). The Ministry of Health, Labor and Welfare in Japan does not allow anyone who lived in the UK for one month or over between 1980 to 1996 to donate blood. This is because during this period there was an outbreak of **BSE** (**Bovine spongiform encephalopathy**), commonly called "mad cow disease," in the UK. Eating meat from infected cows could cause a fatal brain disease called **variant Creutzfeldt-Jakob disease** (vCJD) in humans. This disease causes the brain to become spongiform, in other words, like a sponge. BSE is a zoonosis, but it is unusual in that the pathogen is not a virus, bacteria, fungus, or parasite, but a **prion**. A prion is not a living organism but is a protein. Specifically, it is a type of abnormally folded protein that triggers normal proteins in the brain to also become misfolded (a protein's function depends on its shape, and a protein's shape is determined by how its amino acid chains are folded). Cooking meat to high temperatures is enough to destroy bacteria and other pathogens, but does not destroy prions. Even some sterilization techniques used in hospitals are ineffective at deactivating these abnormal proteins.

5-4 Well, what do you know?

(どのくらいわかるようになったか試してみよう)

Are the following statements true (T) or false (F)?

1. Brushing your teeth can contribute to the prevention of pneumonia.
2. Lung cancer only affects heavy smokers.
3. Gas exchange in the lungs occurs mainly in tubes called bronchi.
4. Cyanosis is a sign of hyperoxia.
5. Histological and other evidence suggests that many victims of the Spanish influenza pandemic died from a secondary bacterial infection of the lungs.

What is the meaning of the underlined WFE?

1. Japanese cedar pollen is the most common causative allergen for seasonal allergic **rhin<u>itis</u>** in Japan.

2. Some congenital heart defects cause a baby to be born with skin that is bluish. This is called **<u>cyan</u>osis**.

3. Until the x-ray, **<u>auscultation</u>** using a stethoscope was the main way to diagnose pneumonia.

4. The pufferfish, called *fugu* in Japanese, is a delicacy in Japan. However, it must be prepared properly because the liver and other internal organs contain a high concentration of the poison tetrodotoxin (TTX). Ingesting this poison can cause paralysis of **<u>respirat</u>ory** muscles.

5. Because of the COVID-19 pandemic, many people had to **post<u>pone</u>** their trip abroad.

6. In Japan, people aged 65 years or older are recommended to get a pneumococcal vaccine. This vaccine gives good protection against **<u>pneumonia</u>** and other infections caused by *Streptococcus pneumoniae*.

Choose a word from below to replace the underlined word(s)

a) weaken   **b)** low blood oxygen   **c)** pleural membranes   **d)** nosocomial
e) sputum   **f)** alveoli

1. I was waiting at a bus stop one day, when an old man, who was smoking a cigarette, spat out some greenish **<u>phlegm</u>** onto the pavement near my feet. It was disgusting.

2. Inflammation of **<u>the membranes that surround the lungs</u>** is called pleurisy.

3. Air pollution can **<u>impair</u>** the respiratory system's defense mechanisms.

4. Chlorine bleach, which is used for household cleaning, can release chlorine gas if it is mixed with certain other agents such as vinegar. Chlorine gas was used during World War I as a choking agent. Exposure to chlorine gas results in bronchial damage and bleeding in the **<u>air sacs</u>**.

5. **<u>Hospital-acquired</u>** infections is a leading cause of morbidity and mortality in the UK.

6. The modern pulse oximeter was developed by Aoyagi Takuo (青柳卓), a Japanese engineer who died in 2020, at the age of 84. A pulse oximeter is placed on a fingertip and measures peripheral (or percutaneous) oxygen saturation (SpO2). Historically, patients were measured by four vital signs: temperature, blood pressure, pulse, and respiratory rate, but thanks to Aoyagi's invention, oxygen level has become the fifth vital sign. With the pulse oximeter, the rapid identification of **<u>hypoxemia</u>** in patients has become much easier.

5-5 May Jo's Health-Podcast

（メイ・ジョーの健康ポッドキャスト）

Podcast presenter May Jo (MJ) and Dr Mike Reed (Dr) are talking about the stigma of lung cancer.

MJ: This month is Lung Cancer Awareness Month. In the studio today we have Dr Mike Reed, an oncologist at Heath Hospital in London. Dr Reed is here to correct a few common misconceptions about lung cancer, the leading cause of cancer death in the UK. Dr Reed, what are these lung cancer misconceptions?

Dr: Well, the biggest misconception is that lung cancer only happens to smokers. Anyone can get it, including never smokers—people who've never smoked.

MJ: What percentage of people who get lung cancer are never smokers?

Dr: In the UK, it's 10% to 20% of cases. It's important to emphasize that smoking is by far the biggest cause of lung cancer, but the incidence in never smokers is increasing.

MJ: Before talking a bit more about never smokers, could you briefly tell the listeners how smoking causes lung cancer.

Dr: Tobacco smoke contains thousands of chemicals, many of which are carcinogenic, and every time you smoke a cigarette, there's a risk that a lung cell will develop a mutation.

MJ: A mutation is a change in the cell's DNA, isn't it?

Dr: That's right. And the more mutations that build up in a cell, the greater the likelihood that it will become cancerous.

MJ: What are the main symptoms of lung cancer?

Dr: Well, in the early stage there may be no symptoms. But as the tumor gets bigger, people often develop a persistent cough.

MJ: How long does a cough have to last to be persistent?

Dr: A rule of thumb is that you should see a doctor if a cough doesn't go away after two weeks or doesn't improve with prescribed antibiotics. One reason for lung cancer diagnosis being delayed is that people often attribute a persistent cough to being run down, or they blame it on a cold or a chest infection. And smokers often assume that they just have a smoker's cough.

MJ: We're going a little bit off topic now, but what causes a smoker's cough?

Dr: It's thought that tobacco smoke paralyzes hair-like cells called cilia that line the airways. These cilia are part of the defense system of the lungs. When this system is working normally, dust, pollen, microbes, and other things that enter the airways get trapped in mucus and are then swept out of the lungs by the cilia. But if the cilia are damaged by cigarette smoke, mucus builds up and causes coughing.

MJ: Apart from a cough, what other symptoms should we look out for?

Dr: Well, there are general symptoms such as feeling tired and a bit out of breath, but people often put such symptoms down to getting old or being out of shape. Other symptoms that may indicate lung cancer are hoarseness, chest pain, and repeated chest infections. Coughing up blood is also quite a common symptom of lung cancer.

MJ: That sounds like an alarming symptom.

Dr: It is. The medical term for it is hemoptysis.

MJ: Let's return to the misconceptions about lung cancer.

Dr: Yes, as I said before, people tend to associate lung cancer with smoking, but over one in ten people who develop lung cancer have never smoked. And this misconception is really harmful.

MJ: Why's that?

Dr: Let me give you an example. One of my patients, let's call her Sue—she's in her early 40s—was diagnosed with lung cancer in 2022. When she told a work colleague about her diagnosis, her colleague said, "I didn't know that you smoked." Another co-worker was sympathetic, but asked, "Didn't you know that smoking could give you lung cancer?"

MJ: So, there's a stereotype that anyone with lung cancer is a smoker or ex-smoker.

Dr: That's right. Because of its association with smoking, there's a view that people with lung cancer deserved to get it. If someone gets breast cancer or pancreatic cancer, for example, its due to bad luck. But people often think that lung cancer is self-inflicted.

MJ: So, because of its association with smoking, lung cancer carries a stigma.

Dr: Yes. And this stigma is not only a burden for lung cancer patients, but it also results in lung cancer receiving less research funding compared to other cancers.

MJ: You mentioned that one of your patients was a woman in her 40s. Many people will assume that lung cancer is a disease of old men.

Dr: That's another myth. Lung cancer is more common in men, but in the UK, while the incidence of lung cancer in men has been falling, it's been increasing in women. Listeners may be surprised to hear that lung cancer is the leading cause of cancer death in women. And a sizeable minority of women who get lung cancer are never smokers.

MJ: Is it known why some never smokers develop lung cancer?

Dr: In a small number of people, it's related to identifiable inherited genetic mutations, but in most cases the cause is not known for certain. However, various environmental factors definitely increase the risk of lung cancer in never smokers.

MJ: Do you mean things like exposure to secondhand tobacco smoke?

Dr: Yes, and also occupational exposure to certain chemicals and long-term exposure to radon, a naturally-occurring radioactive gas. However, the biggest worry for me is air pollution. Your listeners may have heard of PM2.5.

MJ: You're talking about tiny particles in the air from car exhaust, pollutants from factories, and things like that.

Dr: That's right. Many epidemiological studies have shown that breathing in these particles is associated with an increased risk of lung cancer in never smokers. In 2022, Professor Charles Swanton and his team at London's Francis Crick Institute discovered a mechanism by which PM2.5 causes lung cancer.

MJ: If listeners would like to read more about this study, we've put a link to it on our homepage. Dr Reed, thank you helping to bust some myths about lung cancer. The take-home message is that lung cancer is not exclusively a smoker's disease. People who have never smoked get it too, and they should be treated with empathy.

Dr: I just want to add that smokers who get lung cancer should also be treated with empathy. Just because someone has smoked does not mean they should be blamed for their disease. No one deserves to get lung cancer.

MJ: That's a very important point. Anyone diagnosed with cancer deserves our care and support. We have to remember that nicotine, the addictive substance in tobacco, is in some ways as addictive as heroin. It can be very difficult to quit smoking.

Dr: If we want to blame someone, it should be the tobacco companies that spend huge amounts of money on advertising to get young people hooked on cigarettes.

MJ: That's all we have time for. Thanks so much for joining us.

Dr: Thank you very much.

著者紹介

Mark Rebuck

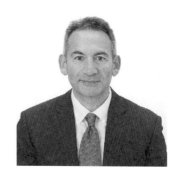

1990 年　バーミンガム大学スポーツ科学部卒業
　[Bachelor of Arts with Honours Class II(Division I)
　(Physical Education)]
1996年　シェフィールド大学大学院東アジア研究科修士
　課程修了
　(Master of Arts in Japanese Studies with Distinction)
2001年　バーミンガム大学大学院英語教授学研究科修士
　課程修了
　[Master of Arts (Teaching English as a Second/Foreign
　Language)]
2001 年　名古屋商科大学外国語学部専任講師
2004 年　名古屋市立大学人文社会学部外国人専任講師
2008 年　名古屋大学大学院国際開発研究科助教
2013 年から現在まで　名城大学薬学部薬学科准教授
現在は名城大学薬学部で医療英語を教える。
プライベートでは 3 人の子どもを育てていて、長女は希少染色体異常（プラダ・ウィ
リー症候群）である。

2023 年 1 月 26 日　　　　　　　初版　第 1 刷発行

医療系のための英語
Medical English and More

著　者　Mark Rebuck　©2023
発行者　橋本豪夫
発行所　ムイスリ出版株式会社

〒169-0075
東京都新宿区高田馬場 4-2-9
Tel.03-3362-9241(代表)　Fax.03-3362-9145
振替　00110-2-102907

ISBN978-4-89641-318-2　C3082

カバーイラスト・章トビライラスト：根岸隆之
カット：藤井笙子
印刷・製本：共同印刷株式会社